Altruism and Health

Altruism and Health

Perspectives from Empirical Research

Edited by
Stephen G. Post

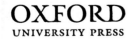

OXFORD
UNIVERSITY PRESS

2007

OXFORD
UNIVERSITY PRESS

Oxford University Press, Inc., publishes works that further
Oxford University's objective of excellence
in research, scholarship, and education.

Oxford   New York
Auckland   Cape Town   Dar es Salaam   Hong Kong   Karachi
Kuala Lumpur   Madrid   Melbourne   Mexico City   Nairobi
New Delhi   Shanghai   Taipei   Toronto

With offices in
Argentina   Austria   Brazil   Chile   Czech Republic   France   Greece
Guatemala   Hungary   Italy   Japan   Poland   Portugal   Singapore
South Korea   Switzerland   Thailand   Turkey   Ukraine   Vietnam

Published by Oxford University Press, Inc.
198 Madison Avenue, New York, New York 10016

www.oup.com

Oxford is a registered trademark of Oxford University Press

Library of Congress Cataloging-in-Publication Data
Altruism and health : perspectives from empirical research /
edited by Stephen G. Post.
    p. cm.
Includes bibliographical references and index.
ISBN 978-0-19-518291-0
1. Altruism.   2. Altruism—Psychological aspects.   3. Psychology.
I. Post, Stephen Garrard, 1951–
BF637.H4A48 2007
610.1'9—dc22   2006010604

Printed in the United States of America
on acid-free paper

PREFACE

This collection of original chapters brings together leadings researchers and interpreters to form the foundation volume for the field of altruism and health studies. The focus is on how altruistic behaviors and emotions impact the health of the *agent* of generosity, rather than the recipient.

Appreciation is due to the Institute for Research on Unlimited Love—Altruism, Compassion, Service, a research institute located at the School of Medicine, Case Western Reserve University. Funded largely through the generosity of the John Templeton Foundation, the institute also enjoys the support of various individuals, including Judith B. and Richard T. Watson, Cathy M. and John F. Lewis, Maria and Samuel H. Miller, Audrey and Albert Ratner, Renee Rizzo, Sanford N. McDonnell, Lindsay and David Morganthaler, Jeanette Grasselli Brown, and Kathy and James Pender.

Might it be the case that altruistic or "other-regarding" behaviors and affections, if properly cultivated, enhance well-being, health, and even longevity? Proverbs reads, "[T]he generous will prosper, and those who refresh others will themselves be refreshed" (11:25). So, too, it is said, "It is better to give than to receive." But does science say it's so? This volume responds to such moral and spiritual exhortation in an objective and scientific manner.

The evidence generally provides a new basis of support for the notion, as old as Plato, that virtue is its own reward. Of course it is good to "do unto others" for purely moral reasons, but it seems also that doing so is a key to well-being. The caveat, certainly, is that it does no one any good to be stressed by a giving that becomes overwhelming, that ignores the necessary care of the self, or that masks self-destructive tendencies. And yet too much focus on phenomena such as "caregiver burnout," or on psychoanalytic and existentialist suspicions of impure motivations, has badly deflected attention from the health benefits of prosocial behaviors and emotions that center on contributing to the lives of others. It seems that human beings are in fact wired to do well by doing good.

Catherine Carlin, my editor at Oxford University Press, was remarkably supportive as the book prospectus was developed and reviewed. Throughout, Ms. Carlin was patient and offered thoughtful guidance. Her creativity and vision are gratefully acknowledged.

The Department of Bioethics at Case Western Reserve University's School of Medicine provided a tolerant environment for this project, which lies outside of the usual range of bioethics. In addition, the numerous students in my graduate seminar "Altruism and Bioethics" provided immense stimulation as we reflected together on many of the topics included in this volume.

Special thanks to Brie B. Zeltner, who has been of immense help in sorting through an extensive literature and summarizing existing research.

Finally, the chapter by Andrea H. Marques and Esther M. Sternberg of the National Institutes of Health includes graphics reprinted from *Physiology & Behavior*, 79 (2003), pp. 351–357.

CONTENTS

CONTRIBUTORS

Peter L. Benson, Ph.D., is president of Search Institute, a not-for-profit research and educational organization dedicated to positive child and adolescent development. Under his leadership, the institute has developed a theoretical and research-based model for mobilizing the engagement of citizens and communities in creating the ecologies and relationships crucial for successful development. Dr. Benson currently serves as the first visiting scholar at the William T. Grant Foundation in New York City; he is the author of 12 books on child and adolescent development and is the general editor of the new Search Institute Series on Developmentally Attentive Communities and Society. He has been a recipient of the William James Award from the American Psychological Association. He has published extensively on the topics of altruism, spiritual development, and positive youth development.

Christopher Boehm, Ph.D., is professor of anthropology and biological sciences and director of the Jane Goodall Research Center at the University of Southern California. He has conducted field research with Navajo Indians, mountain Serbian tribes in Montenegro, and wild chimpanzees in Tanzania. He is a recent recipient of a Simon J. Guggenheim Fellowship and is the author of *Blood Revenge: The Enactment and Management of Conflict in Montenegro and Other Tribal Societies*; *Hierarchy in the Forest*; "Impact of the Human Egalitarian Syndrome on Darwinian Selection Mechanics," in *American Naturalist*; "The Prosocial Side of Moral Communities," in the *Journal of Consciousness Studies*. His current research includes the creation of a comprehensive database on hunter-gatherer social behavior and investigating altruistic behavior among these nomadic foragers.

R. Michael Brown, Ph.D., is a Professor of Psychology at Pacific Lutheran University. His research interests include depression and self-destructive tendencies in non-clinical populations. In particular, his research is devoted to the psychological experience of burden from the perspective of the care recipient. He has identified factors that exacerbate the harmful effects of feeling like a burden to others, such as poor health and difficulties in romantic relationships. He also studies the factors that ameliorate these effects, including making contributions to the lives of others. Dr. Brown is the co-creator of Selective Investment Theory and has collaborated on projects designed to investigate the stress-relieving effects of helping behavior.

Stephanie L. Brown, Ph.D., is currently an assistant professor in Internal Medicine in the Center for Behavioral and Decision Sciences in Medicine at the University of Michigan. She was formerly research investigator at the University of Michigan's Institute for Social Research. Her research interests include the application of evolutionary theory to close relationships and altruism and the health benefits of altruistic forms of behavior. She was recently awarded a 3-year research scientist development award from NIMH to study the benefits of giving for reducing depression among dialysis patients. Currently, Brown is examining emotional and cognitive mechanisms that may regulate whether giving produces health benefits for the giver, such as accelerated recovery from cardiovascular stress.

Lisa D. Butler, Ph.D., is a senior research scholar in the Department of Psychiatry and Behavioral Sciences at Stanford University School of Medicine. Her research examines the effects of traumatic experience and aspects of resilience and thriving across a variety of populations, including medical patients, abuse survivors, and individuals exposed to terrorism. Her other research interests include pathological and normative dissociation, the affective and cognitive determinants of paranoia, and the effectiveness of psychosocial interventions that include hypnosis.

Adah N. Carter is a doctoral student in gerontology at the University of Kentucky. She is currently a recipient of the Lyman T. Johnson Fellowship and Research Challenge Trust Fund Fellowship from the Graduate Center for Gerontology at the University of Kentucky. Her research interests include nonverbal communication and the emotional behavior of African Americans.

C. Sue Carter, Ph.D., became a professor at the University of Maryland in College Park in 1985, and in 1997 she was elected to the rank of distinguished university professor. In 2001, Dr. Carter and her husband, Stephen Porges, moved to the College of Medicine at the University of Illinois at Chicago, where they are currently professors in the Department of Psychiatry and co-directors of the Brain-Body Center (BBC) at the University of Illinois. Dr. Carter is a fellow of the American Association for the Advancement of Science and the International Society for Behavioral Neuroscience and is president-elect of that latter society. She has edited three volumes dealing with the neurobiology of sexual and social behaviors. Dr. Carter is especially known for her work over the last three decades on the biological basis of monogamy and social attachment. She is particularly interested in social support and the mechanisms for the health benefits of social bonds. She has also studied the endocrine changes associated with human behavior, including studies that demonstrate the physiological benefits of lactation to the mother.

E. Gil Clary is professor of psychology at the College of St. Catherine in St. Paul, Minnesota. The majority of his research is devoted to prosocial behavior generally and participation in volunteer work more specifically. In addition, Clary has been engaged in research on other questions concerning the voluntary and nonprofit sector, including the consequences of long-term helpers' philosophies of helping, the socialization of prosocial tendencies, and environmental influences on volunteer activity.

Mihaly Csikszentmihalyi is one of the most distinguished psychologists of his generation. He is renowned for his books on such phenomena as "flow" and creativity. For many years he taught at the University of Chicago before moving to the Claremont Graduate School. He is a major leader in the positive psychology movement, and few researchers have had so much influence on both the scholarly and public worlds.

Deborah D. Danner, Ph.D., is a developmental psychologist with the University of Kentucky's Alzheimer's Research Center. She is interested in the arousal and expression of basic emotional states and how the emotional lives of the elderly affect their quality of life. Her research has focused on how positive emotional expression enhances longevity and how normal aging and degenerative neurological diseases such as Alzheimer's alter emotional arousal and expression. The long-term goals of her studies have been to provide an understanding of what arouses emotion so as to increase the positive emotions of happiness, amusement, and interest and to enhance the relationship between patients and those who provide care. Dr. Danner participated in a recent multisite NIA-funded research project that examined ethical issues involved in informing patients with diminished capacity of the risks and benefits of research participation. She currently is working to implement a grant from the Administration on Aging to increase awareness of signs of dementia and the utilization of diagnostic and family services in the African-American population in the Lexington, Kentucky, bluegrass area.

Michele Dillon, Ph.D., currently is associate professor of sociology at the University of New Hampshire. Dillon is past chair of the Sociology of Religion Section of the American Sociological Association. Her publications include *Catholic Identity: Balancing Reason, Faith, and Power; Debating Divorce: Moral Conflict in Ireland; Handbook of the Sociology of Religion* (editor); and articles on religion and culture published in *Journal for the Scientific Study of Religion, Sociology of Religion, Public Opinion Quarterly*, and *Sociological Theory*. She is currently writing on the historical continuities, life course trajectories, and social implications of religion using longitudinal life course data.

Marivic Dizon is a doctoral candidate in counseling psychology at Stanford University's School of Education. Her research/counseling background is in the area of child development and trauma. Her doctoral research explores how animals can help to promote children's psychological health and well-being through animal-assisted therapy.

Gregory Fricchione, M.D., is director of the Division of Psychiatry in Medicine, Department of Psychiatry, Massachusetts General Hospital. Dr. Fricchione's clinical work has helped to establish the use of lorazepam as a first-line treatment for the catatonic syndrome. He has written extensively about the care of patients with medical and neurological illness. His research in neuroimmunology and neuropsychiatry includes work on macrophage-endothelial cell interaction and led to his appointment to the Dana Farber–Harvard Cancer Center. He is board certified in general psychiatry and has additional qualifications in geriatric psychiatry.

Wallace V. Friesen retired from the University of California, San Francisco, following decades of study of the expression of emotion and underlying neurological correlates. More recently, with Dr. Danner and colleagues of the Nun Study, Dr. Friesen examined the impact of positive emotion on longevity, a study that has provoked reflection on how one appraises life events. In his retirement, Dr. Friesen continues to consult with colleagues in Kentucky and throughout the world.

Bita Ghafoori, Ph.D., of California State University, Long Beach, is past director of research for the University of California, San Francisco, Fresno, Psychiatry Residency Training Program. She is currently a co-principal investigator for a grant funded by the Institute for Research on Unlimited Love entitled Care for the Soul: The Role of Divine and Human Love in the Adjustment to Military Trauma. She is the site principal investigator for an exploratory/developmental project funded by the Mental Illness Research Education and Clinical Centers (MIRECC) entitled Open Trial of Cognitive Behavioral Therapy for the Treatment of Chronic PTSD in Vietnam Combat Veterans. She is also site coordinator for the MIRECC Post Traumatic Stress Disorder Research Project.

Robert Hierholzer, M.D., a psychiatrist, is the associate chief of staff for research and education at the VA-Central California Healthcare System (Fresno) and is a clinical professor at the University of California, San Francisco (UCSF), Department of Psychiatry. His clinical work mainly involves the assessment and treatment of PTSD and geriatric psychiatric conditions. Dr. Hierholzer's research interests parallel his clinical interests. He is especially interested in exploring the cultural, spiritual, and ethical dimensions of psychiatric conditions and practice. He is also an adjunct faculty member at the Mennonite Brethren Biblical Seminary.

Adam S. Hirschfelder, Ph.D., is a principal investigator at the Public Health Institute in Oakland, California, one of the largest statewide public health research firms in the country. His current research focuses on the role of the medical community in promoting volunteerism.

Gail Ironson, M.D., Ph.D., is professor of psychology and psychiatry at the University of Miami and a board-certified psychiatrist. Dr. Ironson specializes in behavioral medicine and served as the president of the Academy of Behavioral Medicine Research in 2002. Her research interests explore stressors, their effects on health and disease, and identifying protective psychosocial and immune pathways. Some of the protective factors identified in her research for the health of people with HIV include optimism, the doctor-patient relationship, spirituality, processing of trauma/emotional expression, and NK cells. In addition to leading or co-leading major projects on long survivors of AIDS and stress management for cancer, HIV, and cardiac patients, she established and co-directs the Trauma Treatment Program at the University of Miami. She is a fellow in the Society of Behavioral Medicine and Academy of Behavioral Medicine Research, on the council of the American Psychosomatic Society, and has been on the editorial boards of four journals. She has published more than 100 articles and chapters in peer-reviewed publications.

Eva Kahana, Ph.D., is the Robson Professor of Humanities, chair of the Sociology Department, and director of the Elderly Care Research Center at Case Western Reserve University. She has published extensively in the areas of stress, coping, and health of the aged. She is principal investigator of NIA-funded studies considering successful aging among old-old individuals confronting the normative stressors of ill health, social losses, and lack of person-environment fit. She has also collaborated with Elizabeth Midlarsky on studies of altruism in late life. She has served on NIH and NIMH peer review committees and on editorial boards of the *Journal of Gerontology, Psychology and Aging, Gerontologist,* and *Annals of Family*

Medicine. The awards she has received include the John S. Diekhoff Distinguished Graduate Teaching Award at CWRU; Gerontological Society of America (GSA) Distinguished Mentorship Award; Polisher Award for outstanding contribution to applied gerontology; Mary E. Switzer Distinguished Fellowship of the National Institute of Rehabilitation; Ohio Distinguished Gerontological Researcher; and Distinguished Scholar Award, Section on Aging & the Life Course of the American Sociological Association (ASA). She received an honorary doctorate of humane letters from Yeshiva University in 1991. She is past chair of the ASA Section on Aging & the Life Course and of the Behavioral and Social Sciences Section of the Gerontological Society of America.

Harold G. Koenig, M.D., is board certified in general psychiatry, geriatric psychiatry, and geriatric medicine and is on the faculty at Duke University Medical Center as a professor of psychiatry and behavioral sciences and associate professor of medicine. He is also a registered nurse (RN). Dr. Koenig is director and founder of the Center for the Study of Religion/Spirituality and Health at Duke and has published extensively in the fields of mental health, geriatrics, and religion, with nearly 250 scientific peer-reviewed articles and book chapters and 26 books in print or in preparation. He is editor of the *International Journal of Psychiatry in Medicine*, a Medline research journal, and is founder and editor in chief of *Science and Theology News*. His research on religion, health, and ethical issues in medicine has been featured on more than 35 national and international TV news programs, 80 national or international radio programs, and more than 250 national or international newspapers or magazines. Dr. Koenig has been nominated twice for the Templeton Prize for Progress in Religion. His latest books include *The Healing Power of Faith, The Handbook of Religion and Health,* and *Spirituality in Patient Care.*

Cheryl Koopman, Ph.D., is associate professor (research) in the Department of Psychiatry and Behavioral Sciences, Stanford University School of Medicine. Her research examines the psychological and health consequences of stress and traumatic life events. She also investigates the effectiveness of psychosocial interventions in improving quality of life and health, particular among persons facing intimate partner violence, sexual abuse, cancer, or HIV/AIDS. She has more than 160 publications on these and related subjects.

Neal Krause, Ph.D., is a professor in the Department of Health Behavior and Health Education in the University of Michigan's School of Public Health. He is also a senior research scientist in the Institute of Gerontology. For the past 25 years, his research has focused primarily on the relationship between stressful events and health in late life, with an eye toward studying the resources upon which older people rely to deal with the problems that confront them. This research as been funded through a series of grants from the National Institute on Aging (NIA). Recently, his work has turned toward assessing the relationship between involvement in religion and health, with a special emphasis on how race or ethnicity may come into play.

Jeff Levin, Ph.D., M.P.H., is a scientist and writer living in Kansas. An epidemiologist by training and a former medical school professor, he left a successful academic career in 1997 to devote his full-time efforts to writing and consulting. He is the author of more than 140 scholarly publications, and author or editor of six books, including *God, Faith, and Health* and *Faith, Medicine, and Science.* He is a former chair of the NIH Working Group on Quantitative Methods in Alternative Medicine, and a Fellow of the Gerontological Society of America. Dr. Levin's most recent work is twofold: empirical investigation of the impact of love on indicators of population health, and exploration of canonical and rabbinic perspectives on the role of divine love in Jewish moral theology. He has served as IRUL research area consultant for the Public Health and Medicine Program Area.

Andrea H. Marques, M.D., Ph.D., is a licensed staff psychiatrist at the Institute of Psychiatry in the Consultation-Liaison Unit and Psychiatric Emergency Unit at the University of São Paulo Medical School. She is currently a postdoctoral fellow at the National Institute of Mental Health, in the Section on Neuroendocrine Immunology and Behavior, where she dedicates her studies to understanding the bidirectional connection between the brain and the immune system and between emotions and disease.

Michael E. McCullough, Ph.D., is associate professor of psychology at the University of Miami. His scholarly work focuses on religion, spirituality, and the virtues, how these aspects of people's lives unfold, and how they are linked to health and well-being. In 2000, he was awarded the Margaret Gorman Early Career Award from Division 36 (Psychology of Religion) of the American Psychological Association, and in 2001 received third prize in the American Psychological Association/John Templeton Foundation award program for research in positive psychology. Dr. McCullough has written more than 60 peer-reviewed journal articles and book chapters. He has also authored or edited four books, including *Forgiveness: Theory Research and Practice, Handbook of Religion and Health,* and an upcoming volume on the psychology of gratitude.

Elizabeth Midlarsky, Ph.D., is professor and director of the M.A. program in the Department of Counseling and Clinical Psychology at Columbia University, Teachers College, and is professor in the Graduate School of Arts and Sciences of Columbia University. Her work on altruism and helping currently focuses on three domains: (1) helping within families, (2) altruism and helping among community-residing older adults, and (3) Holocaust heroism. Dr. Midlarsky's national activities have included appointments to review boards of the National Institute of Mental Health and the National Institutes of Health, where she reviewed for the National Heart, Lung, and Blood Institute, Human Development and Aging, and Mental Health and Aging. She has been in the National Reviewers Reserve and was on the National Bone Marrow Registry Evaluation Panel, which had direct input to the Senate Appropriations Committee. She has been editor of the *Academic Psychology Bulletin*, is on the editorial board of the *Journal of Traumatic Stress*, and has reviewed scientific articles for numerous other journals, including the *Journal of Personality and Social Psychology, Psychological Bulletin, American Psychologist, Psychology of Aging*, and the *American Journal of Orthopsychiatry*. Midlarsky is a fellow of the American Psychological Association, American Psychological Society, American Orthopsychiatric Association, and the Gerontological Society of America.

Marc A. Musick, Ph.D., is an associate professor of sociology and a faculty research associate of the Population Research Center at the University of Texas at Austin. Much of his past research has examined the role of religion in social life, especially related to the health and well-being of adults. Although still active in that field, currently his research examines the predictors of volunteering, how people volunteer, and the effects that the behavior has on individual lives. His work on volunteering has appeared in numerous peer-reviewed journals, including the *American Sociological Review, Social Forces, Social Science and Medicine*, and the *Journal of Gerontology: Social Sciences*. His forthcoming book, *The Volunteer*, is being co-authored by John Wilson.

Doug Oman, Ph.D., is adjunct assistant professor at the School of Public Health of the University of California, Berkeley. His research and professional publications involve theoretical, observational, and experimental studies of spirituality, religion, and health, including epidemiologic studies of religious involvement and mortality, the application of social cognitive theory to religion and spirituality, and studies of effects on health professionals from receiving training in a comprehensive nonsectarian spiritual toolkit. Dr. Oman also serves as instructor and research advisor in the Division of Maternal and Child Health, School of Public Health, University of California, Berkeley. He is the author of a study on the effects of volunteer work on longevity and was recently principal investigator on a grant from the National Institute of Aging to examine the positive effects of volunteer work on physical health. He is currently the principal investigator on a project funded by the Fetzer Institute.

Allen M. Omoto, Ph.D., professor of psychology at Claremont Graduate University, is a social psychologist whose research interests include the social and psychological aspects of volunteerism, interpersonal relationships, HIV disease, and lesbian, gay, and bisexual issues. He has an ongoing program of research on volunteerism and helping relationships, including multiyear studies that are supported by grants from the National Institute of Mental Health, the Fetzer Institute, and the Institute for Research on Unlimited Love. He also has extensive public policy experience, including helping to found and administer a community-based AIDS organization and working in the U.S. Congress as the American Psychological Association's inaugural William A. Bailey AIDS Policy Congressional Fellow.

Stephen G. Post, Ph.D., is a professor in the Department of Bioethics, School of Medicine, Case Western Reserve University, as well as senior research scholar in the Becket Institute at St. Hugh's College, Oxford University. Post has made major contributions to bioethics (e.g., as editor in chief of the definitive *Encyclopedia of Bioethics*, third edition). With regard to altruism and compassionate love in the context of scientific research, philosophy, ethics, and the professions, Dr. Post has written several books on this topic, most recently co-editing a book entitled *Altruism and Altruistic Love: Science, Philosophy, and Religion in Dialogue*. He is the author of more than 120 articles in leading peer-reviewed journals and seven books, and he has edited four reference works, seven books, and two journals. His articles have appeared in *Science, Hastings Center Report, Annals of Internal Medicine, Journal of Religion, American Journal of Psychiatry, Journal of the American Medical Association, Hypatia, Journal of the American Academy of Religion*, and *Lancet*. He is co-author of *Why Good Things Happen to Good People*, with science journalist Jill Neimark.

Sabrina L. Reilly is deputy director of the RespectAbility Initiative for the National Council on Aging (NCOA), a multiyear project focusing on increasing awareness, understanding, and action by policy makers, journalists, and organizational and community leaders to maximize opportunities and reduce barriers to the civic engagement of older adults. She has also worked as a program officer for the National Senior Service Corps (Senior Corps) of the Corporation for National and Community Service and as a staff consultant for community service in the State and National Initiatives Groups at AARP.

Peter C. Scales, Ph.D., senior fellow at the Search Institute, is a developmental psychologist, author, speaker, and researcher who is widely recognized as one of the nation's foremost authorities on children, youth, and families. Specifically, his expertise lies in adolescent development, family life, effective schools, and healthy communities. Dr. Scales conducts research; provides consultation on youth development to schools, youth-serving organizations, and governmental agencies; delivers conference keynote addresses; and publishes widely on youth development and family relations. Dr. Scales serves on the editorial boards for *Middle School Journal* and *Child Welfare* and has published more than 200 articles in scientific and practitioner journals, such as the *Journal of Early Adolescence*,

Applied Developmental Science, Youth Policy, Journal of Health Education, American School Board Journal, and the *Journal of School Health.*

Ashley Schiavone, B.S., graduated from the University of Michigan in Biopsychology in 2004 and is a research assistant at Wayne State University in the Department of Psychiatry and Behavioral Neuroscience. She is currently co-coordinating the BioSocial Health Program at the University of Michigan, in the Center for Behavioral and Decisions Sciences. Her current research focuses on positive psychology interventions, mindfulness techniques, helping-behavior, well-being, emotional states, and their physiological effects.

Michèle M. Schlehofer, M.A., is a fifth-year student in the applied social psychology doctoral program at Claremont Graduate University. Her research interests include health, health care utilization, coping, and religiousness and spirituality.

Carolyn Schwartz, Sc.D., is president of the Delta Quest Foundation. She has been involved in research on psychosocial factors in health for more than 15 years, with an emphasis on developing new measures and new quantitative methods that are patient-centered for chronically and terminally ill patient populations. She co-edited a book published by the American Psychological Association in 2000. She has served on the editorial board of *Psychosomatic Medicine* and is currently on the editorial boards for the *International Journal of Behavioral Medicine* and the *Journal of Happiness Studies.* She is an associate editor for *Quality of Life Research,* a member of the board for the International Society of Quality of Life Research, and a member of the Quality of Life Advisory Group for the American Cancer Society. She holds a faculty appointment as associate professor of medicine at the University of Massachusetts Medical School in Worcester.

Dylan M. Smith, Ph.D., is a research assistant professor in Internal Medicine at the University of Michigan and at the VA Health Services Research & Development Center for Excellence. He received his Ph.D. in social psychology, with an emphasis on intergroup relations and evolutionary psychology. His current focus is on measurement issues in health-related quality of life.

Esther M. Sternberg, M.D., Ph.D., is one of the world's leading scientists at the interface of emotion, neuroscience, and immunology. As chief of the Section on Neuroendocrine Immunology and Behavior, National Institute of Mental Health, and as director of the Integrative Neural Immune Program at NIMH and NIH, Dr. Sternberg has achieved international status in her field. Her recent book, *The Balance Within: The Science Connecting Health and Emotions,* has been universally well received as one of the best books on emotions and health.

George E. Vaillant, M.D., is professor of psychiatry at Harvard Medical School and director of research for the Department of Psychiatry, Brigham and Women's Hospital. Dr. Vaillant has spent his research career charting adult development and the recovery process from schizophrenia, heroin addiction, alcoholism, and personality disorders. He has spent the last 30 years as director of the Study of Adult Development at the Harvard University Health Service. His published works include *Adaptation to Life*, *The Wisdom of the Ego*, and *The Natural History of Alcoholism Revisited*. His summary of the lives of men and women from adolescence to age 80 is entitled *Aging Well*. Dr. Vaillant has been a fellow at the Center for Advanced Studies in the Behavioral Sciences, is a fellow of the American College of Psychiatrists, and has been an invited speaker and consultant for seminars and workshops throughout the world. Dr. Vaillant has received the Foundations Fund Prize for Research in Psychiatry from the American Psychiatric Association, the Strecker Award from the Institute of Pennsylvania Hospital, the Burlingame Award from the Institute for Living, and the Jellinek Award for research in alcoholism. More recently, he received the research prize of the International Psychogeriatric Society.

Miranda R. Waggoner is a graduate student in the Sociology Department at the University of Texas at Austin. Her areas of interest are gender and sexuality, social theory, and aspects of volunteering research, including the intersection of gender, health, and volunteering. Ms. Waggoner has been active in many organizations at the University of Texas, and she has won several academic awards and scholarships. Her current research, titled "College Feminisms: Attitudes of Today's Young Women," focuses on feminism and personal politics among women students at the University of Texas.

David Sloan Wilson, Ph.D., professor in the department of biology at Binghamton University, SUNY, is an evolutionary biologist who studies humans along with other species. He is best known for championing the theory of multilevel selection, in which adaptation and natural selection can occur at all levels of the biological hierarchy. Additional interests include the nature of individual differences and evolutionary processes that involve nongenetic inheritance mechanisms. He publishes in psychology, anthropology, and philosophy journals in addition to his mainstream biological research. His books include *The Natural Selection of Populations and Communities*, *Unto Others: The Evolution and Psychology of Unselfish Behavior* (with Elliott Sober), and *Darwin's Cathedral: Evolution, Religion, and the Nature of Society*.

Paul Wink, Ph.D., is currently a professor in the Psychology Department at Wellesley College and has been a visiting faculty member at the Department of Psychology at the University of Michigan, Ann Arbor. Dr. Wink has published extensively in the areas of adult development, generativity, religiousness and spirituality, and narcissism. Since 1997, he has directed a follow-up study of participants in the Berkeley Guidance and Oakland Growth Studies in late adulthood. Wink's research has been supported by grants from the Open Society Institute, the Lilly Foundation, the Fetzer Institute in collaboration with the Institute for Research on Unlimited Love, and the Templeton Foundation. He is a reviewer for numerous journals, including *Psychology and Aging, Journal of Personality and Social Psychology*, and *Journal for the Sociology of Religion*.

Charlotte V. O. Witvliet, Ph.D., is associate professor of psychology at Hope College. Dr. Witvliet's research interests include the psychophysiology of emotion, trauma, unforgiveness, forgiveness, and justice. With the support of the John Templeton Foundation and a four-year Hope College Towsley Research Scholar Award, she has conducted five empirical studies of forgiveness, published journal articles and book chapters, and given presentations in local, national, and international venues.

Brie Zeltner graduated from Dartmouth College in 2001 with majors in evolutionary biology and environmental studies. Since then, she has been a greenhouse assistant, a medical journalist, and a research consultant to Dr. Stephen G. Post at Case Western Reserve University.

Altruism and Health

General Introduction

Stephen G. Post

This collection presents existing scientific research on the association between altruistic emotions and actions, on the one hand, and the health of the altruist, on the other. The authors are leading researchers on this topic, and their presentations are intended to foster the consolidation of a new field of study.

Altruism, for the purposes of this volume, refers to a fundamental orientation of the agent that is primarily "other-regarding," in contrast to one that is primarily self-regarding. Altruistic (benevolent, kind, compassionate, charitable) individuals, motivated with little or no interest in reciprocity or reputation gain, may enjoy enhanced health, broadly defined. This secondary effect does not constitute motivational selfishness, unless one defines selfishness so broadly that it can only be considered a virtue. Altruism is *not* about so-called selflessness, which is merely a rhetorical exaggeration of the valid ideal of unselfishness and an ontological impossibility. The altruistic self is still a self, although a very different kind of self than the narcissist or solipsist, who relate to others only insofar as the others contribute to their own little agendas.

Reason can help somewhat in creating what Kantians refer to as "the possibility of altruism" by virtue of the logic of equality—there is, after all, no compelling reason to think that my life is more important than that of the other. But in the traditions of the British moralists, such as Adam Smith and David Hume, or of Buddhism, reason is in the final analysis instrumental in the sense that, while it provides guidance to emotional inclinations such as compassion and sympathy, it is not the driving force behind altruism. The very fact that we debate about that action most likely to maximize beneficence is itself due only to the fact that reason can be driven by altruistic emotions. It is our benevolent moral emotions, with reason as their servant, that give rise to altruism.

An immediate caveat is that the behavioral aspect of our focus is strictly on "reasonable" forms of altruism, which are not themselves overwhelming to the point of having adverse health consequences or so perilous as to endanger the agent. Indeed, the fastest way to destroy the moral resources of benevolent emotions and helping behavior is to strain them to the point of burnout. This concern has been implicit in the very language of the "burden of care," which dominates the social science of caregiving. Yet it is possible to speak of altruistic flourishing as well as of altruistic burden.

My purpose here is merely to help open the door to a serious research assessment. Critique is welcomed at this early stage of the field. Indeed, I discussed the contents of this book with the renowned Jerome Kassirer, M.D., for many years the editor of the *New England Journal of Medicine*. Now on the faculty at Case Medical School with an appointment in my own Department of Bioethics, Dr. Kassirer and I warmly disagree over meals and in more formal conversations. A loyal scientific skeptic, Dr. Kassirer refers often to the good feelings that the agent of altruism experiences as an indication of hedonic motive. My response is that this is at best a matter of "indirect effect," in the paradoxical sense of the surprising and unexpected discovery that in the giving of self lies the unsought discovery of self. This is at best a very weak form of hedonism and one that does not pertain to at least initial motivations. Moreover, as I enjoy pointing out to Dr. Kassirer, he is himself the most generative and kindly senior scholar I have encountered in a long while.

Yet I do acknowledge human nature as a mixture of self-conserving and benevolent inclinations, and I am convinced that these need not be viewed as conflictual. In everyday circumstances, benevolent emotions and helping actions are salutary manifestations of an abiding human inclination that will, when expressed, be internally fulfilling. Such expression will often result in reciprocal or reputation gains as well—but the altruist just lets these gains take care of themselves one way or another. Many people do generous things for others with no anticipation of gain whatsoever: Holocaust rescuers, for example, would have been killed if their actions became publicly known at the time. The fact that they felt good about themselves at the end of the day is inconsequential to their original motives.

But these debates about human nature have been thoroughly addressed elsewhere, also through the venue of Oxford University Press, and the skeptics are referred there for a thorough scientific conversation (Post et al., 2002). There will always be those who, while others flock to help those devastated by catastrophic events, such as Hurricane Katrina, will assert from the quiet armchair, "Scratch an altruist and watch an egoist bleed."

This book brings together a total of 23 original chapters involving 41 authors. A modest honorarium was provided for each chapter, but the authors were purposefully not brought together for a working conference, nor was communication between authors across chapters allowed. I wanted these researchers to arrive at their conclusions without any group bias. The only instruction was that they take a hard-nosed perspective on the purported association between altruism and health. This approach hopefully minimized any tendencies to overstate this association through peer pressure. As it turns out, the great majority of these researchers do find such an association.

A number of core questions shape the chapters in part I of the book, "Research on Volunteering and Health." First, does altruism enhance well-being, as characterized by feeling hopeful, happy, and good about oneself, as well as energetic and connected to others? Second, does altruism result in lowered depressive symptoms and greater psychological health? Third, does altruism have physical benefits? The researchers in this section of the book answer affirmatively, by and large, and quite strongly so.

It must always be kept in mind that significant findings regarding health in relation to altruism and other phenomena in population studies are expressed on average and across a given population. Altruism appears to be one of the factors that increases the odds of well-being, better health, or survival in many people; it is no guarantee of good health. This could be said of any ostensibly protective factors, e.g., good diet, low blood pressure, not smoking, good family history, not living in poverty, nontoxic environment, and educational level.

What about cause and effect? If someone is depressed or physically disabled due to illness, it certainly is less likely that he/she will engage in helping behaviors. This probably does partially explain the better health of altruists, but it would be reductive to dismiss the causative potential of unselfish love and benevolent actions. It is much more likely that causality would simultaneously exist in both directions. These researchers tend to see causality going in both directions. This stands the test of common experience in that most of us have suggested to a despondent friend or an unhappy child that they might benefit by going out and helping someone.

Some models are necessary to help explain plausible causality, and so part II, "The Contribution of Altruistic Emotions to Health," is intended to indicate such a framework. Presumably, benevolent emotions are less stressful, or stressful in the very different sense of creating solicitude rather than apathy. Unselfish love and kindness, including manifestations such as forgiveness, displace emotional states such as rage, bitterness, and hatred, all of which cause stress and consequently stress-related illnesses through adverse impacts on immune function. This second section of the book amply supports the first.

Part III moves from emotional models to evolutionary ones and is entitled "Evolutionary Models of Altruism and Health." While it is not appropriate here to make a full case for evolutionary altruism, it can be asserted that the new rise of group selection theory suggests a powerfully adaptive connection between widely diffuse altruism within groups and group survival (Sober & Wilson, 1998).

Members of a successful group would likely be innately oriented to other-regarding behaviors. Anthropologists point out that early egalitarian societies practice institutionalized, or ecological, altruism, where helping others is not an act of volunteerism but a social norm. There appears to be a fundamental human drive toward other-regarding actions. According to the most current evolutionary science, genuine unselfishness does lie within the human repertoire (Sober & Wilson, 1998). Does tapping into this deeply evolved human capacity to love others, as the Golden Rule ("do unto others") prescribes, enhance happiness and health? If so, then "love thy neighbor" might be recommended as a matter of public health, providing an added reason for doing good. Group selection theory provides an impressive evolutionary underpinning for parts I and II, and this is a theory that is on the rise in evolutionary circles.

Part IV, "Altruism, Health and Religion," discusses religion primarily as a form of organized altruism and suggests that this model explains a great deal of the association between religion and health.

Each part of the book begins with an overview of the chapters and a brief statement on their significance. The reader is directed to examine these four introductions with care.

The interpretive models mentioned above suggest that human nature may have evolved emotionally and behaviorally in a manner that confers health benefits as a result of benevolent emotions and helping behaviors. We seem to prosper under the canopy of positive emotions, to have evolved such that these emotions have value to the group in its competition against other groups, and to have immune and endocrine systems that reflect this evolutionary strategy.

There is wisdom in the words of Proverbs: "A generous man will prosper, he who refreshes others will himself be refreshed" (11:25). A general freedom from the narrow concerns of the self may bring us closer to our true and healthier nature, as most significant spiritual and moral traditions prescribe. Perhaps a new definition of altruism is called for: genuine altruism is an action done without assuming reciprocal or reputational gains for the agent, but that by its very inward dynamic enhances well-being and often contributes to health so long as it is not experienced as overwhelming.

REFERENCES

Post, S. G., Underwood, L. G., Schloss, J. R., & Hurlbut, W. B. (2002). *Altruism and altruistic love: Science, philosophy and religion in dialogue.* New York: Oxford University Press.

Sober, E., & Wilson, D. S. (1998). *Unto others: The evolution of unselfish behavior.* Cambridge, MA: Harvard University Press.

PART I

Research on Volunteering and Health

Introduction

Stephen G. Post
Brie Zeltner

This part brings together premier researchers who have been contributing most thoughtfully to the study of volunteerism in relation to health. The authors do not all agree, and they offer differing perspectives on the association under consideration. The reader is invited to consider these carefully written chapters, which are primarily intended to present the currently available research data in an objective manner.

Doug Oman, in "Does Volunteering Foster Physical Health and Longevity?" takes a scientific look at the relationship between formal, unpaid volunteer work and physical health and functioning. First, the author reviews the potential mechanisms that may explain a positive effect of volunteering, the most prominent of which are increased social support and enhanced positive psychological states. He also offers several potential reasons for the specific contribution of volunteer work as opposed to paid work, including the ability to choose the type of work and hours spent performing it and a sense of heightened meaning, which often accompanies work that is sought out and considered to be worthwhile. In terms of motivation for volunteering, Oman believes that the altruistic motive, while not always present initially, may develop during the volunteering experience and may have an important effect on the health benefits derived from the activity. In his empirical evidence review, Oman focuses in particular on six studies that help to clarify causality and concludes that volunteering is consistently associated with reduced mortality rates that cannot easily be explained by confounding variables. There are, however, other explanations that need to be ruled out, the most probable of which is that an established tendency toward healthy behaviors can account for healthier volunteers. In other studies, volunteering was shown to have a positive effect on physical functioning and mobility, self-rated physical health (although there is no evidence here for causality), and improved mental health and health behaviors. Oman believes that the weight of the evidence supports a tentative yes in response to his title question, but that we have a lot more to learn from experimental or intervention-style studies and need to firmly establish which types of volunteering are the most beneficial, and for whom. In conclusion, Oman recommends more studies that include interventions in older adult populations, studies of middle-aged volunteers, and cross-cultural studies to broaden our understanding of the volunteering-health relationship.

Carolyn Schwartz, the author of "Altruism and Subjective Well-Being: Conceptual Model and Empirical Support," is, like Oman, a leading researcher. Historically, psychological research has focused on the health implications of *receiving* support, and it was while doing just such research that Schwartz first found evidence that *giving* support may be just as or more important to human health. Using two very different studies, neither of which was intended to assess the implications of giving support, Schwartz hypothesizes that altruistic social-interest behaviors enhance subjective well-being for both healthy and chronically ill adults. The first study focused on chronically ill patients with multiple sclerosis (MS) and examined the health implications of receiving training in coping strategies accompanied by monthly telephone support versus simply receiving 15-minute phone calls from trained peer supporters (who also had MS) once a month for a year. Data incidentally collected from the five peer supporters revealed that they (the givers) reported improvement on more outcomes and that the effect size of these changes was larger than for the supported patients. Using these findings, Schwartz developed a conceptual model to explain the effect using response shift; that is, the giver is able to escape the self-focus that is a common cause of anxiety and depression, and this outward focus facilitates a change in the internal measures of quality of life. The second study used previously collected data on a large stratified sample of Presbyterians, and Schwartz was able to examine her hypothesis within a remarkably healthy and much larger cohort. Importantly, she found that giving help was a more important indicator of better mental health than receiving it. In conclusion, Schwartz discusses the serious problem of causality within the realm of altruism research and suggests some ways to solve it in terms of experimental design. Last, she relates some personal thoughts on the importance of altruism to developing a larger human community "net" to help and care for the needy and the importance of feeling part of a larger benevolent community to being able to escape self-focus and social isolation.

Paul Wink and Michele Dillon, in their "Do Generative Adolescents Become Healthy Older Adults?" present novel findings based on longitudinal data. The authors address their title question by examining data gathered from two adolescent research cohorts first interviewed in California in the 1930s and subsequently interviewed every 10 years until the late 1990s. *Generativity*, defined as behavior indicative of intense positive emotion extending to all humanity, was measured in three dimensions: givingness, prosocial competence, and social perspective. Using this multidimensional measure of generative behavior, the authors were able to isolate a potential mechanism underlying the generativity-health connection. The results of the study indicated that generative adolescents indeed do become both psychologically and physically healthier adults and that this health effect is more pronounced in the psychological realm. They also found that while parental social class and religiousness were surprisingly unrelated to adolescent generative behavior, positive intrafamilial relationships strongly predicted generativity. Last, the physical health effect appears to be the result only of the prosocial competence dimension of generativity. The authors note that while their measure of generativity was indistinguishable from measures of altruism, their study lends support to the thesis that while givingness and warmth are key emotions underpinning altruism, the ability to put these emotions into practice depends upon the competence to act prosocially. In conclusion, the authors discuss the necessary limitations of the study in terms of sample size and demographic make-up caused by the relative homogeneity of the sample living in San Francisco's East Bay area in the 1930s. Despite these limitations, Wink and Dillon's study lends crucial support to the notions that it is good to be good and that the benefits of altruism accrue across the entire lifespan.

Elizabeth Midlarsky and Eva Kahana, in "Altruism, Well-Being, and Mental Health in Late Life," provide a splendid combination of philosophy and science as they explain the consequences of altruism, in the forms of well-being and mental health, through the prism of the altruistic paradox. "Why should altruism have positive consequences for well-being and for mental health?" they ask. Midlarsky and Kahana have for several decades researched the contributory model of successful aging.

Although such contributory or altruistic helping "is not *motivated* by rewards to the helper, and may be very costly, it is expected to yield benefits to the helper," they hypothesize. Midlarsky and Kahana describe their work over the 24 years during which they have engaged in a program of research relevant to altruism and helping in late life. Their research was initiated in the 1980s to address the extent to which older adults help others, why they do so, and what the psychosocial benefits for altruism and helping are in late life.

Gail Ironson, in "Altruism and Health in HIV," presents her research on altruism and health in the specific context of persons with AIDS. She begins with a review of the literature on AIDS patients who volunteer to help others with the illness. This literature indicates that, as a result of such helping, the volunteers develop a positive sense of self, increase safer sex behaviors, and feel at greater peace with regard to their own future deaths. Ironson then turns to her own research on a group of 79 long-term survivors of AIDS (people who have survived twice as long as expected), who were compared with a group who had AIDS with a normal course of the illness. The long survivors were significantly more likely to have engaged in AIDS volunteerism and had significantly less depression, anxiety, and perceived stress. In her subsequent study on the psychological predictors of slower disease progression, she again found that volunteering, giving to charities, and expressing caring for others are related to better prognosis in AIDS and to less emotional distress.

Marc A. Musick and Miranda R. Waggoner, in "Self-Initiated Volunteering and Mental Health," propose and test a theory that self-initiated volunteers will reap greater mental health rewards than those who volunteer after being invited. The authors first present a literature review of volunteering and health, noting that while there are many studies showing a positive benefit of volunteering to health, they are largely limited to older adults and fail to address the dynamics of the volunteering process, specifically in what ways the how and why of volunteering affect health outcomes. The authors posit that self-initiated volunteering is a more altruistic act than invited volunteering, mainly because of the social contractual or obligatory relationship that arises in the latter. Further, because the mental health benefits of volunteering often come from improved self-esteem and social networking, self-initiated volunteers may reap greater rewards in these areas because their motives are in essence "purer," and they are more likely to be entering an entirely new social circle than are invited volunteers. To address their hypotheses, the authors use the Survey of Texas Adults (2004), a telephone interview–based survey of 1,504 adults on questions of health, community participation, and religion. The two main variables studied were psychological distress and volunteering. Interestingly, the main effects of volunteering were either insignificant or were opposite to the authors' expectations. Musick and Waggoner offer two possible explanations for the discrepancy: First, they need a better measure than self-initiation to access the altruistic motivations behind volunteering (i.e., the hypothesis is true but the measures are faulty), and second, the dynamics of being asked to volunteer and then fulfilling that request may bestow the mental health benefit of fulfilling social expectations rather than causing feelings of guilt or obligation. In conclusion, there is much room for further research on the intricacies of the decision to volunteer and how the nature of that decision can affect the beneficial health outcomes of the act.

Peter L. Benson, E. Gil Clary, and Peter C. Scales, in "Altruism and Health: Is There a Link During Adolescence?" begin by identifying three categories of adolescent health: the obvious domain of physical health, risk behaviors that are the traditional focus of intervention programs, and a newer approach that focuses on both individual and societal well-being as a health measure. The latter includes indicators of adolescent thriving and flourishing, like prosocial orientation, and measures of developmental success. In the next two sections of

the chapter, the authors review the current literature on the relationship between prosocial orientation and risk and thriving measures, and the influence
of community volunteerism on health. Particular attention is given to the Search
Institute's large cross-sectional study of 200,000 students in 318 communities,
which found positive associations between volunteering and thriving measures
and negative associations between volunteering and risk behaviors. In several
intervention-style studies, teens who were given a volunteering opportunity were
then compared to others who did not participate. This research yielded moderate associations of volunteerism with reduced risk behavior. The authors offer
several mechanisms to explain the observed relationships, including the constructive use of time, access to positive role models, development of moral identity, and development of supportive relationships, which volunteerism often
provides. Volunteering may provide access to external assets, such as relationships with adults, parents, school, and community, and internal assets, like
the development of compassion, empathy, and competence. It is important
to recognize the interconnection of internal and external assets in the volunteering experience, as well as the dynamic relationship between prosocial activities and health. In order to further research in this area, the authors recommend
more studies on adolescent cohorts and more studies that follow the scientific method of pre-test evaluation, intervention, and follow-up in order to
better assess the causal relationships among prosocial orientation, volunteerism,
and health.

Adam S. Hirschfelder, with Sabrina L. Reilly, in "Rx: Volunteer: A Prescription for Healthy Aging," look at how physicians might recommend healthy altruistic behaviors in older adults. The authors examine the role that primary
care physicians can play in translating the research on the health benefits of
volunteering into effective interventions and programs that will reach the burgeoning population of older adults in this country. At present, the United States
has the largest and fastest growing population of older adults in its history, primarily due to the aging of the "baby boomer" generation. This group is also
healthier, wealthier, and longer-lived than previous generations and is increasingly seen as a large potential resource for the volunteer sector. While there are
many government and independent agencies recruiting older adults to serve, the
authors believe that there is a missing element in these efforts—the health care
system. There are several reasons that physicians may be effective volunteerism
advocates. First, volunteering tends to drop off after age 65, at the precise time
when its health benefits have been shown to be the most pronounced and when
doctor visits are frequent. Second, studies have shown that older adults in particular are receptive to health advice from their physicians. Last, physicians have
been effective advocates for increased physical activity in older adults, and involvement in volunteering may actually be easier to achieve, given the resistance
of much of this population to exercise programs. In California, the Public Health
Institute has begun an 18-month study to assess patient and physician knowledge

about the health benefits of volunteering, implement a referral service for placing older adults in volunteer positions, and assess a small intervention study in which physicians will mention the positive impact of volunteering during office visits. In conclusion, the authors identify several steps needed to help integrate volunteering advocacy into the medical setting, including specific profiles of which older adults will most benefit from volunteer activity, information about which volunteer activities have the highest mental and physical health benefits, and funding for more intervention studies like the one mentioned above.

1   Does Volunteering Foster
Physical Health and Longevity?

Doug Oman

In the abstract, few ideas generate more widespread agreement than the notion that a high level of citizen volunteering will benefit society. Formal volunteer work and informal helping of diverse kinds are seen as signs of "social capital" and socially healthy civic engagement, supported by both the political Left and the political Right (Putnam, 1993). Approximately half of adults of all ages in the United States engage in formal volunteer work each year (Hodgkinson & Weitzman, 1996). Several authors have presented data or argued that such volunteering may bring health or well-being benefits for youth, mature adults, or older persons. Others describe interventions in school, medical, or other settings to encourage such volunteering (Hirschfelder & Reilly, this volume; Midlarsky & Kahana, 1994). Beneficial effects from volunteering, as this volume suggests, may be part of a larger pattern of benefit from altruistic emotions and altruistic behaviors (e.g., Ironson, this volume; Schwartz, this volume; Sternberg, this volume). In modern societies, where people possess few extended family ties, some argue that volunteering may be especially beneficial (Oman et al., 1999).

Cautionary voices have also been raised. Social critics warn against extreme political approaches that relegate to volunteers the responsibility for activities that are best done by other institutions in society, such as governments (Petras, 1997). Scientific critics question whether the effects of volunteering might be fully explained by other factors, such as social support or social capital. Many point out that the benefits of volunteering are likely to be larger for some persons than for others. For example, the benefits of volunteering may vary according to a person's age, gender, or stage of emotional, cognitive, or spiritual development. *Too much* volunteering—volunteering beyond what is best for an individual —could be unhealthy. An additional question also commonly arises: If volunteering provides benefits beyond paid work, then, if a person receives pay for a job that he or she previously performed as a volunteer, will the job abruptly become less healthy?

The purpose of this chapter is to offer a scientific perspective and to review available evidence on how volunteering affects health and longevity. We focus on formal volunteer work, performed through a school, hospital, library, or environmental, political, or other organization. Formal volunteer work stands in contrast to more casual or unorganized helping activities, often termed "informal helping," such as giving directions to a stranger or serving as a caregiver for a family member or a neighbor (Wilson, 2000). Volunteering must also be distinguished from paid work. Formal volunteering has been the topic of a great deal of social scientific study, although most previous research has examined predictors of volunteering rather than its consequences (Wilson, 2000).

This chapter's primary focus is on physical health outcomes, although I will also cite evidence linking volunteering with improved mental health and subjective well-being. First, I describe mechanisms by which volunteering might affect physical health, as well as moderating factors that might strengthen or weaken these influences. Next, I review empirical evidence suggesting that volunteering may indeed provide physical and mental health benefits. I conclude by discussing some practical implications and needs for further research.

MECHANISMS LINKING VOLUNTEERING TO HEALTH

Scholars from several different academic disciplines have described mechanisms by which formal volunteering may bring health benefits. Volunteering-health mechanisms have been theorized, for example, in the professional literatures of sociology (Musick et al., 1999), psychology (Oman et al., 1999), and gerontology (Morrow-Howell et al., 2003). Although scholars trained in different disciplines use distinct languages, they tend to identify similar potential mechanisms. Some note that performing volunteer work may foster enhanced physical activity (Luoh & Herzog, 2002). But job requirements for physical activity are often minimal and offer an insufficient explanation for observed patterns.

Across disciplines, two additional suggested mediating pathways are enhanced social support and enhanced positive psychological states (e.g., mental health). The first of these widely proposed pathways, social ties and support, is well established as a protective factor for physical health. Precisely how social support translates into physical health remains unclear, however, despite much research (Cohen et al., 2000). Potential benefits from possessing social support may include access to better health information (such as how to access health services), more instrumental and tangible support (e.g., child care, food, money, access to jobs), being subjected to social pressure toward healthy behavior, and improved mental health. Most types of volunteer work appear likely to foster larger and more supportive social networks by encouraging positive interactions with coworkers and clients.

The second widely cited pathway is improved mental health and psychological states, which are also increasingly well established as a protective factor for physical health. This factor may translate into improved physical health in at least two ways. First, improved psychological states may prevent or reduce maladaptive health behaviors (e.g., reduce the impulse to smoke or to engage in other substance abuse). Second, improved psychological states and mental health may foster reduced distress-related wear and tear on the body ("allostatic load"), translating into improved physical health through psychoneuroimmunologic or psychoendocrinologic pathways (McEwen, 1998). Volunteer work may foster improved mental health through several mechanisms, including reduced maladaptive self-absorption and enhanced experience of meaning. Importantly, social support and mental health are mutually reinforcing factors, in the sense that a person who enjoys a higher level of one of these factors will typically find it easier to get or maintain a high level of the other factor.

It is obvious yet noteworthy that volunteer work and paid work share many common protective features (Luoh & Herzog, 2002). For example, volunteering may provide a stable role in life when one or more other roles are missing (Greenfield & Marks, 2004). Like many kinds of work, formal volunteering may also provide a healthy opportunity for challenge. As useful skills are learned or maintained, volunteering may foster perceived self-efficacy and competence and support an active, "agentic" self-identity (Shmotkin et al., 2003). By engaging the volunteer in a collective effort with other persons, volunteer work may also foster enhanced meaningfulness and purpose. Being engaged in a larger purpose may beneficially distract a volunteer from his or her own troubles, protecting against maladaptive self-absorption (Matthews & Wells, 1996). If perceived as benefiting society or other persons, work may satisfy a perceived or dispositional need to feel "useful" and to contribute to the welfare of others (Luoh & Herzog, 2002). These are common potential benefits shared by many jobs, both paid and volunteer.

Specific Contributions of Volunteer Work

But because their work is voluntary, some protective mechanisms may operate more intensely among formal volunteers, in comparison to paid workers. For example, volunteers are generally more able to seek out jobs that are meaningful and not excessively stressful (Luoh & Herzog, 2002). Volunteers are often freer to set upper and lower limits to their work hours and to pursue the work at a comfortable pace. Volunteers may also more freely direct their efforts toward tasks and causes that they perceive as truly beneficial to society (in contrast, for example, to some paid work that generates profits by selling unneeded or harmful products). Heightened meaning in work may in turn offer intensified protection against maladaptive self-absorption (Matthews & Wells, 1996). More generally, a heightened experience of meaning in life may promote mental and physical health because "a number of aspects of meaning may be critical in people's adjustment to stress" (Park & Folkman, 1997, p. 115). Thus, compared to paid workers, volunteers may often be positioned to experience more of a variety of psychological benefits that work can provide.

However, nothing suggests that volunteer work is *uniformly* better than paid work. Everything else being equal, for example, much evidence confirms that a higher income is related to better health. Furthermore, receiving payment for work could be seen as confirmation of a worker's worthiness, leading to better mental health or a wider set of future opportunities.

Can the advantages of paid and volunteer work be combined? The observation that both volunteer work and paid work tend to possess specific advantages suggests that from a life course development perspective, each may offer distinct contributions. While paid work offers more financial benefit, volunteer work may offer other specific advantages, such as exploring and acting upon what is most meaningful.

Research confirms that people engage in volunteer work for diverse, sometimes altruistic, motives. Self-reports of altruistic motives need not be dismissed scientifically. Empirical evidence confirms that altruistic motivations, understood as other-oriented emotional responses "elicited by and congruent with the perceived welfare of someone else," cannot be reduced to or explained away as disguised selfishness (Batson et al., 2002, p. 486). Clary and colleagues (1998) found consistent evidence for six motives for volunteering: gaining social support, career advancement, growth in understanding, protection against negative feelings, personal enhancement, and the altruistic value of serving others. Individual volunteering occurs in many cases for a combination of motives.

Potential developmental benefits and health influences from volunteer work are not limited to benefits that a volunteer consciously understands or envisions. For example, a person may initially volunteer through a desire for sociability and experience benefits from enhanced social support. The volunteer work experience may also foster a reduced maladaptive self-centered focus on "me, my and mine" (Oman et al., 1999). Over time, if such a person develops a desire to "give back" to society, or develops spiritual strivings to serve humanity, such a person may volunteer for primarily selfless motives, but still experience heightened social and emotional support by volunteering.

The Contribution of Altruistic Motives

These considerations suggest that volunteer work may influence health in part by facilitating exploration, at various stages in a person's life course, of commitments to altruistically and prosocially motivated personal strivings. Thus, the potential contribution of volunteer work and altruistic behavior to health may depend in part upon the role played by altruistic motives in optimal human development and in optimal mental health.

At present, no scientific consensus exists regarding the precise role of altruistic motives in optimal human development or functioning. Uncertainty about altruism is related to a broader set of scientific and philosophical questions about how human nature evolved and is constituted. For example, views differ about how human beings may be related to higher or divine powers, how human nature evolved and is shaped by its evolutionary history and genome, and the extent to which human beings can or should aim to transcend selfishness (Miller, 2005; C. Smith, 2003). Modern daily living, too, is shaped by competing and contradictory views of human nature. For example, the mass media in the United States strongly project individualistic, consumerist, and hedonistic views of human developmental needs. On the other hand, many modern laypersons and scientists draw practical guidance from other sources, including spiritual and religious wisdom traditions, which emphasize overcoming selfishness as a primary task of optimal human development (H. Smith, 1991).

What seems plausible and likely to generate considerable consensus is that becoming committed to and enacting prosocial and altruistic motives plays at least *some* part—perhaps paramount or perhaps circumscribed—in optimal human development. Such a view is consistent with observed linkages between positive mental health and prosocial qualities such as generativity and informal helping (e.g., Schwartz, this volume; Wink & Dillon, this volume). That is, most individuals may experience periods in life—perhaps brief or perhaps prolonged or enduring—when a key developmental task, harmful if neglected, requires intensifying in some way the person's prosocial and altruistic commitments. Successfully intensifying or adopting a novel personal commitment is often quite challenging. Thus, some have suggested that overcoming selfishness and cultivating altruistic love is a lifelong task for most persons (H. Smith, 1991). If so, then volunteering, as a way of cultivating selfless concern, might offer benefits to many persons throughout the life course.

Who Benefits Most?

People clearly differ from each other and change over time in their immediate developmental needs and personal motivations. Accordingly, the perspective outlined above suggests that the specific benefits of being a volunteer may vary according to the nature of the volunteer work, as well as a person's background and upbringing, personal qualities, and stage in life. A newly retired executive, for example, might find a life-restorative sense of purpose through volunteer tutoring, whereas a decade earlier, amid 60-hour weeks, the prospect of volunteering might have appeared to be a distressing burden.

Oman and Thoresen (2000) suggest that benefits from volunteering may be greatest when volunteering is complemented by activities that support reshaping personal goals for meeting urgent or important life tasks (whatever these may be). For example, goal change may be beneficial for adolescents to become personally independent, or for older adults to cope, perhaps through religion, with heightened awareness of their physical decline and mortality:

> By experientially engaging a person in activities that are congruent with both old and new goals, volunteering may help people to loosen their ties to older goals and to contemplate as well as to commit themselves to new goals. By providing affirmation of a person's emerging changes in personal goals . . . other activities, such as religious involvement, may help the person to consolidate their engagement with new goals and motives. (Oman & Thoresen, 2000, pp. 65–66)

Theory also suggests that *motivation* could influence the health consequences of volunteering. For example, volunteering solely for the sake of career advancement could result in distressing self-consciousness about job performance, reinforcing rather than reducing destructive levels of self-preoccupation. On the other hand, we cannot expect altruistic motivations to be purely advantageous for health. For example, an altruistically motivated volunteer might experience reduced social support if he or she is seen as unusual in a setting where others volunteer for the sake of career concerns.

Clearly, many factors may potentially influence the degree to which volunteer work is beneficial for an individual. Much individual variation will be present, leading to unpredictability in individual cases. But human beings are endowed with a common human nature—whatever precisely it may be—and thus possess broadly similar developmental needs across the life course. Thus it seems quite possible that, across populations, many patterns may exist in how much health benefit people derive from volunteer work, and in who benefits most. An important function of empirical research is to search for and document such patterns.

EMPIRICAL EVIDENCE

Dozens of studies over several decades have examined relationships between volunteer work and health-related outcomes. Most studies have shown positive volunteering-health associations. Among youth, evidence suggests that volunteer work is associated with a plethora of positive developmental outcomes, such as academic achievement, civic responsibility, and life skills that include leadership and interpersonal self-confidence (Astin & Sax, 1998). A major experimental study reveals that volunteer work may exert favorable causal effects on health-related behaviors among youth. Allen, Philliber, Herrling, and Kuperminc (1997) randomly assigned 695 high school students at 25 sites nationwide to either a control condition or to participate in a "developmentally focused" intervention that included volunteer work as a primary component. Compared to nonvolunteers, adolescent volunteers had significantly lower rates of teen pregnancy and school dropout 9 months later. Consistent with theoretical perspectives suggested above, Allen and colleagues noted that the most successful program sites for adolescent volunteers offered a second intervention component consisting of classroom activities that helped the students to "cope with important [psychosocial] developmental tasks" of adolescence (1997, pp. 731–732).

Very few studies have examined volunteering and health relationships among middle-aged adults. Much more plentiful evidence is available on older adults. More than a dozen studies, for example, have examined volunteering and mental health among older adults (Wheeler et al., 1998). Multiple studies have also explored the consequences of older volunteering for longevity, physical functioning, and self-rated health (a strong independent predictor of longevity). The remainder of this section therefore reviews evidence about older volunteers.

Individual and collective limitations in available studies, however, place corresponding limits on what we may infer. For example, studies of older volunteers have assessed volunteer work in diverse ways, sometimes yielding differing results, making it unclear which features of volunteering matter the most for health. Studies that focused on mental health or subjective well-being outcomes have usually failed to document whether these psychological advantages translate into better physical health. Many studies used correlational designs that assessed volunteer work and health at the same moment in time. Such cross-sectional studies cannot easily determine causal direction, i.e., distinguish between the possibility that volunteering causes people to become more healthy or, alternatively, that people who begin with better health are more likely to volunteer. To provide persuasive evidence of causality, a study must guard against the effects of such selection of volunteers according to prior health status.

But selection by health status is only one of many threats to valid causal inference. Another difficulty is confounding by unrelated demographic factors. For example, additional education might lead people to adopt better health behaviors, as well as making people more likely to volunteer. Even if volunteering had no independent causal influence on health, the mutual influence from education would lead to a positive correlation of volunteering with health. Thus, to guard against such threats to valid causal inference—and to provide persuasive evidence about causality—a study must guard against confusing the effect of volunteering with the effect of prior health, prior education, or other such potential confounding variables.

Volunteering and Longevity

Six recent studies about volunteering and longevity provide relatively strong, although far from conclusive, evidence about causal direction. Major features of these recent studies are summarized in Table 1.1. All of these studies performed statistical adjustments to eliminate the effects of selection by prior health status or other potential confounding variables.

As can be seen in Table 1.1, five of these studies took place in the United States, and the other occurred in Israel. All but one of the U.S. studies examined nationwide probability samples, suggesting that their findings can be generalized to the nation as a whole. All six studies focused on older adults, both men and women, with the minimum age varying from 55 to 75 years. Each study began following its participants, consisting of both volunteers and nonvolunteers, when they were dwelling in the community. Sample sizes varied from about 1,200 to almost 16,000. The mortality status of participants was tracked for periods that ranged from 2 to 8 years. Four of the six studies used Cox proportional hazards regression, a rigorous and sophisticated analytic technique, to compare the risks of death among participants who volunteered more with those who volunteered less or not at all.[1] Volunteering was assessed by self-report, drawing upon four strategies: (1) dichotomous, i.e., any volunteering versus none; (2) the number of organizations for which the person volunteered; (3) the average number of hours volunteered over a period of time, e.g., per year; or (4) the use of a more or less subjective measure of frequency ("never," "rarely," "sometimes," "frequently").

As can be seen in Table 1.1, column 4, all of these studies reported that volunteers tended to live statistically significantly longer than those who did not volunteer. For example, the study by Oman and colleagues shows that compared with nonvolunteers, those who volunteered for one organization or two or more organizations experienced unadjusted reductions in mortality of 26% and 63%, respectively. Across all studies in Table 1.1, compared to those who did not volunteer, unadjusted mortality rates among volunteers were reduced by between 26% and 63%.[2]

Only the study by Musick and colleagues (1999) reported evidence suggesting that larger amounts of volunteering—in this case, more than 40 hours per year, or for two or more organizations—might produce less benefit than smaller amounts of volunteering. In contrast, two studies showed trends, sometimes statistically significant, for larger amounts of volunteering to be associated with larger benefits (Harris & Thoresen, 2005; Oman et al., 1999).

Table 1.1. Characteristics and Findings From Major Studies of Volunteer Work and Mortality

Authors (Year)	Sample and Follow-up Period	Measure of Volunteering	Risk Reduction (%)		Adjustment Variable[a]			
			Unadjusted	Adjusted	Prior Health	Health Behaviors	Social Support	Moderators[b]
Rogers (1996)	Ages 55+ (U.S.), 1984–1991, N = 15,938	Any volunteering in past year vs. none	50[c]	19	Lives with others for health reason, Household ADL[d]		Married, Family structure, Attends shows, Religious services, Visits relatives, Visits friends	(unexplored)
Musick et al. (1999)	Ages 65+ (U.S.), 1986–1994, N = 1,211	# Organizations (1 vs. 0, 2+ vs. 0), Hours/year (< 40 vs. 0, 40+ vs. 0)	60, 35, 54, 42	40, ns[e], 30, ns[e]	Chronic illness, Mobility	Physical activity	Lives with others, Informal social interaction	↓Informal social interaction, ↑Lives with others
Oman et al. (1999)	Ages 55+ (Calif.), 1990–1995, N = 1,972	# Organizations (1 vs. 0, 2+ vs. 0), Hours/week (< 4 vs. 0, 4+ vs. 0)	26, 63[g], 31, 51[g]	ns[e] 44, —, —	Chronic illness, Mobility, Perceived health, Depressed	Exercises, Smokes, Alcohol[h], Sleep[h]	Married, Religious services, Social connections	↑Religious services, ↑Religious groups
Shmokin et al. (2003)	Ages 75+ (Israel), 1989–1997, N = 1,343	Any volunteering at present vs. none	—	33	Perceived health, Cognitive function, Depressed, Life satisfaction	Physical activity	Close relationships	↑Everyday activities

(continued)

Table 1.1. (continued)

Authors (Year)	Sample and Follow-up Period	Measure of Volunteering	Risk Reduction (%)		Adjustment Variable[a]			
			Unadjusted	Adjusted	Prior Health	Health Behaviors	Social Support	Moderators[b]
Harris & Thorensen (2005)	Ages 70+ (U.S.), 1984–1991, N = 7,496	Volunteering in past 12 months (rarely, sometimes, frequently vs. never)	41, 42, 53	ns, ns[e] 19	Chronic illness Mobility Activity limits Perceived health	Exercises	Married Living arrangements Visits friends Visits relatives Religious services Attends shows	↑Religious services ↑Visit friends
Luoh & Herzog (2002)	Ages 70+ (U.S.), 1998–2000, N = 4,860	Hours/year (100+ vs. <100)	67[i]	60[i]	Chronic illness Perceived health ADL[d] Cognitive function Depressed Psychological problem	Smokes Exercises	Married Social contacts Importance of religion[h] Employed	(unexplored)

[a]All studies adjusted for demographics (age, gender, ethnicity) and socioeconomic status (education and sometimes income and wealth).
[b]Arrows indicate that greater longevity increases associated with volunteering correspond to higher (↑) or lower (↓) levels of the moderator.
[c]Computed from information supplied in Table 1 of Rogers (1926).
[d]ADL = activities of daily living.
[e]ns = not significant.
[f]Significant at only p < .10). (other moderators are significant at p < .05).
[g]Adjusted for age and gender in Oman et al. (1999).
[h]Text indicates that adjustment for this variable had little effect, although it is not included in final adjusted estimates.
[i]Approximately 60% reduction in chance of death versus being in good to excellent health

Could these patterns of advantage among volunteers be attributable not to causal health benefits from volunteering, but to potential confounding variables? Each of these studies adjusted for demographic variables, such as age, gender, and ethnicity, and the Israeli study also adjusted for place of origin. Each study also adjusted for measures of socioeconomic status, including education and sometimes income and wealth. As seen in column 6, each study also adjusted for one or more measures of health status, as measured before the beginning of the follow-up period. For example, Oman and colleagues (1999) adjusted for number of chronic diseases and a measure of physical mobility. They also adjusted for self-perceived health status and depression.

Most of these studies adjusted for two other classes of potentially confounding variables: measures of health behaviors and of social connections/support. For example, high levels of volunteering and good health behaviors might both be attributable to a preexisting trait or disposition (e.g., a tendency to be conscientious). Therefore, a conservative estimate of the causal relationship between volunteering and health should adjust for prior health behaviors (see column 7). Except for the early investigation by Rogers (1996), an adjustment for physical activity or exercise was included in every study. However, only two studies included a measure of smoking, and only one included a measure of alcohol consumption. These omissions raise the possibility that the favorable correlations are explained by a volunteer's previously developed healthy habits, rather than by the effects of volunteering.

A similar issue exists with regard to social support. High levels of volunteering and abundant forms of social support might both be attributable to a preexisting trait or disposition (e.g., extroversion). Therefore, most studies included adjustments for prior social connections and support (column 8). Most studies included a measure of marital status or close relationships. Most studies also adjusted for religious involvement, usually with a measure of attendance at religious services. Several studies also adjusted for measures of social connections with family or friends.

Table 1.1, column 5 ("adjusted" effect), indicates the overall protective effect of volunteering among all participants, after the adjustments for demographics, prior health, health behaviors, and social support. Across studies, the most active volunteers experienced statistically significant mortality rate reductions of between 19 and 44%,[3] when compared to nonvolunteers. An exception to this pattern is the report by Musick and colleagues that participants most active in volunteering were not significantly protected, whereas statistically significant reductions of 30–40% occurred among *moderately* engaged volunteers.

Although these studies do not agree in the precise details of their findings, the overall pattern seems clear: Volunteering is associated with substantial reductions in mortality rates, and these reductions are not easily explained by differences in demographics or socioeconomic status, or by prior health status or other types of social connections and social support, or by prior levels of physical activity and exercise. Greater longevity among volunteers also does not appear attributable to prior levels of smoking, although smoking was examined in only two studies. Only one study examined preestablished patterns of alcohol consumption and sleep, neither of which explained volunteer longevity.

Which volunteers are most likely to experience additional longevity? The final column of Table 1.1 indicates that four of the six studies reported statistically significant patterns in who received added longevity. The benefit tended to be greatest among those with *higher* levels of other psychosocial support indicators, such as religious involvement and social connections and interactions. That is, these other forms of psychosocial support appeared to complement volunteering and boost its value, rather than substitute for it or make it unnecessary. For example, after adjusting for all potential confounders, Oman and colleagues reported that volunteering was associated with a (significantly larger) 60% reduction in mortality among persons who frequently attended religious services. Similarly, after all adjustments, Harris and Thoresen reported that volunteering was associated with 30% lower mortality among those attending services, but the protection associated with volunteering was not statistically significant among nonattenders. The only exception to this general pattern was reported by Musick and colleagues, who found that volunteering was associated with more benefit among volunteers with *less* social interaction.

Physical Functioning and Mobility

Volunteers apparently live longer—but are they healthier? Several studies have examined relationships between volunteering and physical functioning. Moen, Dempster-McClain, and Williams (1989) studied 427 women who resided in upstate New York and were both wives and mothers in 1956. Over the next 30 years, compared to nonvolunteers, women who did any volunteering had better physical functioning in 1986, after adjusting for baseline health status, level of education, and number of life roles. Similarly, Luoh and Herzog (2002) found that, compared to nonvolunteers or those volunteering less than 100 hours, those who were volunteering 100 hours or more in 1998 were approximately 30% less likely to experience physical functioning limitations, even after adjusting for demographics, socioeconomic status, baseline functioning limitations, health status, paid employment, exercise, smoking, and social connections. Morrow-Howell and colleagues (2003) examined data collected between 1986 and 1994 from more than 1,500 U.S. adults, finding that volunteering predicted significantly less functional disability 3 to 5 years later, after adjusting for demographics, socioeconomic status, marital status, and informal social integration. Protective effects were significantly stronger among older volunteers.

Self-Rated Physical Health

Self-rated physical health is a strong predictor of longevity, independent of numerous established predictors, including demographics, specific health status indicators, and social support (Idler & Benyamini, 1997). Three of the studies in Table 1.1 examined baseline cross-sectional relationships between volunteering and perceived health, and in each case more volunteering was associated with better perceived health (Harris & Thoresen, 2005; Oman et al., 1999; Shmotkin et al., 2003). But since these relationships were studied cross-sectionally, these studies do not address the possibility that people who perceive their health as better are more likely to volunteer (selection effects).

Stronger longitudinal evidence about perceived health is provided by Luoh and Herzog (2002) and by other studies not included in Table 1.1. Van Willigen (2000) studied 2,867 U.S. adults aged 25 and older, finding that (any) volunteer work in 1986 was associated with significantly better perceived health in 1989 for participants of all ages, with effects especially pronounced among persons over age 60. Advantages for volunteers remained significant after adjusting for demographics, socioeconomic status, baseline levels of perceived health, social integration and support, and marital, parental, and paid employment status. When individuals over 60 years of age in this cohort were followed until 1994, volunteers continued to report better self-rated health, after similar adjustments (Morrow-Howell et al., 2003). Using a different data set, Luoh and Herzog (2002) found that volunteering for 100 or more hours per year in 1998 was associated with approximately 30–40% reduction in the odds of rating one's health as fair or poor, in contrast to good or excellent, in 2000 after adjusting for numerous potential confounders, including demographics, socioeconomic status, baseline perceived health, health status, paid employment, exercise, smoking, and social connections. One study, however, did not find a relationship: Among 427 women recruited in 1956, Moen, Dempster-McClain, and Williams (1989) found no significant differences in perceived health between volunteers and nonvolunteers 30 years later in 1986, after multiple adjustments.

Health Behaviors

Do volunteers practice better health behaviors? Several of the studies in Table 1.1 present evidence of positive cross-sectional relationships between volunteering and beneficial health behaviors. After adjusting for age, Oman and colleagues (1999) found that higher levels of volunteering were significantly related to exercising and refraining from smoking. Furthermore, Musick and colleagues (1999), Shmotkin and colleagues (2003), and Harris and Thoresen (2005) each found statistically significant associations between volunteering and greater physical activity.

Mental Health

Recently, Musick and Wilson (2003) studied volunteering and depression from 1986 to 1994 among 3,617 U.S. adults aged 25 or older. Depression was assessed with a widely used self-report scale originally developed by the Center for Epidemiologic Studies. Consistent volunteering (e.g., in 1986, 1991, and 1994) was associated with reduced depression among all age groups at the end of the study, but was most beneficial for persons aged 65 or older. These results held after adjusting for baseline levels of depression, demographics, employment, socioeconomic status, health and functioning status, health behaviors, and attendance at religious services. Among persons over 65, volunteering for a religious organization was significantly more beneficial than other types of volunteering.

Much additional evidence, most of it cross-sectional, suggests consistent positive relationships between volunteering and better mental health and subjective well-being. Wheeler and colleagues (1998) analyzed 29 studies of the impact of volunteering and voluntary association membership by older adults on well-being outcomes, such as life satisfaction, happiness, lack of alienation, and self-actualization. They found that those who engaged in direct helping (e.g., volunteer work, 12 studies) derived significantly greater rewards than others engaged in indirect or less formalized helping roles. Furthermore, "nearly eight of every ten such formally helping older volunteers scored higher on quality of life measures than the average non-volunteer" (p. 75).

A rare if not unique experimental study of the health effects of volunteering by older adults examined self-esteem as an outcome. Midlarsky and Kahana (1994) randomly assigned 60 community-dwelling older adults to a control group and 60 to receive a strong and individualized persuasive appeal to volunteer. Those receiving the intervention were significantly more likely to volunteer and to do other forms of helping. They also scored higher on a subsequent measure of self-esteem.

Weight of the Evidence

What does this evidence tell us about the effects on physical health of volunteer work and of altruistic motives? The available studies are fairly consistent in suggesting that volunteering is associated on average with longer life, better self-rated health, and better physical functioning, even after adjusting for numerous potential confounding variables. However, the studies do not present a consistent picture regarding which features of volunteering—the time spent, the number of organizations served, or merely occupying the volunteer role—are most strongly associated with benefit. Conclusions must be also tempered because relatively few experimental studies are available, and the most persuasive experimental evidence applies only to adolescents (Allen et al., 1997). Furthermore, despite numerous adjustments, most studies have failed to examine other potentially relevant confounding variables, such as smoking and alcohol consumption. Thus, although these data are quite compatible with the possibility that volunteering causally benefits health in the ways discussed earlier, other explanations cannot yet be firmly ruled out.

Does volunteering foster better health behaviors? Several studies confirm that volunteers are more physically active, and a few studies indicate other risk-profile advantages (e.g., less smoking). These results are consistent with suggestions that volunteering supports better health behaviors, although the present evidence does not address the underlying causal direction.

Do all volunteers benefit equally? Available mortality studies (Table 1.1) seem to agree that longevity benefits are *not* shared equally by all volunteers. After adjustments, four of the six mortality studies report that some volunteers enjoy more added longevity than others. The greatest apparent benefit is generally not received by volunteers who are socially isolated or inactive. Rather, of the seven statistically significant moderating variables reported by these studies, all but one indicate that volunteering is associated with more benefit among volunteers who have higher levels of other psychosocial connections. This phenomenon appears in populations from Israel, California, and two different nationally representative U.S. samples, suggesting it is not merely accidental. The phenomenon seems consistent with the suggestion made above that volunteer work is most beneficial when complemented with resources for coping with important life tasks. That is, many social connections among older persons may supply assistance in coping with important life tasks, which for older persons may involve finding renewed meaning and purpose in the face of declining health and increasing reminders of physical mortality. Additional research seems warranted to test this hypothesis as well as other possible explanations for unequal benefit.

In sum, therefore, the available evidence is consistent with most or all of the mechanisms suggested above, by which volunteering may be theorized to causally benefit health. However, other explanations may in many cases be possible, and the nature of the existing data does not permit firm causal inferences.

Also unclear is the specific health contribution of altruistic motives for volunteering. But the numerous observed moderating effects are consistent with the possibility that volunteering fosters benefit in part through increased personal commitment to altruistic and prosocial motives and through reduced rumination and self-absorption.

CONCLUSIONS

Causal health benefits from volunteering in general, and from altruistic volunteering in particular, are quite plausible when viewed in light of the large amount of evidence and theory presented here and elsewhere in this book. For laypersons who need to decide today how they will lead their lives, such evidence may be sufficient to further confirm them in personal belief systems that have celebrated altruism and love through the ages (e.g., C. Smith, 2003; H. Smith, 1991). However, a rigorous scientific investigation of unresolved questions about effects from volunteering will require much additional work. To obtain cross-cultural insight, studies of U.S. samples should be complemented with many more studies of European or non-Western cohorts. Other valuable contributions might include:

- Experimental intervention studies among older persons, perhaps testing whether benefits are enhanced by providing concurrent psychosocial support for accomplishing developmental life tasks.
- Studies of relationships between volunteering and a wider spectrum of physical health variables, including incident disease as well as physiological measures of immune and endocrine function (e.g., cortisol).
- Additional studies of volunteering and health behaviors among adolescents and middle-aged adults, especially longitudinal studies of change over time.
- Qualitative, quantitative, and theoretical studies to explain why some volunteers reap greater health benefits than do others.

Much work still remains, but the studies reviewed here offer a promising and highly suggestive beginning. Longevity enhancements for older adults as large as those observed here merit serious social attention and individual reflection. Adolescents, too, the evidence suggests, may reap large benefits from appropriate volunteering. A fuller and cross-culturally grounded understanding of the dynamics and consequences of volunteering could help extend such benefits globally to individuals of all ages.

NOTES

1. The study by Luoh and Herzog (2002) used multiple logistic regression, and the study by Rogers (1996) used discrete-time hazard rate models.
2. Note that the 67% reduction from Luoh and Herzog (2002) is not strictly comparable to other studies: It represents a 67% reduced chance, among volunteers for 100 or more hours, of dying versus enjoying "good to excellent" health.
3. See note 2 regarding the study by Luoh and Herzog (2002).

REFERENCES

Allen, J. P., Philliber, S., Herrling, S., & Kuperminc, G. P. (1997). Preventing teen pregnancy and academic failure: Experimental evaluation of a developmentally based approach. *Child Development, 68,* 729–742.

Astin, A. W., & Sax, L. J. (1998). How undergraduates are affected by service participation. *Journal of College Student Development, 39,* 251–263.

Batson, C. D., Ahmad, N., Lishner, D. A., & Tsang, J.-A. (2002). Empathy and altruism. In C. R. Snyder & S. J. Lopez (Eds.), *Handbook of positive psychology* (pp. 485–498). New York: Oxford University Press.

Clary, E. G., et al. (1998). Understanding and assessing the motivations of volunteers: A functional approach. *Journal of Personality and Social Psychology, 74,* 1516–1530.

Cohen, S., Underwood, L., & Gottlieb, B. H. (2000). *Social support measurement and intervention: A guide for health and social scientists.* New York: Oxford University Press.

Greenfield, E. A., & Marks, N. F. (2004). Formal volunteering as a protective factor for older adults' psychological well-being. *Journals of Gerontology: Psychological Sciences and Social Sciences, 59B,* S258–S264.

Harris, A. H. S., & Thoresen, C. E. (2005). Volunteering is associated with delayed mortality in older people: Analysis of the longitudinal study of aging. *Journal of Health Psychology, 10,* 739–752.

Hodgkinson, V. A., & Weitzman, M. S. (1996). *Giving and volunteering in the United States, 1996.* Washington, DC: Independent Sector.

Idler, E. L., & Benyamini, Y. (1997). Self-rated health and mortality: A review of twenty-seven community studies. *Journal of Health and Social Behavior, 38,* 21–37.

Luoh, M. C., & Herzog, A. R. (2002). Individual consequences of volunteer and paid work in old age: Health and mortality. *Journal of Health and Social Behavior, 43,* 490–509.

Matthews, G., & Wells, A. (1996). Attentional processes, dysfunctional coping, and clinical intervention. In M. Zeidner & N. S. Endler (Eds.), *Handbook of coping: Theory, research, applications* (pp. 573–601). New York: Wiley.

McEwen, B. S. (1998). Protective and damaging effects of stress mediators. *New England Journal of Medicine, 338,* 171–179.

Midlarsky, E., & Kahana, E. (1994). Helping and volunteering in late life: The results of an experimental intervention. In E. Midlarsky & E. Kahana (Eds.), *Altruism in later life* (pp. 189–220). Thousand Oaks, CA: Sage.

Miller, W. R. (2005). What is human nature? Reflections from Judeo-Christian perspectives. In W. R. Miller & H. D. Delaney (Eds.), *Human nature, motivation, and change: Judeo-Christian perspectives on psychology* (pp. 11–29). Washington, DC: American Psychological Association.

Moen, P., Dempster-McClain, D., & Williams, R. M. (1989). Social integration and longevity: An event history analysis of women's roles and resilience. *American Sociological Review, 54,* 635–647.

Morrow-Howell, N., Hinterlong, J., Rozario, P. A., & Tang, F. (2003). Effects of volunteering on the well-being of older adults. *Journals of Gerontology: Psychological Sciences and Social Sciences, 58B,* S137–S145.

Musick, M. A., Herzog, A. R., & House, J. S. (1999). Volunteering and mortality among older adults: Findings from a national sample. *Journals of Gerontology: Psychological Sciences and Social Sciences, 54B,* S173–S180.

Musick, M. A., & Wilson, J. (2003). Volunteering and depression: The role of psychological and social resources in different age groups. *Social Science and Medicine, 56,* 259–269.

Oman, D., & Thoresen, C. E. (2000). Role of volunteering in health and happiness. *Career Planning and Adult Development Journal, 15,* 59–70.

Oman, D., Thoresen, C. E., & McMahon, K. (1999). Volunteerism and mortality among the community-dwelling elderly. *Journal of Health Psychology, 4,* 301–316.

Park, C. L., & Folkman, S. (1997). Meaning in the context of stress and coping. *Review of General Psychology, 1,* 115–144.

Petras, J. (1997). Volunteerism: The great deception. *Economic and Political Weekly, 32,* 1587–1589.

Putnam, R. D. (1993). The prosperous community: Social capital and public life. *American Prospect, 4,* 35–42.

Rogers, R. G. (1996). The effects of family composition, health, and social support linkages on mortality. *Journal of Health and Social Behavior, 37,* 326–338.

Shmotkin, D., Blumstein, T., & Modan, B. (2003). Beyond keeping active: Concomitants of being a volunteer in old-old age. *Psychology and Aging, 18,* 602–607.

Smith, C. (2003). *Moral, believing animals: Human personhood and culture.* New York: Oxford University Press.

Smith, H. (1991). *The world's religions: Our great wisdom traditions.* San Francisco: Harper San Francisco.

Van Willigen, M. (2000). Differential benefits of volunteering across the life course. *Journals of Gerontology: Psychological Sciences and Social Sciences, 55B,* S308–S318.

Wheeler, J. A., Gorey, K. M., & Greenblatt, B. (1998). The beneficial effects of volunteering for older volunteers and the people they serve: A meta-analysis. *International Journal of Aging & Human Development, 47,* 69–79.

Wilson, J. (2000). Volunteering. *Annual Review of Sociology, 26,* 215–240.

2   Altruism and Subjective Well-Being: Conceptual Model and Empirical Support

Carolyn Schwartz

Although the benefits of giving support have long been acknowledged among spiritual and religious texts as a key to living well, the predominant focus in psychological research on social support has been on the benefits one enjoys when one receives social support. There is, however, emerging evidence that giving support to others provides as much or perhaps more reward to the giver than to the recipient. On the basis of two serendipitous sets of findings, I believe that altruistic social interest behaviors enhance subjective well-being for both healthy and chronically ill adults. In this chapter, I will briefly describe these findings and how they fit with a conceptual model of altruistically induced response shifts. I will conclude with some musings for the broader implications of this work and issues that have yet to be addressed in altruism research.

A GLIMPSE INTO THE SCIENTIFIC PROCESS: STUMBLING ONTO THE BENEFITS OF HELPING OTHERS

Given the predominant focus of social support literature, a natural focus for behavioral scientific work aimed at helping people with chronic illnesses would be on the benefits of receiving social support. Indeed, my first study of altruism was intended to compare the effects of two different approaches to helping people with chronic illnesses. The chronic illness we chose to study was multiple sclerosis (MS), a progressive neurological disease often characterized by cycles of flares, or exacerbations, and improvements ("relapsing-remitting" in medical jargon). My clinical experience suggested that patients' abilities to cope with the disease and its ramifications on their lives had a substantial impact on their physical, mental, and social well-being.

Building on prior work that posited that flexible coping was salutogenic, I implemented a randomized controlled trial comparing a group intervention that taught coping flexibility (Schwartz & Rogers, 1994) to a control condition in which participants received monthly phone calls from someone else with MS (Schwartz, 1999). This "peer supporter" was trained to engage in active listening, a technique from Rogerian psychotherapy where the listener helps the speaker to deepen his or her level of introspection and dialogue by asking questions that probe the emotional experience. Often, the active listener will simply repeat or paraphrase the last statement with an intonation of questioning, thereby encouraging the speaker to delve further into the topic. The study's peer supporters were explicitly requested not to shift the focus of the conversation onto themselves or experiences they might have had that were similar to the other person. They were also encouraged not to share information about the extent of their own disabilities, which ranged across the full spectrum from no obvious disability, to being constrained to an electric wheelchair and only able to control one finger to manipulate the wheelchair.

Both interventions in the trial were considered active for 1 year. The coping skills group participants attended eight weekly group sessions, usually with a spouse or friend. They were then assigned coping partners from the group and asked to call each other at least monthly for the next 10 months. The telephone support group received 12 monthly calls of 15 minutes in length. Both groups then completed follow-up questionnaires for another year, and then again 5 years after their participation in the intervention (Schwartz, Sprangers, Carey, & Reed, 2004). Results of 2-year follow-up showed significant and lasting effects of the coping skills group on role performance and well-being (Schwartz, 1999) and response shifts at 5-year follow-up that may have obfuscated the detection of any longer-term effects of the interventions (Schwartz et al., 2004).

Data were also collected from the five peer supporters, perhaps to help them relate better to the study participation experience of their "case load," perhaps because it is difficult for a behavioral scientist to resist collecting data on willing patients. Regardless, this supplementary data collection effort facilitated a fortunate serendipity: stumbling upon a stunning effect.

Over the course of 2 years during the randomized trial, the peer supporters met monthly with the principal investigator (PI) of the study (myself, Carolyn Schwartz). These meetings were intended to help the PI monitor the safety of study participants (e.g., regular checking in on all participants to ensure that no one was highly distressed or otherwise in need of a referral to a psychological professional) and to ensure that the peer supporters were following the study's protocol (i.e., maintaining calls for all people on their case load, talking for only

15 minutes, and, most important, retaining a focus on the other person, not on themselves). A notable change in the supporters became evident over this 2-year period: They seemed to be blossoming. Although it was certainly possible that this blossoming was merely the effect of everyone becoming increasingly comfortable with and fond of one another, my colleagues and I decided to look at the data we had collected to see if this effect was empirically substantiated.

As it turns out, it was. In a comparison of the effects of *receiving* either of the two helping interventions and *giving* the nondirective support, we documented that the peer supporters reported improvement on more outcomes as compared to the supported patients and that the effect size of these changes tended to be larger (Schwartz & Sendor, 1999). They reported about 4 times the benefit on psychosocial role performance (e.g., social interaction, alertness, emotional behavior, and communication), 3.5 times the benefit on adaptability (i.e., coping ability), and 7.6 times the benefit on well-being (e.g., depression, anxiety, satisfaction, happiness). Further, the impact of providing support was increasingly beneficial to the helpers over the course of their participation (Figure 2.1).

TRIANGULATING THE BENEFITS OF PEER SUPPORT: RESULTS FROM A QUALITATIVE EXPLORATION

With great curiosity to understand these findings better, we conducted a focus group with the peer supporters approximately 3 years after they had completed their role in the randomized trial (Schwartz & Sendor, 1999). This focus group queried the supporters about changes they had noticed over the course of their participation as peer supporters. For example, we asked about changes they had noticed in themselves; life changes they had initiated; changes in mood, values, relationships with others, sense of the future, and sense of the past, among others (see Schwartz & Sendor, 1999, for more detail). The focus group was recorded, transcribed, and content analyzed to identify the major themes and experiences reported by the peer supporters.

The qualitative data yielded a fuller sense of the impact of giving on the peer supporters. They reported a sense of dramatic change in their lives in a number of areas as a result of going through the experience of being a peer supporter. Five major themes emerged from the content analysis: (1) helper role as self-transcendent; (2) improved listening skills; (3) stronger awareness of the existence of a higher power; (4) increased self-acceptance; and (5) enhanced self-confidence. Whereas the first three themes appear to reflect outer-directedness, the last two seem to be self-referential. The role of peer supporter itself shifted their focus away from themselves and toward others. Their affect was attuned not to the potentially negative content of what they heard, but to the fact that they were helping someone else. They reported becoming more open and

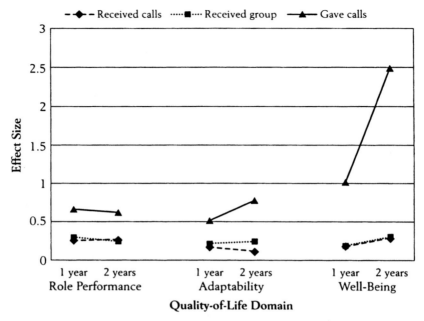

Figure 2.1. A comparison of effect size over time by group. To ease interpretation, average effect size for the three domains of quality-of-life outcome was computed using the absolute value of effect size for each of the subscales or scales within each domain (role performance, adaptability, and well-being). This figure shows that people who gave support reported more gain in outcome at both 1- and 2-year follow-up (baseline minus 1-year follow-up; baseline minus 2-year follow-up) and that the impact of providing support was increasingly beneficial to the helpers over the course of their participation.

tolerant of others and a sense of inner peace that allowed them to listen to others without judgment or interference. Some also reported an enhanced awareness of the existence of a beneficent higher power. Along with the changes in external focus were changes in self-reference, reflecting a stronger sense of self-confidence and self-acceptance. For example, supporters mentioned an increased sense of confidence in their ability to manage life's vicissitudes, as well as developing a meaningful context within the constraints of their MS condition.

A CONCEPTUAL MODEL OF ALTRUISM AND QUALITY OF LIFE

On the basis of the quantitative and qualitative data described above, we began to formulate a conceptual model of how altruistic practice influenced quality of life. We built on the foundation of the Sprangers and Schwartz (1999) model of response shift, which describes a dynamic feedback loop by which perception of quality of life is maintained despite health state changes (catalyst). This homeostasis is hypothesized to be due to the interaction of antecedent dispositional factors and psychosocial mechanisms, which can induce changes in internal standards, values, or conceptualizations of quality of life (response shifts). The central themes revealed in the focus group discussions point to a possible mechanism within the broader framework of the Sprangers and Schwartz model (shaded box in Figure 2.2).

We posited that the role of peer supporter allowed these people to disengage from patterns of self-reference and thereby facilitated an openness to changing internal standards, values, and conceptualizations of quality of life. They could consequently develop a new means of self-reference. Altruistic practice may establish an internal feedback loop which induces response shift. This loop involves projecting outward; disengagement from fixed patterns of self-reference; an openness to changes in internal standards, values, and conceptualization of quality of life; and a consequent reintegration of the antecedent condition (i.e., MS) and its personal meaning.

The peer support study whetted my curiosity about altruism, but I knew that the limitations of the study were substantial. Most important, there were only five peer supporters, and these five people had been selected because of their personal qualities. Additionally, their perseverance in the helper role reflected other positive, adaptive qualities that could have accounted for our striking find-

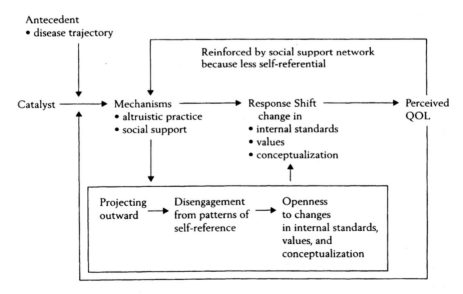

Figure 2.2. A theoretical model of response shift effects in peer support. Adapted with permission from Schwartz and Sendor (Schwartz et at., 1999), copyright Elsevier.

ings, regardless of the altruistic practice. On the basis of this first study, I could only attest to a potentially interesting set of findings that generated hypotheses for subsequent, better-controlled research. Given the difficulty I experienced getting grant funding for altruism research, I had to rely on happenstance to present me with another opportunity to study the health benefits of altruism.

SCIENTIFIC OPPORTUNISM: LESSONS LEARNED FROM A SECONDARY ANALYSIS OF PRESBYTERIANS

This situation arrived a couple of years later, when my colleagues and I were collaborating on a study of religion and health with Janice Meisenhelder. Dr. Meisenhelder facilitated our access to a large panel study of Presbyterians that has been implemented by the Presbyterian church for a number of years. We were allowed to implement secondary analysis of this data set to explore our research questions. The advantages of this data set were numerous, including a large, stratified, random sample ($N = 2,016$) with high-quality data on physical and mental health (using the SF-36; Ware & Sherbourne, 1992), prayer activities, religious coping, stressful events, sociodemographic characteristics, and, of great interest to us, questions about giving and receiving help and about feeling overwhelmed by others' demands. It should be noted that the mental health dimension investigated in this work was composed of the anxiety and depression that plague most people (i.e., the vicissitudes of adult life), rather than more pathological mental illness.

In this study, altruistic social interest was operationalized as giving help to others by summing two Likert-scaled questions that asked how often ("never" to "very often") the person had "made others feel loved and cared for" and "listened to others' concerns." Receiving help was operationalized by summing answers to two questions that asked how often the "congregation made me feel loved and cared for" and if the "congregation listened to you talk about private concerns." Higher summary scores indicated more giving or receiving more help. The balance between giving and receiving help was evaluated using a ratio of the two summary scores. Feeling overwhelmed by others' demands was evaluated by summing answers to two questions that asked how often the congregation "made too many demands on you" and "has been critical of you and the things you have done." Higher overload scores reflected feeling more overwhelmed.

We computed a series of multivariate regression analyses to examine the effects of giving versus receiving help on physical and mental health, after adjusting for possible confounding variables. We found that although giving and receiving help were associated with reported physical function, these relationships were caused by the association of these factors with age and gender and thus disappeared when we adjusted for these confounders. In this sample, older people and females reported lower physical functioning.

In contrast, both giving and receiving help were associated with better mental health, even after adjusting for other possible confounders. Although balance was not associated with mental health, feeling overwhelmed was associated with worse mental health. Our final statistical model demonstrated that giving help and feeling overwhelmed were significantly associated with reported mental health, after adjusting for demographics, prayer activities, and prayerful coping. Giving help was associated with better mental health, whereas reporting overload was associated with worse mental health.

These analyses suggested that giving help was a more important predictor of reported mental health than was receiving help. Given the moderate association between giving and receiving help ($r = .68$), we investigated whether this selection of variables in the final model was a statistical artifact or was meaningful and thus could be interpreted. We performed a conditional regression analysis, looking at the association of one score of mental health within each level of the other score. This analysis revealed that the association of mental health was stronger with the giving help score than with the receiving help score, which confirmed that the greater importance of giving help is not a statistical artifact caused by shared variance but rather reflects a substantial difference in the patterns of association.

Because giving help was such a salient predictor of mental health, we sought to understand what sociodemographic aspects, prayer activities, and religious coping behaviors were associated with this construct. A final multivariate model identified prayer activities, satisfaction with prayer life, positive religious coping, age, female gender, and being a church elder (i.e., lay leader of the congregation) as significant predictors of giving help (see Schwartz, Meisenhelder, Ma, & Reed, 2003, for more detail).

These findings suggest that helping others is associated with higher levels of mental health, above and beyond the benefits of receiving help and other known psychospiritual, stress, and demographic factors. Giving beyond one's resources is, however, associated with worse reported mental health. Our findings also suggest that role expectations and a positive belief system underlie and reinforce altruistic social interest behaviors. For example, church elders, females, older people, and more religious people would all have social role expectations of giving to others. These role expectations would likely be reinforced by a positive belief system, as reflected by positive religious coping, engaging in more prayer activities, and being satisfied with one's prayer life.

Our findings are particularly notable because the sample studied was quite physically and mentally healthy, and thus may have had less of the requisite variability for demonstrating such relationships. Additionally, although the panel data did include 2-year follow-up on the outcomes of interest, the study sample was remarkably stable, and thus there was little change in physical or mental health. This lack of variability made it statistically impossible to predict change and thus to test causal hypotheses about the benefits of helping others. The study was also limited by the post hoc nature of the operationalization of altruism (i.e., not an ideal measure of altruism) and by the fact that the sample consisted solely of volunteers from the Presbyterian church. The external validity of our findings would need to be tested among people not so closely identified with a single religion.

THE CATCH-22: DO YOU HAVE TO BE HEALTHY TO GIVE?

On the basis of the MS study and the Presbyterian study, I can say that helping others appears to be associated with better psychosocial well-being and/or mental health. Both studies did, however, have limitations that prevent broad statements about altruistic social interest behaviors *causing* better psychosocial well-being and/or mental health. Indeed, this catch-22 is a substantial bind for altruism research. Does one have to be healthy in order to have the internal resources to give to others and to glean the health benefits of giving? The results of the MS study would suggest that one does not have to be *physically* healthy, since the peer supporters displayed a broad range of disabilities. The results of the Presbyterian study would suggest that even among a relatively healthy cohort, the mental health benefits of helping others are measurable and significant. One is still left with a niggling doubt, however. In both studies, we were investigating people who volunteered their time and/or attention. It is possible that people who volunteer such commodities are well off in these regards, relative to the general population. The third-variable problem that plagues much of quasi-experimental research also plagues these two studies. To address more definitively the causal role of helping others, one would likely have to randomize people to giving or receiving help, and then measure the impact on physical and mental health. Ideally, one would randomize people with chronic health conditions where there is some room for improvement or deterioration. One could thus investigate the impact on physical and mental health outcomes. It is my hope that, despite the limitations of these initial two studies, behavioral researchers will be encouraged to investigate more comprehensively the health benefits of altruism.

REFLECTIONS FROM PERSONAL EXPERIENCE: CREATING COMMUNITY BY GIVING TO OTHERS

From an intuitive perspective, it seems clear that reaching out to others and providing caring, empathetic attention seems to help the helper. It also seems credible that helping others allows one to transcend a self-centered *zeitgeist* and subsequently to achieve a refreshed view of oneself and one's place in the world, a view that enhances one's life satisfaction and sense of well-being. This response shift model focuses, however, on perceived quality of life, a fundamentally individual outcome. I wonder what the implications of helping others might be for broader, more communal concepts.

I believe that this line of research has substantial implications for how we understand the concept of "community," what it provides to people, and what the most effective therapeutic strategies might be for improving subjective well-being. When one engages in altruistic social interest behaviors, one is reaching out beyond one's limited microcosm and weaving a connection to other microcosms and eventually to a larger world. As this behavior pattern goes on, the helper finds him- or herself touching more people in a way that is at the same time personally significant (i.e., providing help that is targeted to others' very personal needs) and nonspecific (i.e., motivated by a general orientation of benevolence or generosity of spirit). Over time, this reaching out and weaving of benevolent connections would likely lead to a sense of a benevolent net that links the helpers to a broader cosmos that extends beyond themselves, their families, or even their known friends. This net catches the needy and protects or buffers them from isolation and harm. It is a continually expanding community.

An example might serve to ground these far-reaching and perhaps romantic terms in reality. Some time ago, I underwent a highly invasive surgery for a potentially life-threatening medical condition. Upon my return home for the extended recuperation from the surgery, members of my religious community brought meals to help my family and myself to deal with the initial period of convalescence. The people who brought these meals were doing this generous act because they wanted to help other people in need, not because they knew me intimately or had a strong personal connection to my family. They chose to help because of a nonspecific generous inclination, and this help was personally meaningful to myself and my family. Henceforth, upon seeing these people at various religious events over time, our relationship has remained polite, sometimes friendly, but remote rather than growing more intimate. When I see them, I am reminded by the comfort they provided in making me feel cared for. I am also aware, however, that when we convene as a congregation, these benevolent people look out and see the many people they helped over the years and feel warmed by the sense that they made a difference in someone else's life. Thus, those faces create a net that connects the helper to an increasingly broader community.

Engaging in behaviors that increase one's community can enhance well-being by reducing the sense of isolation. There is a substantial body of research that suggests that social isolation has substantial health consequences (House, Landis, & Umberson, 2003). It is unfortunate that social isolation is often concomitant with technological advancement (e.g., reduced day-to-day contact among coworkers due to telecommuting or even simply relying on e-mail rather than in-person meetings), "sandwich generation" responsibilities (i.e., caring for young children and aging parents while working full time), and increasing expectations of what is a standard work week (e.g., overtime expected on a continual basis). The documented high prevalence of depressive disorders among Americans (Bloom, 2004;

Simon, Fleck, Lucas, Bushnell, & LIDO Group, 2004) speaks to a problematic lifestyle that has become the norm. If more people regularly engaged in altruistic social interest behaviors, would the prevalence of depression decrease? What are some feasible approaches for introducing social interest behaviors into normal daily practice for broad segments of society? As one's sense of community grows, what other attitudes and outcomes are affected by altruistic practice?

The mechanisms underlying the health benefits of altruism merit substantial scientific attention, not only to understand the conceptual relationships and physiological mechanisms underlying the individual-level benefits, but also as an antidote for societal ills that have emerged as a result of technological, sociodemographic, and cultural changes over the past several decades. My colleagues and I believe that conceptualizing the gain at both an individual and a communal level will be useful to enhancing our understanding of how altruism affects change and for creating positive change.

REFERENCES

Bloom, B. S. (2004). Prevalence and economic effects of depression. *Managed Care, 13*, 9–16.

House, J. S., Landis, K. R., & Umberson, D. (2003). Social relationships and health. In P. Salovey & A. J. Rothman (Eds.), *Social psychology of health: Key readings in social psychology* (pp. 218–226). New York: Psychology Press.

Schwartz, C. E. (1999). Teaching coping skills enhances quality of life more than peer support: Results of a randomized trial with multiple sclerosis patients. *Health Psychology, 18*, 211–220.

Schwartz, C. E., Meisenhelder, J. B., Ma, Y., & Reed, G. (2003). Altruistic social interest behaviors are associated with better mental health. *Psychosomatic Medicine, 65*, 778–785.

Schwartz, C. E., & Rogers, M. (1994). Designing a psychosocial intervention to teach coping flexibility. *Rehabilitation Psychology, 39*, 61–76.

Schwartz, C. E., & Sendor, M. (1999). Helping others helps oneself: Response shift effects in peer support. *Social Science and Medicine, 48*, 1563–1575.

Schwartz, C. E., Sprangers, M. A. G., Carey, A., & Reed, G. (2004). Exploring response shift in longitudinal data. *Psychology and Health, 19*, 51–69.

Simon, G. E., Fleck, M., Lucas, R., Bushnell, D. M., & LIDO Group. (2004). Prevalence and predictors of depression treatment in an international primary care study. *American Journal of Psychiatry, 161*, 1626–1634.

Sprangers, M. A., & Schwartz, C. E. (1999). Integrating response shift into health-related quality of life research: A theoretical model. *Social Science and Medicine, 48*, 1507–1515.

Ware, J. E., Jr., & Sherbourne, C. D. (1992). The MOS 36-item short-form health survey (SF-36): I. Conceptual framework and item selection. *Medical Care, 30*, 473–483.

3   Do Generative Adolescents
Become Healthy Older Adults?

Paul Wink
Michele Dillon

There is growing evidence that adolescents who engage in prosocial activities do better academically and personally in school (e.g., Eccles & Barber, 1999) and subsequently in college (e.g., Barber, Eccles, & Stone, 2001). Research with middle-aged and older adults also documents a positive relation between volunteerism and physical (e.g., Oman, Thoresen, & McMahon, 1999) and psychological health (e.g., Thoits & Hewitt, 2001). Little is known, however, about the long-term relation between caring behavior in adolescence and health in late adulthood. We bridge the gap between these two literatures by using long-term longitudinal data to investigate the relation between generativity in adolescence and physical and psychological health in late adulthood, a time interval of more than 50 years.

In this chapter, we focus on four questions critical to understanding the long-term connection between generativity and health. First, we examine whether adolescents who manifest generative behavior in high school (see the next section for the definition of generativity and its relation to altruism) grow up to be physically and psychologically healthy older adults. Second, we disentangle the different dimensions of concern for others. Sustained engagement in behavior that benefits others involves a *giving disposition*, but it also includes empathy with those being helped (*social perspective*) and *competence* that enables the individual to plan and execute caring activities (e.g., Colby & Damon, 1992; Penner, 2002). These three characteristics draw on different personal resources, each of which may be related to maintaining good health over time. We are particularly interested, therefore, in finding out whether good health in older age is better predicted by the givingness dimension of generativity or whether it is more strongly related to a competence that enables individuals to make sound personal choices in adulthood. Our third aim is to investigate whether the generativity–health connection is related to sociodemographic background and, in particular, to religiousness and social class, both of which have been related to volunteering (e.g., Putnam, 2000) and health (e.g., Cartwright, Wink, & Kmetz, 1995; Koenig, McCullough, & Larson, 2001). Finally, we explore the factors associated with generativity in adolescence in order to find out what personal and family characteristics are likely to promote a giving attitude toward others and secure long-term health benefits for the giver. After discussing the meaning of generativity and its relation to altruism, we describe our sample and measures, report on the long-term relations between generativity and physical and mental health, and discuss our findings in regard to the potential mechanisms explaining the association. We conclude with a discussion of some of the implications of our findings.

GENERATIVITY AND ITS RELATION TO ALTRUISM

Erik Erikson (1963) coined the term *generativity* to refer to the individual's concern for the welfare of future generations and for the world at large (see Dillon & Wink, 2004). According to Erikson, generative concerns become particularly salient in middle adulthood, a time in the life course when individuals typically occupy dominant social roles and consequently care for future generations not only as parents but also as mentors to younger adults at work and in volunteer organizations. Even though generative concerns may peak in middle adulthood, Erikson's (1963) developmental model assumes that they are present at all stages of the life cycle. The concept of generativity is closely related to Pitrim Sorokin's (1954/2002) notion of compassionate love or altruism because both constructs assume an *intense* positive emotion toward others that *extends* to all of humanity and that is *realized*, or actualized, in behavior. The main difference is that contemporary researchers assume that generative behavior can be driven by a variety of motives, including a selfless concern for others, a desire to outlive the self or have impact on others, and creativity (e.g., Kotre, 1996). In contrast, compassionate love (Sorokin, 1954/2002) and altruism (e.g., Oliner & Oliner, 1988) assume the presence of a pure or selfless motive for behavior, although in everyday practice it may be difficult to infer the exact reasons for particular actions.

THE IHD STUDY AND SAMPLE

The longitudinal data we use come from the intergenerational studies established by the Institute of Human Development (IHD) at the University of California, Berkeley, in the 1920s. The original sample was a representative sample of newborn infants in Berkeley in 1928–1929 (the Berkeley Guidance Study; GS) and of preadolescents (ages 10–12, born in 1920–1921) selected from elementary schools in Oakland, California (the Oakland Growth Study; OGS). The GS and OGS samples were combined into a single IHD study in the early 1960s (Eichorn, 1981) and subsequently followed up when the participants were in their 30s (assessment in 1958), 40s (assessment in 1970), mid-50s/early 60s (assessment in 1982), and late 60s/70s (assessment in 1997–2000). Since age 18, the attrition in the IHD study has been very low. Of the participants who were alive and contactable, close to 90% (N = 184) were interviewed in late adulthood. Prior analyses indicated very little bias due to sample attrition other than a slight tendency for lower participation rates among individuals with lower levels of education (Eichorn, 1981; Wink & Dillon, 2002).

The sample is equally divided among men and women and age cohort, although due to higher mortality among the older cohort (40% compared to 10% for the younger cohort), two thirds of the participants in late adulthood came from the younger cohort. Most of the participants are White, reflecting the racial composition of the Bay Area in the 1920s when the sample was drawn. Of the participants' fathers, 32% were upper-class professionals or executives, 27% were administrative personnel or small business owners, 16% had clerical or sales jobs, and 25% were skilled or unskilled workers. In late middle adulthood, 59% of the participants (or their spouses) were upper middle-class professionals or executives, 19% were lower middle class, and 22% were working class. In late adulthood, 71% (85% of men and 55% of women) were living with a spouse or partner (paralleling same-age national census data). Sixty-nine percent of the sample's couple households had an annual income over $40,000—higher than the comparable figure (49%) for same-age married households nationwide. In late adulthood, the study participants resided primarily in Northern (69%) or Southern (12%) California, and the western or southwestern states (12%). The majority of the sample (73%) grew up in Protestant families, and most were affiliated with mainline denominations (e.g., Presbyterian, Episcopal), renowned for their emphasis on social concerns and volunteering (e.g., Thuesen, 2002). Sixteen percent grew up Catholic, 5% grew up in mixed religious households, and 6% came from nonreligious families.

A distinct features of the IHD study is that all of the assessments during adolescence and adulthood included lengthy, in-depth interviews during which the participants discussed all of the major aspects of their lives, including family relations, work, religion, health, leisure and volunteer activities, personal interests, and social and political attitudes. They also completed self-administered questionnaires. The presence of interview material adds depth to the study and allows for the evaluation of attitudes and behaviors that go beyond self-report ratings. The extensively detailed interview data have been summarized using the California Adult Q-set (CAQ; Block, 1971). This observer-based measure enables trained expert raters to describe the personality and social behavior of the interviewee using a deck of 100 sentence descriptors that they sort into nine forced-choice categories ranging from "extremely characteristic" to "extremely uncharacteristic." Independent panels of between two and four raters used the interview material for adolescence and for the four adulthood interviews to provide composite CAQ ratings for each participant at each of the interview time periods. In this study, we use CAQ-sort ratings based on the data gathered when the participants were in late adolescence; the older cohort was assessed at ages 15–18 in 1936–1938, and the younger cohort was assessed at ages 15–18 in 1944–1946. The adolescent Q-sorts were completed by expert raters in the early 1960s (Block, 1971).

The CAQ Measure of Generativity

We measured generativity with the well-validated CAQ Generativity Scale (CAQ-GS; Peterson & Klohnen, 1995), which assesses three dimensions central to Erikson's conceptualization. As shown in Table 3.1, the first dimension, *givingness*, measures whether the person engages in behaviors that are judged to be giving, sympathetic, considerate, and characterized by warmth, compassion, and reassurance. The second dimension, *prosocial competence*,

Table 3.1. The Three Subscales of the California Adult Q-sort (CAQ) Generativity Prototype

CAQ Items
Givingness
Behaves in a giving way toward others (regardless of motivation involved)
Behaves in a sympathetic or considerate manner
Is protective of those close to him or her
Has warmth, is compassionate
Is turned to for advice and reassurance
Prosocial Competence
Is productive, gets things done
Tends to proffer advice
Is a genuinely dependable and responsible person
Social Perspective
Is socially perceptive of a wide range of interpersonal cues
Is concerned with philosophical problems, e.g., religion, values, the meaning of life
Has a wide range of interests

assesses whether the person is productive, dependable, and engaged with others in ways that are conducive to showing concern for others. The third dimension, *social perspective*, reflects the presence of a broad range of interests and a social perceptiveness that is sensitive to and empathetic with the needs of other individuals and groups. The subscales reflecting the three dimensions of generativity are highly correlated with the overall CAQ-GS (*r*'s ranging from a low of .70 for social perspective to a high of .88 for givingness in adolescence), but are only moderately correlated with each other (*r*'s ranging from a low of .44 to a high of .54 in adolescence), indicating that each subscale assesses a distinct facet of generativity.

Because we are interested in establishing not only the relation between adolescent generativity and physical and psychological health in late adulthood but also in exploring its underlying mechanisms, we include the overall CAQ-GS and its three subscales in all of the analyses. This allows us to identify whether a positive relation between generativity and health is driven by overall generativity and/or whether it is more specifically related to interpersonal givingness and warmth, competence in dealing with everyday life, or breadth of social perspective.

The Relation Between Generativity and Background Variables

In adolescence, the CAQ-GS was unrelated to gender, religiousness, religious denomination (being mainline Protestant, other Protestant, or Catholic), and mother's and father's social class. Members of the older cohort, however, were more generative than the younger cohort. In addition, highly generative adolescents tended to grow up in families characterized by positive interactions (as assessed by expert ratings of transcripts of interviews conducted separately with the study participants and their parents in the 1930s and 1940s). Among the three generativity subscales, the only deviations from the pattern of findings characteristic of the overall CAQ-GS was a negative relation between givingness and mother's and father's social class and a positive relation between social perspective and father's social class (data available from the authors). This means that adolescents from high social status backgrounds were less giving than others, and those whose fathers were of high status were more likely than others to be socially perceptive.

Adolescent generativity was positively associated in early adulthood (1958; age 30s) with social class, educational attainment, religiousness, and IQ. Among the three subscales, high social class, educational attainment, and IQ were characteristic of both prosocial competence and social perspective, and high religiousness was associated with givingness and prosocial competence.

Generativity in Adolescence and Health in Late Adulthood

We now turn to the central question of whether there is a positive relation between adolescent generativity and physical and psychological health in late adulthood. In other words, we use longitudinal data to test whether adolescent generativity can predict outcomes over a time interval of 60 years for the older cohort (ages 16–18 to ages 76–78) and of 52 years for the younger participants (ages 16–18 to ages 68–70). As shown in Table 3.2, the CAQ-GS in adolescence was related positively to an interview-based rating of physical health (4 = no physical complaints; 1 = presence of one or more chronic illnesses resulting in serious disability and/or threat to life) and a self-report rating of physical functioning (the ability to perform physical activities without limitations due to health) in late adulthood. The CAQ-GS was unrelated to self-reported general health (5 = excellent health; 1 = poor health that is likely to get worse). Among the subscales of the CAQ-GS, prosocial competence was related positively to all three measure of physical health, but the two other subscales were unrelated to physical health outcomes in late adulthood.

Adolescent generativity was related to all three measures of psychological health in late adulthood. Thus generative adolescents tended, more than 50 years later, to report feeling satisfied with life; being peaceful, happy, and calm (i.e., having good mental health); and not being depressed as older adults. Each of the three subscales of the CAQ-GS was related positively to life sat-

Table 3.2. Relation Between Generativity in Adolescence and Physical and Mental Health in Late Adulthood

Characteristics in Late Adulthood	Adolescence			
	Generativity	Givingness	Prosocial Competence	Social Perspective
Physical Health				
Ratings of Physical Health	.20*	.13	.26**	.11
SF-36 General Health	.13	.08	.19*	.07
SF-36 Physical Functioning	.23*	.17	.24**	.15
Psychological Health				
Life Satisfaction	.34**	.21*	.40**	.27**
SF-36 Mental Health	.24**	.14	.33**	.20*
Depression	−.18*	−.12	−.24**	−.11

Note: $N = 139$ for the rating of physical health, and $N = 123$ for all other measures. Physical health rated by two experts using health section of in-depth interview; SF-36 scales come from the self-report MOS survey (Ware, 1993); life satisfaction = Diener et al.'s (1985) self-report Satisfaction With Life Scale; depression = self-report CES-D Scale (Radloff, 1977)
*p < .05; **p < .01.

isfaction, but only prosocial competence and social perspective were correlated with mental health and only prosocial competence was related negatively to depression.

Generativity in Adolescence and Health Practices in Middle Age

What are the mechanisms underlying the positive relation between adolescent generativity and physical and psychological health in late adulthood? We first present data on the association between adolescent generativity and health practices in middle age, and then discuss the moderating effect of early adulthood social class, IQ, and religiousness on the long-term generativity–health relation.

Adolescent generativity was positively related in late middle adulthood (1982; age early 50s/early 60s) with having an adequate health plan (covering all medical expenses) and negatively with smoking and, at a trend level, with the number of cigarettes smoked (see Table 3.3). Although adolescent generativity was unrelated to the frequency of drinking alcohol in late middle age, it was negatively related to the number of drinks consumed per drinking episode. Among the components of generativity, prosocial competence was related positively to frequency of physical check-ups and to the adequacy of the individual's health plan and was related negatively to smoking and the number of alcoholic drinks consumed, though not to frequency of drinking. The givingness and social perspective aspects of generativity were not related to any of the health practices in late middle adulthood.

Table 3.3. Relation Between Generativity in Adolesence and Health Practices in Late Middle Adulthood

Characteristics in Late Middle Adulthood	Adolescence			
	Generativity	Givingness	Prosocial Competence	Social Perspective
Frequency of physical check-ups	.12	−.01	.20*	.15
Adequacy of health plan	.18*	.06	.28**	.10
Smoking on a regularbasis	−.28**	−.15	−.37**	−.16
Number of cigarettes smoked	−.19	−.09	−.22*	−.17
Frequency of drinking	−.06	−.02	−.08	−.11
Number of drinks per episode	−.19*	−.10	−.23 *	−.13

Note: N ranges from 109 to 133 with the exception of number of cigarettes smoked, N = 83. Health practices in late middle adulthood assessed with self-report rating scales.

*p £ .05; **p < .01.

PREDICTING HEALTH OUTCOMES IN LATE ADULTHOOD FROM GENERATIVITY, CONTROLLING FOR CHARACTERISTICS IN EARLY ADULTHOOD

Although there was no association in adolescence between generativity and the individual's social class background, IQ, and religiousness, the study participants who were highly generative during adolescence tended by early adulthood (1958; age 30s) to belong to a high social class, to have high IQ, and to be moderately or highly religious. In addition, we found that members of the older age cohort were more generative than were members of the younger cohort. Because all of these variables may affect the relation between generativity and health, we regressed, in separate equations, our strongest measures of physical health (interview-based ratings of physical health) and psychological health (Diener et al.'s [1985], self-report Satisfaction With Life Scale) on the CAQ-GS in adolescence while controlling for cohort and for early adulthood social class, IQ, and religiousness (Model 1). In Model 2, we substituted adolescent prosocial competence, the CAQ-GS subscale that was most consistently related to health outcomes in late adulthood, for the overall CAQ-GS.

In the two models predicting physical health in late adulthood, we found that after controlling for cohort and early adulthood characteristics, the relation between generativity and physical health was no longer significant, and the relation between prosocial competence and physical health was significant at a trend level only. The only consistent predictor of physical health was cohort with the older participants having poorer health (see Table 3.4). In the two models predicting psychological health in late adulthood, both the CAQ-GS and its prosocial competence subscale continued to be significant predictors of life satisfaction in late adulthood even after controlling for cohort and for early adulthood social class, IQ, and religiousness.

Finally, as will be recalled, we found a positive association in adolescence between generativity and warm family relations. Because positive family relations in adolescence proved to be related to good physical and psychological health in late adulthood, we recomputed the relation between adolescent generativity and health in late adulthood while controlling for positive family relations. We found that generativity continued to be a significant predictor of both physical and psychological health. (Data not shown but available from the authors.)

DISCUSSION AND CONCLUSIONS

Our analyses of longitudinal data investigating the relation between adolescent generativity and physical and psychological health in late adulthood (ages late 60s/70s) uncovered three main findings. First, we found that adolescents who

Table 3.4. Multiple Linear Regressions Predicting Health in Late Adulthood
From Generativity in Adolescence and Background Variables in Early Adulthood

| | Late Adulthood | | | |
| | Physical Health Rating | | Life Satisfaction | |
Predictors	Model 1	Model 2	Model 1	Model 2
Cohort	.21*	.20*	.15	.14
Early Adulthood				
Social Class	.16	.11	.08	.01
Religiousness	.09	.09	.09	.12
IQ	.01	.01	.00	.02
Adolescence				
Generativity	−.10	——	.39**	——
Prosocial Competence	——	.18	——	.40**
R^2	.10*	.12*	.19**	.19**
Degrees of Freedom	(6,118)	(6,118)	(6,104)	(6,104)

Note: For cohort, 2 = member of OGS, and 1 = member of GS; social class assessed with the
Social Class Index (Hollingshead & Redlich, 1958); religiousness measured with an interview-
based rating scale (Dillon & Wink, 2004).
*$p < .05$; **$p < .01$.

were judged to be generative grew up to be in better physical and psychological
health than their less generative peers. In particular, generative adolescents
experienced fewer incapacitating chronic illnesses and limits placed on their
activities by poor physical health in old age. They also reported higher life satisfaction; felt more peaceful, happy, and calm; and were less depressed. The
effects we found were relatively small in magnitude (accounting for around 4%
of the variance in physical health and up to 16% of the variance in psychological health). Nevertheless, when measurement error and the length of time between the baseline and the outcome (an interval of between 50 and 60 years)
are taken into account, the findings are impressive and offer strong support for
the main premise of this volume that concern for others has a positive effect on
physical and psychological health; in other words, it is good to be good.

The second main finding concerns the mechanisms underlying the long-term
association between generativity and health. Because we used the overall CAQ
Generativity Scale and its three subscales, we were able to establish which component of generativity was primarily responsible for the generativity-health connection. In particular, we were interested in whether the beneficial effects of
generativity on health would be associated with giving behavior and interpersonal

warmth or whether they would be related more strongly to prosocial competence or the ability to plan and execute goal-directed behavior. Our findings on physical health are unequivocal. All of the positive physical health findings for late adulthood were associated with adolescent prosocial competence, and none of them were related to adolescent givingness. What accounts for the significant association between adolescent prosocial competence and physical health in late adulthood? Our data suggest that the most likely mechanism involves the cumulative effect of sound judgment, choices, and habits. Although adolescents who were high in prosocial competence did not come from economically privileged backgrounds, by the time they reached early adulthood (age 30s), they tended to be of higher social class than their peers who were low in prosocial competence. We also found that in midlife, individuals who were prosocially competent in adolescence tended not to be smokers or excessive drinkers. The damaging effects of smoking on health were less well known in the 1940s and 1950s, when our study participants were young adults. Nonetheless, it is a testimony to the foresight and good judgment associated with prosocial competence that the prosocial adolescents in our study refrained from developing such risky behavioral habits as smoking. In addition, the fact that prosocially competent adolescents tended to attain higher social class status as adults meant that they also had more money and thus had access to good health care, which also, of course, contributes to increasing their odds of maintaining good physical health in old age.

Although we found a similar positive relation between generativity and psychological health as we did for physical health, there were also important differences. In particular, adolescent generativity was more strongly related to psychological than to physical health in late adulthood. Psychological health was also positively related to each of the three facets of generativity rather than being primarily associated with prosocial competence, as was the case for physical health. Specifically, in late adulthood, life satisfaction was related to all three subscales of the CAQ-GS; and the absence of depression, and self-reported feelings of peace, happiness, and calmness (as measured by the SF-36) were characteristic of the study participants who in adolescence were prosocially competent and who manifested a broad social perspective. Finally, the relation between adolescent generativity and life satisfaction in late adulthood was, unlike physical health, not affected by background characteristics in early adulthood (especially not by social class). This finding suggests that psychological health is less dependent than physical health on the cumulative effect of day-to-day personal habits such as smoking and drinking and/or on the affordability of health care. Rather, psychological health in old age is more directly related to an early propensity to feel and to show concern for others.

Does the finding that physical and psychological health in late adulthood was related more strongly to adolescent prosocial competence rather than to givingness challenge the claim that it is good to be good? We would like to argue that it does not. First, most of the health outcomes in late adulthood were associated with both prosocial competence and the overall CAQ-GS, thus indicating a general beneficial effect of generativity on physical and psychological health. Second, all three facets of generativity were positively correlated as well as being highly related to the overall CAQ-GS. This means that although the three dimensions of generativity are analytically separate, they nonetheless tend to hang together in real life. Finally, it is important also to emphasize that prosocial competence as a construct measures not only an individual's productivity, dependability, and sense of responsibility, but also taps into the individual's concern for others as indicated, for example, by a willingness to give advice. Accordingly, givingness partially inheres in prosocial competence. Our findings do, however, affirm the thesis that being generative or altruistic involves both having the desire to give to others and the ability to act prosocially in the execution of that desire. Importantly, it is the competence to act prosocially that is particularly beneficial, especially to physical but also to psychological health in the long term. As crystallized in the wisdom of an old proverb, good intentions alone do not ensure good outcomes.

The third main finding pertains to the characteristics conducive to the early development of generativity. Given that adolescent generativity is a significant predictor of health in old age, it is important to identify the circumstances conducive to its emergence. To our surprise, adolescent generativity was unrelated to adolescent religiousness and social class, characteristics that we (Dillon & Wink, 2007; Dillon, Wink, & Fay, 2003) and others (e.g., Putnam, 2000) have found to be positively related to volunteerism and to prosocial activities in adulthood. This discrepancy in findings may reflect the fact that religious involvement in adolescence is partly dictated by parents who are concerned about the religious socialization and moral development of their children. And, among religious adolescents, the social aspects of church may exert a stronger hold than any theological emphasis on concern for others. Additionally, given the array of social and psychological tasks associated with adolescence, the high school years may not developmentally be the right time to manifest the noblesse oblige expected in families with high social status.

We did, however, find a significant connection between adolescent generativity and the experience of positive intrafamily relations. This finding supports Erikson's (1963) claim that generativity, or concern for others, is based on the early childhood ability to develop trusting relations with others (and trust in oneself). In other words, growing up in a relatively harmonious and giving family environment may predispose the individual to develop a positive regard for others, a broad perspective on social issues including a sensitivity to inequality, and a sense of competence that facilitates effectiveness in the pursuit of generative goals.

The IHD sample consists of a relatively small number of men and women who, although representative of the population of San Francisco's East Bay in the 1920s, are predominantly White and mainline Protestant. It is clearly important for our results to be replicated using data from samples that have greater racial and ethnic diversity. Similarly, given the dominance of mainline Protestants in our study, and especially in light of the fact that historically the mainline has stressed social activism and care for others, it is important that our findings be replicated with samples that have a greater range of religious traditions. By the same token, the participants in our study were born in the 1920s and consequently are members of the long civic generation of older Americans (cf. Putnam, 2000). Research with later-born cohorts may reveal a different set of patterns in regard to the generativity-health domain. Finally, although we have found generativity to be indistinguishable from altruism, it is important for future research to further explore the relation between these two constructs and to bridge the gap between these two research traditions. This chapter, nonetheless, offers the first evidence of a positive association between a generative concern for others in adolescence and good physical and psychological health in old age. Our findings indicate that when concern for others translates into giving or generative behavior it is not only beneficial on a communal level but also offers tangible, long-term rewards to the giver. Thus there are good individual and societal reasons to encourage young people to show concern for others in daily life and to provide them with the opportunities for acting on their altruistic impulses.

REFERENCES

Barber, B. L., Eccles, J. S., & Stone, M. R. (2001). Whatever happened to the jock, the brain, and the princess? *Journal of Adolescent Research, 16,* 429–455.

Block, J. (1971). *Lives through time.* Berkeley, CA: Bancroft.

Cartwright, L., Wink, P., & Kmetz, C. (1995). What leads to good health in midlife women physicians? *Psychosomatic Medicine, 57,* 284–292.

Colby, A., & Damon, W. (1992). *Some do care: Contemporary lives of moral commitment.* New York: Free Press.

Diener, E., Emmons, R. A., Larsen, R. J., & Griffin, S. (1985). The satisfaction with life scale. *Journal of Personality Assessment, 49,* 71–75.

Dillon, M., & Wink P. (2004). Religion, cultural change, and generativity in American society. In E. de St. Aubin & D. P. McAdams (Eds.), *The generative society* (pp. 153–174). Washington DC: American Psychological Association Press.

Dillon, M., & Wink, P. (2007). *In the course of a lifetime: Tracing religious belief, practice, and change.* Berkeley: University of California Press.

Dillon, M., Wink, P., & Fay, K. (2003). Is spirituality detrimental to generativity? *Journal for the Scientific Study of Religion, 42,* 427–442.

Eccles, J. S., & Barber, B. L. (1999). Student council, volunteering, basketball, or marching band: What kind of extracurricular involvement matters? *Journal of Adolescent Research, 14,* 10–43.

Eichorn, D. (1981). Samples and procedures. In D. Eichorn, J. Clausen, N. Haan, M. Honzik, & P. Mussen (Eds.), *Present and past in middle age* (pp. 89–116). New York: Academic.

Erikson, E. (1963). *Childhood and society* (2nd ed.). New York: Norton.

Hollingshead, A. B., & Redlich, F. C. (1958). *Social class and mental illness.* New York: Wiley.

Koenig, H., McCullough, M. E., & Larson, D. B. (2001). *Handbook of religion and health.* New York: Oxford University Press.

Kotre, J. (1996). *Outliving the self* (2nd ed.). New York: Norton.

Oliner, S. P., & Oliner, P. M. (1988). *The altruistic personality.* New York: Free Press.

Oman, D., Thoresen, E., & McMahon, K. (1999). Volunteerism and mortality among the community-dwelling elderly. *Journal of Health Psychology, 4,* 301–316.

Penner, L. (2002). Dispositional and organizational influences on sustained volunteerism: An interactionist perspective. *Journal of Social Issues, 58,* 447–467.

Peterson, W., & Klohnen, E. (1995). Realization of generativity in two samples of women at midlife. *Psychology and Aging, 10,* 20–29.

Putnam, R. (2000). *Bowling alone.* New York: Simon & Schuster.

Radloff, L. S. (1977). The CES-D scale: A self-report depression scale for research in the general population. *Applied Psychological Measurement, 3,* 385–401.

Sorokin, P. (2002). *The ways and power of love.* Philadelphia, PA: Templeton Foundation Press. (Original work published 1954)

Thoits, P. A., & Hewitt, L. N. (2001). Volunteer work and well-being. *Journal of Health and Social Behavior, 42,* 115–131.

Thuesen, P. (2002). The logic of mainline churchliness: Historical background since the Reformation. In R. Wuthnow & J. Evans (Eds.), *The quiet hand of God* (pp. 27–53). Berkeley: University of California Press.

Ware, J. E. (1993). *SF-36 health survey: Manual & interpretation guide.* Boston: Health Institute, New England Medical Center.

Wink, P., & Dillon, M. (2002). Spiritual development across the adult life course: Findings from a longitudinal study. *Journal of Adult Development, 9,* 79–94.

4 Altruism, Well-Being, and Mental Health in Late Life

Elizabeth Midlarsky
Eva Kahana

Giving is more joyous than receiving, not because it
is deprivation, but because in the act of giving lies
the expression of my aliveness.
—Erich Fromm

Blood donors and community service volunteers are recruited with posters announcing that by giving to others, they will receive even more than they give. Is this true? Will those who help others to benefit themselves obtain the rewards that they expect? In this chapter, we begin with the background of and theory on altruism. We then focus on our own research on older helpers, emphasizing work on Holocaust heroes, who are now quite elderly. A basic premise of this chapter is that the consequences of altruism, in the form of well-being and mental health, can be viewed through the prism of the altruism paradox.

The paradox of altruism is based on the law of effect, wherein human beings pursue pleasure for themselves, and avoid pain. How, then, can we explain "pure" altruism, which is motivated by concern for the well-being of another, despite the costs or risk to the self? Although such pure altruism is considered to be a *rare* phenomenon (Batson & Powell, 2003; Midlarsky, 1968; Midlarsky & Kahana, 1994) both within and between individuals, it is worthy of investigation for both theoretical and practical reasons. When we genuinely comprehend the behaviors of the most altruistic among us (and altruism in ourselves), then an important facet of humanity can be understood. We will also consider behaviors variously referred to as volunteering, rescuing, prosocial behavior, generativity, and compassion. What these terms have in common is that none assumes that altruism motivates the behavior.

BACKGROUND AND THEORY

Why should altruism have positive consequences for well-being and for mental health? The first conceptions of altruism and its consequences are found in the domains of philosophy and theology, rather than in science. The earliest recorded theories about altruism and its consequences were promulgated by the Chinese philosopher Mencius, in the philosophies of the Greeks (*agape*) and Romans (*philanthropia*), in the Torah (*tzedaka*), and in the New Testament, just to name a few sources (Batson, 1991; Midlarsky & Kahana, 1994). In 1851, Auguste Comte coined the term *altruism* from *altrui*, an Italian adjective meaning "of or to others, or someone else," which he used to characterize unselfish as opposed to egoistic tendencies. In this doctrine, the goal of all conduct, and the source of happiness, is a life lived for others. Comte wrote that the two primary impulses are the egoistic, or self-oriented, and the altruistic, or social. In human life, one of these must be dominant; a balance is impossible. Both individual and social well-being can only be achieved by subordinating self-love to the love of others (Lewes, 1904).

According to Tenzin Gyatso, the Fourteenth Dalai Lama of Tibet, the most certain way to attain happiness, and particularly inner tranquility, is by developing the capacities for love and compassion. Indeed, much human misery results from an egoism in which one pursues one's own self-interest at the expense of others. Conversely, most of our joy and security results from emotions and thoughts suggesting that the well-being of others should be cherished (Piburn, 1990). The paradox here is that it is only when we develop empathy for all organisms that we can secure our own well-being.

The sociologist Pitirim Sorokin was one of the first to bring altruism into the social sciences, arguing that generosity to others leads to increased mental and physical health (Sorokin, 1954/2002). Among Freudian psychoanalysts, on the other hand, genuine altruism is theoretically impossible, because human beings are viewed as intrinsically hedonistic and self-centered. Any behavior that may appear altruistic is viewed by psychoanalysts as either egoistic or masochistic. For the psychosocial neo-Freudians, the emphasis is on the relationship between social interactions and personality development. For Alfred Adler, social interest was important for the fully functioning adult (Schwartz, Meisenhelder, Ma, & Reed, 2003). According to Erich Fromm, we all crave love, and love is not emotion but behavior. Love for Fromm is based on giving rather than receiving and is conceptualized in a manner similar to conceptions of altruism. Erik Erikson's eight stages were designed to replace Sigmund Freud's stages of psychosexual development. The seventh stage involves a conflict between generativity and stagnation. The generative individual, destined to mature into the eighth stage, is an adult who works to give support to the next generation. Thus, in Erikson's theory, maturity is equated with generosity.

When empirically oriented psychologists began to investigate altruism and helping, much of the work within psychology was devoted to the question of whether altruism can exist and to the causes of helping behavior (Penner, Dovidio, Piliavin, & Schroeder, 2005). An important goal was to determine factors that could promote the development of altruism in children. It was not until very recently that helping in later life was recognized as valuable for the older adult and for society. Instead, explanations of social behavior in late life focused almost entirely on theoretical models—dependency, autonomy, and exchange—that did not allow for the possibility of altruism (Kahana, Midlarsky, & Kahana, 1987).

In the *dependency model*, the elderly are depicted as recipients of aid and, indeed, as a sick and handicapped group, to the extent that aging is viewed as "a terminal illness that uniformly begins in the sixties" (Sankar, 1984, p. 251). The presumption of the dependency model is that when helping behavior occurs in a social interaction involving older adults, helping flows from the younger (including middle-aged) to the older people. The older the individual, the more likely it is that he or she will be a helpless, dependent recipient (Settersten, 1999).

A second model, the *autonomy model*, reflects the assumption by developmental theorists that independence is a hallmark of adult development. Disengagement theory (Cumming & Henry, 1961), a related perspective, historically was the lens through which late life was viewed. According to Cumming and Henry, people become less amenable to social demands and obligations as they age. This motive to limit involvement with others as either helper or recipient is combined with a desire to fulfill one's own egoistic needs. What is predicted, in turn, is a lesser involvement in helping by older people and fewer benefits, including satisfaction, from helping others.

The *exchange orientation*, rooted in economic theory and in behaviorism, assumes that all social interaction is governed by the motive to maximize rewards and to minimize costs. Because human behavior is governed by the norm of reciprocity according to the exchange model, older adults would give help only to reciprocate for resources received or expected or to earn resources from others. Helping may occur under these circumstances, but altruism is not a possibility in this model.

To this panoply of theoretical orientations, we added a fourth model, the *contributory model of successful aging* (Kahana, Midlarsky, & Kahana, 1987). This model presents altruistic or contributory helping, which is prompted by concern for the other and/or by moral or religious motives. In contrast to the dependency and autonomy models, the contributory model depicts older adulthood as a period in which altruistic motivation is probable, rather than improbable.

In contrast to the exchange model, the contributory model depicts altruistic helping as behavior that is based on moral dispositions, such as empathetic concern and altruistic moral judgment, rather than on reciprocation or on expectations of extrinsic rewards. Although altruistic helping is not *motivated* by rewards to the helper, and may be very costly, it is expected to yield benefits to the helper. In contrast to models of older adulthood as a period in which people are primarily consumers of social support, older adults can therefore be viewed as an important resource to others. Our model of contributory behavior in late life may also serve as a counterpoint to views in which older adults are depicted as costly and burdensome.

What positive consequences can accrue to older adults when they help others? One possibility is that helping behaviors may ameliorate the impact of the normative stresses of aging (Kahana, Kahana, & Kercher, 2004). If altruism and helping do buffer stress, what mechanisms can account for this effect? One possible explanation is attributable to the importance of the volunteer role, especially for older people who have suffered role losses. In role theory, role accumulation has positive effects on well-being because social roles provide meaning, status, and a sense of purpose (Thoits & Hewitt, 2001). In a similar vein, Pillemer, Wethington, and Glasgow (2000) emphasize the role of volunteering in promoting social integration by older adults, a model supported by findings about the impact of helping in families and in the community (Midlarsky & Kahana, 1994) and about the link between generativity (helping that is designed to maintain the next generation and civic society) and social integration (Keyes & Ryff, 2000). In addition to the enhancement of social integration, helping others has been linked to competence, mastery, and perceived control (Midlarsky, 1984). Others propose that helping results in elevations in mood. For example, social psychologists, such as Cialdini and his associates, have argued that people are socialized to reward themselves when they help others. Helping should therefore lead to decreases in depression and increases in happiness, a proposition that has been supported by research with older helpers (Cialdini & Fultz, 1990; Piliavin & Callero, 1991).

In a model of helping as a useful means for coping with stress, Midlarsky (1991) proposed that several mechanisms combine to account for any positive consequences of helping that may be experienced by the helper. Helping may benefit the helper because helping may (1) increase self-evaluations and perceived competence, (2) distract the helper from focusing on other troubles and stresses, (3) enhance the sense of meaning and value of life by indicating that he or she "matters," (4) increase positive moods, and (5) facilitate social integration. Snyder, Clary, and Stukas (2000) have been conducting research on six functions that are theoretically served by volunteering behavior, some of which are similar to the mechanisms proposed by Midlarsky (1991) as responsible for the beneficial effects of helping for the helper. These functions are social, knowledge, enhancement, career, value-expressive, and defensive.

In sum, then, the theoretical perspectives reviewed here suggest that altruism is a unique form of helping or motive for helping and that both altruism and helping can theoretically yield benefits for the older helper as well as for the recipient. In the following section, we turn to our research findings about altruism and helping and their association with well-being and mental health in later life.

RESEARCH FINDINGS

During the past 24 years, we have engaged in a program of research relevant to altruism and helping in late life. Our research has focused on altruism and helping across several studies, employing diverse methodologies. Participants have ranged from older adults residing in age-heterogeneous and age-homogeneous community settings, who are generally engaged in more normative volunteering and helping, to older Gentiles who courageously rescued Jews during the Holocaust. We have also conducted experimental studies to determine the impact of situational influences on patterns of prosocial behavior in late life. In general, the results of our research provide evidence of links between helping, on the one hand, and both well-being and mental health, on the other.

Community-Residing Older Adults

Our program of research was initiated in the 1980s and was designed to address several questions: (1) Do older adults help others? (2) If so, why do they help? What are their motives for helping? (3) Is late-life helping related to psychosocial being? (4) Are there psychosocial benefits for altruism and helping in *very* late life?

Do Older Adults Help Others?

In the mid-1980s, we were planning a series of naturalistic experiments on factors that could increase the rates of donation behavior. We chose shopping centers, malls, and parks as the locations in which to assess the effects of employing a young woman who was or was not visibly pregnant as the solicitor of donations on behalf of children with birth defects. All age groups were exposed to this appeal, but we expected the primary donors to be young through middle-aged adults.

In the pilot study, we waited for the expected younger adults to approach the donation booth. However, it was the older adults who approached, one after the other, while searching for cash and grumbling about not having more to give.

This was *not* what we expected, as we were aware of the prevailing view of older adults as people who were more likely to need help than to help others.

We then completed two naturalistic experiments on donation behavior, which were designed to assess donation throughout the lifespan (Midlarsky & Hannah, 1989). In both experiments, the independent variables were the solicitor's condition (pregnant or nonpregnant) and the age of the donor (ages 5–75+). In the first experiment, in which cash donations were requested, there was a linear increase with age in numbers of people donating, with the people aged 65 and over the most frequent and most eager to donate. However, the amounts of money donated by the older, retired adults were lower than the monetary amounts donated by the younger adults. In the second experiment, which served as a replication and extension of the first, the donations consisted of time and effort, rather than money. In this second experiment, the older adults were the most generous on all measures. These findings pointed to the important influences of personal resources and other situational influences in shaping social behavior in late life. We thus concluded that older adults are eager helpers when resources permit them to provide aid to others.

In a cross-sectional survey research study of 400 Detroit area older adults (Midlarsky & Kahana, 1994), about a quarter of the elderly respondents spent a great deal of time helping others, and the helping was more likely to be spontaneous than planned (59% reported that they provided assistance on the spur of the moment). In contrast to the dependency, autonomy, and exchange models of earlier gerontological work (Kahana, Midlarsky, & Kahana, 1987), these older adults described helping as a highly valued activity and said that they greatly preferred to give help over receiving help from others.

In a second set of naturalistic studies, we found that the number of people participating in a fee-based CPR course was significantly related to age, and this relationship accounted for 22% of the variance (Midlarsky & Kahana, 1994). People aged 65 and older had the highest rates of participation. Furthermore, unlike younger participants, there were no significant differences in participation by older adults that were attributable to variations in the course fee ($0, $3, or $10). Several people commented that any amount of money was worth learning ways to help people in life-and-death emergencies.

Why Do Older People Help Others?

In the naturalistic study in which CPR training was provided, participants were asked why they enrolled. Many of the people aged 18 to 64 (54%) said that they were curious about how CPR and first aid are administered. About one third (36%) wanted to use the class to discover whether they were interested enough to consider careers in the health professions. About 34% said they took the class to learn how to help people in need. Among the older adults, on the other hand, the vast majority, 85%, said that their only reason was to learn how to help others during a health-related emergency, and 62% said that their goal was to learn how to save lives in a crisis. These findings suggest that older adults tend to value more intrinsic rather than extrinsic reasons for helping.

In our survey of 400 community-dwelling older adults (Midlarsky & Kahana, 1994), the perceived importance or value of helping and two "moral" motives—the sense of social responsibility and empathy—were significant predictors of helping. The preponderance of respondents, 75%, cited motives that included the desire to give help because it was "the right thing to do," their "duty," a religious obligation, or because someone they knew was obviously in need. An additional 10% said that they helped to feel useful or to alleviate their own distress at seeing another person suffer. About 5% indicated that extrinsic motives, including specific forms of reciprocal help, material payments, acknowledgment by others, gratitude, or a good reputation, served as motives. These findings indicate that, for most of the older adults in our study, altruistic motives prevailed. In considering the anticipation of extrinsic rewards that motivated a few respondents, most were given by people who appeared to be more needy and less independent.

Results of the quantitative analyses provided support for the central hypotheses, i.e., that helping would be related to morale, subjective social integration, and self-esteem. A result that was unexpected but interesting is that empathy is *negatively* related to morale after helping is entered into the equation. A possible explanation of this finding is that empathetic older adults may experience serious distress if exposed to others' pain and suffering, which helping may not alleviate. This suggests that exposure to severe, long-term illnesses and other forms of suffering may result in adverse reactions by caring older adults.

Is Helping Related to Well-Being?

In the community survey of 400 older adults, 220 reported that they found helping others to be especially rewarding. Of this number, 182 people (83%) cited rewards that are intrinsic. These included a sense of inner satisfaction (55%); the feeling that they were socially integrated (22%); the perception of usefulness, competence, and "mattering"; increased self-esteem (10%); and a feeling that they had done the right thing (10%). As one 88-year-old respondent said, "Even though there are things I can no longer do, I can still bring a smile to my neighbor's face." In the words of an 86-year-old respondent, "Helping others confirms one's own existence and integration." Correlational data indicated that those reporting intrinsic motives for helping (e.g., empathetic concern, social responsibility, and altruistic moral judgment) were most likely to report that altruism was rewarding for them. The finding that the rewards were intrinsic in nature was made intelligible by the theoretical perspectives identified above. That is, helping may be rewarding by "enhancing the sense of meaning" (Midlarsky, 1991) and by serving a "value-expressive" function (Snyder, Clary, & Stukas, 2000).

An additional study, an experimental follow-up to the original survey (Midlarsky & Kahana, 1994), was then conducted to investigate the possibility that helping positively affects psychosocial well-being. In our study, 120 of the people who had been interviewed in the survey research project 4 years previously either were (N = 60) or were not (N = 60) exposed to a powerful intervention soliciting their participation in volunteer activities, an intervention that we expected would promote the helping of others.

Results indicated that the intervention did significantly affect the helping of family and neighbors and in volunteer roles. Unexpectedly, the intervention had a direct effect on self-esteem. Many respondents were gratified and reassured about their potential usefulness when "so much trouble" was taken to tell them that their efforts were valuable for their community. The helping of family and neighbors and volunteering all affected well-being. However, only volunteering significantly affected all four indices of well-being: positive affect, morale, self-esteem, and subjective social integration.

Are Altruism and Helping Related to Well-Being in Very Late Life?

In a survey by Kahana, Feldman, Lechner, Midlarsky, and Kahana (2004), 366 old-old people (mean age 85 years), living independently in a Florida retirement community, were asked about their altruism, volunteer behavior, and well-being. Altruism was operationally defined, here, as scores on a measure which included such items as "I place the needs of others ahead of my own," and "I try to help others, even if they don't help me." Helping was defined as the frequency with which people volunteered during the past year, on a 5–point scale ranging from "rarely or never" to "several times a day." Indices of well-being were life satisfaction, positive affect, and depressive symptomatology. The aim was to determine whether altruistic attitudes predicted psychosocial well-being: altruistic attitudes or volunteer activities. We also assessed the degree to which volunteering mediated the relationship between altruism and well-being.

After controlling for age, gender, marital status, and chronic illness, people with high levels of altruism were higher in life satisfaction, were happier, and had fewer symptoms of depression. On the other hand, formal volunteering did not serve as a mediator between altruism and well-being. It should be noted, though, that among these very old adults, only about one third were involved in volunteer activities during the past year. These findings suggest that among the very old, altruistic attitudes are significantly related to well-being even when increasing frailty prevents them from engaging in volunteer activities. Expanded opportunities for prosocial engagement requiring less physical exertion may benefit the growing population of old-old adults who seek to express altruistic attitudes in acts of helping.

Elderly Holocaust-Era Rescuers

In our studies of helping in community-residing elderly, we explored altruistic helping on the basis of self-reported helping and on discrete helping behaviors in field experiments. A second approach consisted of investigating correlates and consequences of helping by people identified as genuine altruists by others. Therefore, as part of our research program on altruism and aging, we conducted empirical research on the late-life helping and well-being of rescuers during the Holocaust in comparison with a group of bystanders (Midlarsky, Fagin Jones, & Nemeroff, in press; M. Midlarsky, 2005).

The sample for our study consisted of 153 people who had lived in Europe during World War II. In contrast to other studies of Holocaust era rescuers (Fogelman, 1994; Oliner & Oliner, 1988), the sample was *not* selected from people currently residing in Europe. Instead, it included 80 rescuers and 73 bystanders who migrated to the United States or Canada between 1945 and 1950. Studying people who are long-term residents of the United States and Canada and who are reasonably acculturated English speakers allowed us to employ measures that had been used in other studies of altruism (Midlarsky & Kahana, 1994).

These 80 rescuers were people who had intentionally helped one or more Jews despite great risk, and with no extrinsic reward for themselves. They were discovered and verified by the research team for the first time and had never been previously interviewed or honored for their wartime activities. The 73 bystanders consisted of people who lived in Nazi-occupied Europe during the war, were not perpetrators, and did not participate in the rescue of Jews. The bystanders were randomly selected from lists of people who lived in the same geographic areas as the rescuers during the war—indeed, they were typically the rescuers' next-door neighbors in Europe. Following the war, they migrated and were now living in the same communities as the rescuers, once again quite often as next-door neighbors. The bystanders interviewed here were people who reported that they offered no help even when asked for help.

Who Were the Rescuers?

We first asked whether the personality and motivational variables identified in the experimental literature on altruism, which investigates determinants of relatively low-cost, short-term helping behavior, would also characterize Holocaust rescuers (cf. Midlarsky, Fagin Jones, & Corley, 2005). A hierarchical discriminant function analysis (HDFA) identified one function that correctly categorized 93.2% of the participants. The rescuers were higher than the bystanders on altruistic moral reasoning, social responsibility, empathetic concern, risk taking, and autonomy. When asked why they helped, they typically answered that there was no choice—"It was the only decent thing to do"—or there was no other way to respond to the fear and pain all around them. Thus, the results of this analysis suggest that the rescuers were indeed extraordinary in the degree to which they manifested prosocial personality dispositions in comparison with the other study participants, even a half century after their wartime rescue activities.

Current Helping Behavior

When asked about their helping of others in the past 6 months, the rescuers said that they gave greater amounts of help and spent more time and effort helping others than did the bystanders. Asked how important helping others is to them, 97.4% of the rescuers versus 45.2% of the bystanders said that helping others is an "important" or "very important" activity. At the other extreme of agreement, none of the rescuers said that helping others is "unimportant," compared to 19% of the bystanders. All differences were significant at $p < .0001$.

When asked about their current helping, rescuers dismissed their postwar helping as "minor" and of little consequence in comparison with their activities during the Holocaust when people *really* needed help. In fact, though, they were found to be more generous than the bystanders with time, money, and effort and in all domains—with neighbors, friends, and family and in volunteer activity. Even in regard to helping behaviors that are infrequent in older adults—such as blood donation—these people often generously participated. One rescuer, for example, mentioned that since she was too old for her own blood to be valuable, she donated money and encouraged others to donate their blood during blood donation drives. It is also noteworthy that significantly more rescuers (44%) than bystanders (12.4%) had signed an organ donor card to have their organs donated after their deaths.

Mental Health and Well-Being

The rescuers emerged as a highly empathetic group, with the sensitivity accompanying that personality trait. Probably as a consequence of their extreme sensitivity, the rescuers (but not the bystanders) told the interviewers that they participated in the interview with a combination of positive feelings and trepidation; some later reported that they had flashbacks and trouble sleeping after the interviews. They shared memories of the good times: the hours spent delivering a hidden Jew's baby, the jokes and tender moments that they shared, the feeling of being engaged together in a critically important enterprise, the feelings of love and warmth. On the other hand, they spoke of the constant vigilance and fear, often over a period stretching for years, not hours or days. Some had been found out and seriously punished. One person, who had sheltered and saved the lives of 12 people, still cried about one Jewish child who had wandered out of the cellar and been shot almost instantly. No feelings or memories of this kind were shared by the bystanders.

When asked about mental health problems that they had experienced during their lives since the war, approximately 20% of the rescuers and none of the bystanders reported that they had experienced anxiety—especially during the period in which they left their home countries and migrated to the United States or Canada. Close to 60% of the bystanders and none of the rescuers reported that they had serious problems with alcoholism and/or depression, which continued to the present. The differences in mental health were significant at $p < .001$.

In regard to well-being, the rescuers reported that they were generally more satisfied with life than did the bystanders. They also reported greater satisfaction when they reminisced about their lives. These differences were obtained although the rescuers were, on the average, 4 years older than the bystanders and had more health problems. They also reported far higher levels of contentment with their family lives and with the friendships that they had made.

The rescuers did not report higher levels of overall happiness, health, or wealth than the bystanders. On the average, they were far less affluent. However, they differed significantly in the aspect of life satisfaction that is termed *value congruence*, which is defined as a sense of deep inner contentment derived from the sense that one's life has been lived in accord with one's own values. The people who were higher in congruence than any other group were rescuers who were high in both altruistic attitudes and altruistic moral judgment (Midlarsky & Kahana, 1994).

DISCUSSION AND CONCLUSION

Theoretical approaches to altruism have a very long history, evolving as they have from philosophy and theory. Research on altruism and helping is relatively recent, and the study of altruism in late life and its consequences is even more recent. In reporting the findings of our program of research, based on diverse samples and methods, some coherent patterns emerge. Older adults, as a group, are apparently committed to the values of helping, but they are sometimes deterred by barriers based on limited resources or opportunities for helping. When barriers are removed and opportunities for helping arise, older adults not only rise to the occasion but may outperform younger persons in prosocial activities. These findings call attention to the value of placing prosocial behaviors in late life in an ecological context (Lawton, Windley, & Byerts, 1982). They also suggest that it is not age per se, but age-associated limitations that may contribute to perceptions of older adults as being less prone to helping than their younger counterparts (Kahana & Kahana, 1983).

Our findings relevant to the question "Do the aged help?" have resulted in affirmative conclusions. In addressing questions about the motivational antecedents and the well-being sequelae of helping, our studies posit the value of simultaneously considering the motivational context and the well-being outcomes of helping in late life. Our data across diverse studies of older adults support expectations concerning the mental health and psychological well-being benefits of helping, which have also been reported in the gerontological literature (Brown et al., 2005). Of special interest, however, are our findings about the unique positive sequelae of altruistic helping.

For those older adults who report altruistic orientations in our studies of the old-old, as well as for older adults who actually engaged in altruistic helping as rescuers earlier in their lives, benefits accrue beyond traditional mental health indicators. Altruistic helpers derive existential benefits related to mattering and experience meaning in their lives without needing to involve secondary gains from engagement in helping, such as keeping busy, making friends, or obtaining reciprocal help from others. Altruism appears to be its own reward even when actual helping acts are no longer possible. Indeed, altruistic motives may continue to result in a sense of meaning and value congruence, regardless of levels of volunteering or other helping acts.

We can also gain insights into late-life altruism by assuming a life course perspective (Settersten, 1999) and recognizing that altruism early in life can serve as both prelude to and rehearsal for late-life altruistic behaviors. Such early and enduring altruism may actually result in modesty and an underestimation of one's helping acts. Older adults who do *not* give in order to get may experience lives rich in meaning and contentment, based on their empathy and love for others.

Support for the research reported in this chapter was provided by grants awarded by the National Institutes of Health and by the AARP Andrus Foundation.

REFERENCES

Batson, D., & Powell, A. (2003). Altruism and prosocial behavior. In T. Millon & M. J. Lerner (Eds.), *Handbook of psychology* (Vol. 5, pp. 463–484).

Brown, W., Consedine, N., & Magai, C. (2005). Altruism relates to health in an ethnically diverse sample of older adults. *Journals of Gerontology, 60B*(3), P143–P152.

Cialdini, R., & Fultz, J. (1990). Interpreting the negative mood/helping literature via meta-analysis. *Psychological Bulletin, 107*, 210–214.

Cumming, E., & Henry, W. E. (1961). *Growing old: The process of disengagement.* New York: Basic.

Fogelman, E. (1994). *Conscience and courage: Rescuers of Jews during the Holocaust.* New York: Anchor.

Kahana, E., Feldman, K., Fechner, C., Midlarsky, E., & Kahana, B. (2004, November). *Altruism and volunteering: Effects on psychological well-being in the old-old.* Paper presented at the Gerontological Society of America meetings, Washington, DC.

Kahana, E., & Kahana, B. (1983). Environmental continuity, discontinuity, futurity and adaptation of the aged. In G. Rowles & R. Ohta (Eds.), *Aging and milieu* (pp. 205–228). New York: Academic.

Kahana, E., Kahana, B., & Kercher, K. (2004). Emerging lifestyles and proactive options for successful aging. *Aging International, 28*(2), 155–180.

Kahana, E., Midlarsky, E., & Kahana, B. (1987). Beyond dependency, autonomy, and exchange: Prosocial behavior in late life adaptation. *Social Justice Research, 1*(4), 439–459.

Keyes, C. L., & Ryff, C. D. (2000). Generativity in adult lives. In M. Lewis & J. M. Haviland-Jones (Eds.), *Handbook of emotions* (pp. 227–257). New York: Guilford.

Lawton, M. P., Windley, P., & Byerts, T. (1982). *Aging and the environment: Theoretical approaches.* New York: Springer.

Lewes, G. H. (1904). *Comte's philosophy of the sciences: Being an exposition of the cours de philosophie positive of Auguste Comte.* London: George Bell.

Midlarsky, E. (1968). Aiding responses: An analysis and review. *Merrill-Palmer Quarterly, 14*(3), 229–260.

Midlarsky, E. (1984). Competence and helping: Notes toward a model. In E. Staub, D. Bar-Tal, J. Karylowski, & J. Reykowski (Eds.), *Development and maintenance of prosocial behavior: International perspectives* (pp. 291–308). New York: Plenum.

Midlarsky, E. (1991). Helping as coping. In M. S. Clark (Ed.), *Review of personality and social psychology: Vol. 12. Prosocial behavior* (pp. 238–264). Newbury Park, CA: Sage.

Midlarsky, E., Fagin Jones, S., & Corley, R. (2005). Personality correlates of heroic rescue during the Holocaust. *Journal of Personality, 73*(4), 1–28.

Midlarsky, E., Fagin Jones, S., & Nemeroff, R. (in press). Heroic rescue during the Holocaust. In R. Bootzin & P. McKnight (Eds.), *Strengthening research methodology.* Washington, DC: American Psychological Association.

Midlarsky, E., & Hannah, M. E. (1989). The generous elderly: Naturalistic studies of donations across the life span. *Psychology and Aging, 4*(3), 346–351.

Midlarsky, E., & Kahana, E. (1994). *Altruism in later life.* Newbury Park, CA: Sage.

Midlarsky, M. (2005). *The killing trap: Genocide in the twentieth century.* Cambridge: Cambridge University Press.

Oliner, S. P., & Oliner, P. (1988). *The altruistic personality: Rescuers of Jews in Nazi Europe.* New York: Free Press.

Penner, L., Dovidio, L. F., Piliavin, J., & Schroeder, D. (2005). Prosocial behavior: Multilevel perspectives. *Annual Review of Psychology, 56*, 365–92.

Piburn, S. (Ed.). (1990). *A policy of kindness: Anthology of writings by and about the Dalai Lama*. Ithaca, NY: Snow Lion.

Piliavin, J., & Callero, P. (1991). *Giving blood*. Baltimore: Johns Hopkins University Press.

Pillemer, K., Moen, P., Wethington, E., & Glasgow, N. (Eds.). (2000). *Social integration in the second half of life*. Baltimore: Johns Hopkins University Press.

Schwartz, C., Meisenhelder, J., Ma, Y., & Reed, G. (2003). Altruistic social interest behaviors are associated with better mental health. *Psychosomatic Medicine*, 65, 778–785.

Settersten, R. (1999). *Invitation to the life course: A new look at old age*. Amityville, NY: Baywood.

Snyder, M., Clary, E. G., & Stukas, A. (2000). The functional approach to volunteerism. In G. R. Maio & J. Molson (Eds.), *Why we evaluate: Functions of attitudes* (pp. 365–393). Hillsdale, NJ: Erlbaum.

Sorokin, P. A. (2002). *The ways and power of love*. Conshohocken, PA: John Templeton Foundation Press. (Original work published 1954)

Thoits, P. A., & Hewitt, L. N. (2001). Volunteer work and well-being. *Journal of Health and Social Behavior*, 42, 106–118.

5 Altruism and Health in HIV

Gail Ironson

For several months while I was really having
symptoms of HIV, I helped my mother care for
him [a dying relative] at her home. He would look
at me with an unspoken knowledge that he now
understood my feelings. Me, my sister, and my
mother held his hands at the hospice unit and he
said he saw his [deceased] mother, and he knew
that his time had come, and I told him he was
a good man and I would see him soon. It was
so peaceful, so beautiful. When he died, I
cried because he was in a better place. So
what started as stressful actually helped me
deal with certain fears I had.
—AIDS patient, healthy despite very low CD4
counts (under 50)

In the midst of a devastating epidemic, there are those who rise to the occasion and help others despite their own suffering and concerns, as illustrated
above. Society's response to the AIDS epidemic is abundant with examples
of people, including those with HIV/AIDS, helping others. While the most
visible examples include an increase in volunteerism (Snyder & Omoto, 1992)
and caregiving for those with HIV/AIDS, there are other forms that altruism
may take.

Is altruism good for the altruistic person? What motivates people to donate their time or money to help others, or to become a volunteer or caregiver? What are the positive and negative consequences to the giver? What are the dangers of burnout, and how can they be avoided? This chapter is divided into three sections that will cover what is known about these questions (1) in the context of the literature on volunteering, (2) in the context of the literature on caregiving, and (3) in the context of some of my own work with people who are HIV-positive. I will focus on several aspects of what may be considered altruism: volunteering, ratings of care and concern for others as expressed in essays, giving to charities, and altruism as a personality variable.

VOLUNTEERISM

Reasons for Volunteering

Part of society's response to the HIV epidemic was an outpouring of volunteerism (Snyder & Omoto, 1992). What makes people volunteer? In a longitudinal study of AIDS volunteers at the Gay Men's Health Crisis Network in New York (Cassel, 1995), altruism was only one of the reasons for volunteering. Another type of volunteer is a "getter," who seeks to gain experiences and personal growth by volunteering. In a parallel study of 587 volunteers at the Gay Men's Health Crisis organization, Ouellette, Cassel, Maslanka, and Wong (1995) identified six basic reasons for volunteering: joining the AIDS cause, personal growth, social contact, helping the gay family, coping with AIDS, and career. Motivation to volunteer was also studied in a different context, an ecumenical AIDS ministry (Christensen, Reininger, Richter, McKeown, & Jones, 1999). In this context, motivation to volunteer came from previous contact with a person with AIDS, altruism, and influences from the volunteer's faith community.

Benefits of Volunteering

What do volunteers get out of volunteering? How does volunteering affect the volunteer? Empirical evidence in a general sample suggests that volunteering is associated with both better mental and better physical health (Grzywacz & Keyes, 2004). Post (2005) reviews more generally the benefits of a broader construct, altruism, and notes that the benefits include both positive mental and physical health, including longevity, providing the altruism is not overwhelming.

More specific to HIV, Ramirez and Brown (2003) found that volunteers develop a positive sense of self, a sense of empowerment, change HIV-preventive behavior such as increasing safer sex behavior, and help to make a positive change in the community. Cassel (1995) notes that benefits include a feeling of gratification and personal growth. The AIDS patient quoted at the beginning of this chapter benefited from helping his mother with the dying relative by feeling more at peace with his own future death.

There are health benefits as well. Ironson et al. (2002) found that being a volunteer was associated with long survival with HIV. Two other studies, in populations not specific to HIV, have shown an association between being the *recipient* of volunteer efforts and lower mortality. In a sample of coronary by-pass patients, those who received hospital support visits from fellow bypass patients had lower subsequent mortality rates (Thoits, Hohmann, Harvey, & Fletcher, 2000). More recently, terminally ill patients in a hospice who received volunteer visits lived longer (Herbst-Damm & Kulik, 2005). Thus, volunteers may benefit by believing their behavior may possibly have an impact on the longevity of those they help.

Not all experiences for volunteers are positive, however. Sometimes the expectations of volunteers are too high: Omoto describes AIDS volunteers finding that their experiences were less satisfying than expected, that they had less in common with the person with AIDS than anticipated, and that the relationship was of lower quality than expected (Omoto, Gunn, & Crain, 1998). Others (Bennett, Ross, & Sunderland, 1996) note that there are both recognition/rewards and burnout in AIDS volunteerism.

Burnout, Sustaining Involvement

Working intensively with AIDS patients can be satisfying but may also lead to burnout. *Burnout* encompasses emotional exhaustion, depersonalization, and a lack of felt personal accomplishment and is a significant issue in both volunteers and professional AIDS care workers (Maslach & Ozer, 1995). Some of the stresses that AIDS care workers face that are often associated with burnout include intense staff-patient relationships over long periods of time during which the health of the AIDS patient declines, self-identification with patients, unremitting involvement in high-intensity tasks, anxieties over safe working conditions and fear of contagion, and lack of support within volunteer organizations (Miller, 1995a). Ross, Greenfield, and Bennett (1999) found several predictors of dropout over 2 years in AIDS volunteers who were members of an interfaith religious organization. These were total stress, the Maslach Burnout Inventory score on depersonalization intensity, and scores on three other subscales measuring stress (client problems and role ambiguity, emotional overload, and organizational factors). Some researchers have related burnout and satisfaction to the reasons for volunteering. Cassel (1995) found that "self-sacrificers" had the least amount of burnout, partly because, although behaviorally engaged, they are able to be emotionally disengaged relative to other volunteers. Andrews (1997) and Omoto and Snyder (2002) found that the context of caregiving has an impact on the burden and satisfaction of the volunteer caregiver. Christiensen,

Reininger, Richter, McKeown, and Jones (1999) found that several conditions fostered sustained involvement: a support system, the expression of faith, support of a faith community, and help with coping with the death of a care partner. Interestingly, Asante (2000) found that time spent providing direct service contact was not related to burnout, while social support and religiosity were protective. Miller notes four strategies for preventing stress in AIDS care workers: professional supervision, emotional support/therapeutic counseling, stress reduction, and context management (Miller, 1995a). Miller also suggests that in order to keep volunteers engaged, staff support and giving a realistic picture of what may be expected from volunteer work should be provided (1995b). Bennett, Ross, and Sunderland (1996) suggest that rewards in the form of gratitude from clients and recognition and support from management might be helpful.

CAREGIVING

Caregiving is an important behavior that, at least in part, may be motivated by altruism. There are obviously other motivations, such as a feeling of obligation. In HIV, caregivers may be less likely to be family members than in other diseases since many people with HIV do not have traditional families or may have been rejected by their families of origin. Caregiving makes the process of illness much more bearable for the recipient, and it saves society an enormous amount of money. Most of the literature on caregiving refers to caregivers of those with Alzheimer's disease. In that context, a major review showed that caregiving negatively affects both mental and physical health (Vitaliano, Zhang, & Scanlan, 2003). The situation in AIDS caregiving is complicated by the fact that many of the caregivers are HIV-positive themselves and are therefore looking at their future as they go through the pain of the person for whom they are caring. Thus, they are faced with the ongoing threat to their own health and well-being (Folkman, Moskowitz, Ozer, & Park, 1997). HIV clients are facing multiple hardships in addition to HIV: poverty, drug use, discrimination, and losses (Schoen, 1998). The major caregiver groups for people with AIDS (PWAs) include partners of gay men (Folkman, 1997; Folkman et al., 1997; Leblanc, 1997), women (Bennett, Casey, & Austin, 1996; Wight, Leblanc, & Aneshensel, 1998), and the elderly (Levine-Perkell, 1996; Linsk & Poindexter, 2000). While many of the issues surrounding illness and dying will be similar across groups, certain issues can be very different for each of these groups. For example, many minority women are facing poverty, worry about who will take care of their children, and fear that a boyfriend upon whom they depend for financial support will leave them (Bennett, Casey, & Austin, 1996). The elderly caregiver may be facing their own health decline as well as stigma and discomfort surrounding the disclosure of a child's HIV and/or gay status. They may also be dealing both with taking care of their adult child and raising their grandchildren. Gay men may be dealing with lack of recognition by the medical establishment and hospitals of their partnership status.

Positive and Negative Correlates of Caregiving

Post (2005) notes that altruism is good as long as it is not overwhelming. Folkman (1997) has pioneered the idea that there are both positive and negative aspects to caregiving. Despite the extreme and chronic stresses of caregiving, some men were able to find events that were meaningful and positive (Folkman et al., 1997). Four types of coping were associated with positive states (Folkman et al., 1997): positive reappraisal, goal-directed problem-focused coping, spiritual beliefs, and the infusion of ordinary events with positive meaning. Positive moods were also associated with perceived support (Soskolne, Acree, & Folkman, 2000). Negative effects have also been found in AIDS caregiving, including both physical (Leblanc, London, & Aneshensel, 1997) and mental health (Irving, Bor, & Catalan, 1995; Land, Hudson, & Stiefel, 2003). For example, depression is one of the common effects associated with HIV caregiving (Irving et al., 1995; Land et al., 2003). Several researchers have investigated factors associated with the occurrence of depression in caregivers. Land notes that younger age, low self-esteem, poorer health, and financial concerns are common predictors of depression in caregivers (Land et al., 2003). Furthermore, negative moods in gay male caregivers have been associated with perceived stress, social conflict, lack of received support, and lack of a family confidant (Soskolne et al., 2000). Mental health in gay male caregivers has also been found to be affected by deteriorating health, perceptions of AIDS alienation or stigma, internalized homophobia, overload, and financial worry (Wight, 2000). Additionally, Leblanc, London, and Aneshensel (1997) found that depression and prior health were strong correlates of physical symptoms in AIDS caregivers. Thus, both positive and negative aspects of caregiving have been identified.

Interventions

There is much in the literature that can be used to suggest what might be done to ease the burden of coping with caregiving. These include utilizing social support, including perceived support (Soskolne et al., 2000), social coping (Billings, Folkman, Acree, & Moskowitz, 2000), and family support when available (Wight, Aneshensel, & Leblanc, 2003); finding meaning (Carlisle, 2000); enjoying the positive aspects of interactions on a daily basis (Folkman et al., 1997); spirituality (Folkman, 1997); and goal-directed problem-focused coping (Folkman, 1997). Having protected time for relief from caregiving may be important as well. One group that has specifically addressed the question of designing interventions to prevent burnout in AIDS caregivers is Pakenham, Dadds, and Lennon (2002). They compared a dyad intervention, a caregiver-only intervention, and a wait list control and found that the dyad intervention produced the most changes on global distress, dyadic adjustment, and target problems, although both dyadic and caregiver-only intervention participants showed improvement compared to the wait list control on all dependent variables except social adjustment.

RESULTS FROM OUR POSITIVE SURVIVORS RESEARCH CENTER

We have been engaged in several analyses of variables relevant to altruism in HIV. Described below are our studies of volunteerism, altruism measured unobtrusively (essay-rated care and concern for others), a behavioral measure of altruism (giving to charities), and a personality measure (altruism as measured on the NEO Personality Inventory Revised [NEO PI-R]).

Our first finding was that volunteering was related cross-sectionally to long survival with HIV (Ironson et al., 2002). In this analysis, a group of 79 long-term survivors of AIDS (people who had survived more than twice as long as expected after getting a serious AIDS-defining symptom) were compared with a group of people who had HIV with a normal course of the illness (n = 200). Those in the long survivor group were significantly more likely to have volunteered (mostly helping other people with HIV) than those in the normal course comparison group ($r = .18$, $p < .01$). Interestingly, those who volunteered had better mental health: Volunteering was significantly associated with less depression ($r = -.22$, $p < .01$), less anxiety ($r = -.17$, $p < .05$), and less perceived stress ($r = -.21$, $p < .01$).

Our subsequent efforts have been looking at psychological predictors of slower disease progression over time in a longitudinal study. For these studies, a sample of 177 people with HIV were intensively studied at baseline (with both psychological and immune measures taken) and have been followed every 6 months with indicators of their emotional and physical (CD4 and viral load) well-being measured. Our sample is diverse with respect to gender (70% male, 30% female) and race (31% Caucasian, 36% African American, 28% Hispanic, 5% other). It is unusual in that the sample at baseline included only people in the midrange of the disease (CD4s between 150 and 500, never had a serious AIDS-defining symptom) and excluded people who were drug dependent at entry to the study. As the disease progresses (i.e., gets worse), CD4s decrease over time and viral load increases over time. Prospective psychological predictors of disease progression (i.e., CD4 and viral load change) have been examined by us (Ironson, O'Cleirigh, et al., 2005; Ironson, Balbin, et al., 2005), and these papers have a more complete description of the sample and methodology.

Data Analysis for Longitudinal Data

For the subsequent analyses of the longitudinal data to determine whether the altruism variables would predict to change over time in CD4 or viral load, we used a statistical technique called hierarchical linear modeling (HLM). HLM has a couple of major features: (1) One can predict to slope rather than a measure at a single time point; and (2) one can control for the effect of changing variables. In the case of HIV, this can be used for medications at every time point. In HLM, level 1 equations are used to model individual growth, which is represented as repeated measure observations nested within persons. Level 2 equations model interindividual differences with between-person predictors, such as education and psychological variables. Thus, systematic variability of the slopes and intercepts at level 1 are modeled with the predictors at level 2. All longitudinal analyses described used the standard covariates noted in the literature. Level 1 control variables were time since baseline and antiretroviral medications (none, combination therapy without Highly Active Anti-Retroviral Therapy [HAART], combination therapy with HAART); level 2 control variables were age, gender, race, and education. Baseline disease progression markers were controlled for in the model as well. A more detailed description of the model can be found in Ironson, O'Cleirigh, et al. (2005).

Measures and Findings of Our Longitudinal Studies

In an effort to measure altruism in an unobtrusive way, essays written by the research participants about stressful situations were rated for indications of care and concern for others. More specifically, research participants were asked: "Think of the most stressful or traumatic situation or feelings you have had to deal with since finding out you were HIV positive, including finding out you were HIV positive. We would like you to write a short essay (1–2 pages) regarding your feelings on this topic. Take about 20 minutes to do this." The essays were scored for indications of concern for others and actual caring behavior for others. An example of concern for others is a person with HIV who didn't tell his grandmother that he is HIV-positive because the grandmother is in poor health; another example is a person with HIV being concerned about who will care for her children when she dies. Caring for others was scored if the person indicated actually doing something for someone, and in this sample the most frequent example was taking care of a partner who was sick or dying. Interestingly, indications in one's essay of *caring* for others predicted slower disease progression over 2 years (both slower loss in CD4 and slower increase in viral load (log), $t(168) = 2.25$, $p = .026$; $t(168) = -2.05$, $p = .042$, respectively), but expressing *concern* for others did not predict either CD4 or viral load change. That is, people who said in their essays that they did something for others were more likely to have maintained CD4s at the end of 2 years and more likely to have better control of the HIV virus than those who did not display caring behaviors.

Our next measure related to altruism was giving to charities. As part of the questionnaires given to participants, people were asked the number of charities to which they routinely give. The measure used was whether they gave to any or not. Giving to charities predicted better control of viral load over 2 years ($t(149) = -2.14$, $p = .034$). Thus, people who contributed to charities were significantly more likely to be doing well physically (better control of the HIV virus as indicated by lower viral load) over 2 years than those who did not contribute. Since giving to charities may depend partly on income, we controlled for income in addition to the control variables noted above. Giving to charities still predicted better control of the HIV virus even after taking income into account ($t = -2.15$, $p = .033$). However, giving to charities was not predictive of changes in CD4 number over time.

The next variable relating to altruism in our data set was altruism conceptualized as a personality style measured on the NEO PI-R (Costa & McCrae, 1992). Examples of adjectives describing this construct include tolerant, generous, and kind. Although self-reports of positive attributes are always subject to bias, this subscale correlated significantly with peer ratings ($r = .33$, $p < .001$, $N = 250$) and spouse ratings ($r = .57$, $p < .001$, $N = 68$), as reported in the NEO PI-R manual. In our sample, altruism was associated with better control of the HIV virus in the longitudinal study over 4 years That is, altruism measured as a personality variable was significantly associated with a slower increase in (log) viral load (slope) over 4 years (using HLM, $t = -4.05$, $p < .001$), controlling for the covariates noted above. However, similar to charities, altruism was not significantly related to changes in CD4 number. Possible reasons for this may include (1) a greater sensitivity of viral load to psychological influences compared to CD4. This is consistent with our prior work (Ironson, O'Cleirigh, et al., 2005), where we have found that decline ratios comparing CD4 changes for those high on variables such as depression versus those low on depression (i.e., at the 75th versus the 25th percentile) were of less magnitude than the increase ratios for viral load. (2) Viral load may respond more quickly to stress or other psychological variables than CD4 does. Conversely, it may respond more quickly to positive psychological influences than CD4 does. Further investigation of associations between the full NEO-PI-R and disease progression in HIV may be found in Ironson et al. (under review, 2006). The relationship of altruism to other biological measures, namely stress hormones, was also explored. Altruism correlated significantly with both lower cortisol concentration ($r = -.19$, $p < .05$) and with lower norepinephrine concentration ($r = -.18$, $p < .05$), both measured in the urine.

Finally, cross-sectional correlations were computed for the above variables to determine whether the indicators of altruism were related to better mental health. Both volunteering (as noted above) and giving to charities correlated significantly with all three indicators of mental health/stress, and they correlated the highest of all of the altruism variables considered. Giving to charities was significantly related to less depression ($r = -.23$, $p < .01$, $N = 156$), less anxiety ($r = -.18$, $p < .05$, $N = 156$), and lower perceived stress ($r = -.22$, $p < .01$, $N = 156$). It is interesting to note that the two altruism variables correlating most highly with better mental health (volunteering and giving to charities) are both behavioral. Expressions of caring and concern for others were only significantly related to lower perceived stress ($r = -.18$, $p < .05$, $N = 176$; $r = -.24$, $p < .01$, $N = 176$). None of the relationships reached significance for the personality variable of altruism.

Thus, there is some indication that volunteering, giving to charities, and displaying caring for others are related to indicators of better physical health (i.e., long survival, higher CD4, lower VL) and less distress in HIV. In addition, altruism measured as a personality variable was associated with better control of viral load over 4 years. The behaviorally oriented variables appear to have the stronger relationships (i.e., caring for others rather than concern for others).

CONCLUSION

Altruism is unquestionably a virtue. But does it confer health protection? Actions of altruism such as volunteering, giving to charities, essay indications of caring for others, and the personality variable of altruism are all associated with better prognosis in HIV. Another interesting finding using the analysis of the essays suggests that health outcomes are more strongly related to the report of actual behaviors rather than concern alone. Thus, it is more about what you do than what you say. Volunteering has also been associated with a variety of health outcomes and less distress, although it may not always give the benefits hoped for. More extensive caregiving can be beneficial but may also be a stressor and cause strain. Thus, both the literature and our own work suggest that with a few caveats, altruism can be beneficial for both physical and mental well-being. The main caveat is making sure that the caregiving is not overwhelming. Important conditions for volunteering or caregiving to be beneficial are to provide proper preparation, orientation, and support. Monitoring for early signs of depression and burnout in caregivers may help to avoid the potential negative effects of caregiving. Screening could also be used to determine who is most at risk and who would benefit most from volunteering. Thus, much could be done to ensure that altruistic actions would be most likely to be beneficial.

Altruism is such a potentially powerful positive force that considerable effort should be directed at understanding it better. Findings may then be applied to provide maximum benefit for both the caregiver and the receiver.

This research was supported by NIMH R01 MH053791; R01 MH066697; the intramural program of the National Institute on Aging of NIH; Action for AIDS; and the Metanexus/Templeton Foundation. The author also wishes to thank Elizabeth Balbin, Rick Stuetzle, Kelly Detz, Conall O'Cleirigh, Annie George, Paul Costa, and Joe Paroulo.

REFERENCES

Andrews, G. H. (1997). The effect of context of caregiving on burden and satisfaction among volunteer caregivers of persons living with HIV and AIDS. *Dissertation Abstracts International: Section B: Sciences and Engineering, 57*(12-B), 7715.

Asante, A. J. (2000). Factors impacting burnout: HIV/AIDS volunteers. *Dissertation Abstracts International: Section B: Sciences and Engineering, 60*(8-B), 4200.

Bennett, L., Casey, K., & Austin, P. (1996). Issues for women as carers in HIV/AIDS. In C. Hankins & L. Sherr (Eds.), *AIDS as a gender issue: Psychosocial perspectives* (pp. 177–190). Philadelphia, PA: Taylor & Francis.

Bennett, L., Ross, M. W., & Sunderland, R. (1996). The relationship between recognition, rewards and burnout in AIDS caring. *AIDS Care, 8*(2), 145–153.

Billings, D. W., Folkman, S., Acree, M., & Moskowitz, J. T. (2000). Coping and physical health during caregiving: The roles of positive and negative affect. *Journal of Personality and Social Psychology, 79*(1), 131–142.

Carlisle, C. (2000). The search for meaning in HIV and AIDS: The carers' experience. *Qualitative Health Research, 10*(6), 750–765.

Cassel, B. J. (1995). Altruism is only part of the story: A longitudinal study of AIDS volunteers. *Dissertation Abstracts International: Section B: Sciences and Engineering, 56*(5B), 2937.

Costa, P., & McCrae, R. R. (1992). *Professional manual for the revised NEO Personality Inventory (NEO PI-R) and NEO Five-Factor Inventory (NEO-FFI)*. Lutz, FL: Psychological Assessment Resources.

Folkman, S. (1997). Positive psychological states and coping with severe stress. *Social Science and Medicine, 45*(8), 1207–1221.

Folkman, S., Moskowitz, J. T., Ozer, E. M., & Park, C. L. (1997). Positive meaningful events and coping in the context of HIV/AIDS. In B. Gottlieb (Ed.), *The plenum series on stress and coping* (pp. 293–314). New York: Plenum.

Grzywacz, J. G., & Keyes, C. L. M. (2004). Toward health promotion: Physical and social behaviors in complete health. *American Journal of Health Behavior, 28*(2), 99–111.

Herbst-Damm, K. L., & Kulik, J. A. (2005). Volunteer support, marital status, and the survival times of terminally ill patients. *Health Psychology, 24*(2), 225–229.

Ironson, G., Balbin, E., Stuetzle, R., Fletcher, M. A., O'Cleirigh, C., Laurenceau, J. P., Schneiderman, N., & Solomon, G. (2005). Dispositional optimism and the mechanisms by which it predicts slower disease progression in HIV: Proactive behavior, avoidant coping, and depression. *International Journal of Behavioral Medicine, 12*(2), 86–97.

Ironson, G., O'Cleirigh, C., Fletcher, M. A., Laurenceau, J. P., Balbin, E., Klimas, N., Schneiderman, N., & Solomon, G. (2005). Psychosocial factors predict CD4 and viral load change in men and women in the era of HAART. *Psychosomatic Medicine, 67*(6), 1013–1021.

Ironson, G., O'Cleirigh, C., Costa, P., & Weiss, A. (2006). *Personality and health in HIV: The relationship between NEO PI-R domains, facets, and profiles and change in CD4 cell number and HIV-1 viral load over 4 years.* Manuscript submitted for publication.

Ironson, G., Solomon, G. F., Balbin, E. G., O'Cleirigh, C., George, A., Kumar, M., Larson, D., & Woods, T. E. (2002). The Ironson-Woods spirituality/religiousness index is associated with long survival health behaviors, less distress, and low cortisol in people with HIV/AIDS. *Annals of Behavioral Medicine, 24*(1), 34–48.

Irving, G. A., Bor, R., & Catalan, J. (1995). Psychological distress among gay men supporting a lover or partner with AIDS: A pilot study. *AIDS Care, 7*(5), 605–617.

Land, H., Hudson, S. M., & Stiefel, B. (2003). Stress and depression among HIV positive and HIV negative gay and bisexual AIDS caregivers. *AIDS & Behavior, 7*(1), 41–53.

Leblanc, A. J., London A. S., & Aneshensel, C. S. (1997). The physical costs of AIDS caregiving. *Social Science and Medicine, 45*(6), 915–923.

Levine-Perkell, J. (1996). Caregiving issues. In M. K. Nokes (Ed.), *HIV/AIDS and the older adult* (pp. 115–128). Philadelphia, PA: Taylor & Francis.

Linsk, N. L., & Poindexter, C. C. (2000). Older caregivers for family members with HIV or AIDS: Reasons for caring. *Journal of Applied Gerontology, 19*(2), 181–202.

Londono-Mcconnell, A. (1998). Sexual risk taking behaviors, attachment styles, independent decision making, and psychosocial development in a college student population. *Dissertation Abstracts International: Section A: Humanities and Social Sciences, 58*(8-A), 3020.

Maslach, C., & Ozer, E. (1995). Theoretical issues related to burnout in AIDS health workers. In D. Miller & L. Bennett (Eds.), *Health workers and AIDS: Research, intervention and current issues in burnout and response* (pp. 1–14). Amsterdam, Netherlands: Harwood Academic.

Miller, D. (1995a). Stress and burnout among health-care staff working with people affected by HIV. *British Journal of Guidance and Counselling, 23*(1), 19–31.

Miller, D. (1995b). The UK Multicentre Occupational Morbidity Study (MOMS): Issues of methodology, volunteer bias and preliminary findings on preferences for staff support in HIV/AIDS health staff. In D. Miller & L. Bennett (Eds.), *Health workers and AIDS: Research, intervention and current issues in burnout and response* (pp. 213–228). Amsterdam, Netherlands: Harwood Academic.

Omoto, A. M., Gunn, D. O., & Crain, A. L. (1998). Helping in hard times: Relationship closeness and the AIDS volunteer experience. In V. J. Derlega & A. P. Barbee (Eds.), *HIV infection and social interaction* (pp. 106–128). Thousand Oaks, CA: Sage.

Omoto, A. M., & Snyder, M. (2002). Considerations of community: The context and process of volunteerism. *American Behavioral Scientist, 45*(5), 400–404.

Ouellette, S. C., Cassel, B. J., Maslanka, H., & Wong, L. M. (1995). *AIDS Education and Prevention, 7,* 64–79.

Pakenham, K. I., Dadds, M. R., & Lennon, H. V. (2002). The efficacy of a psychosocial intervention for HIV/AIDS caregiving dyads and individual caregivers: A controlled treatment outcome study. *AIDS Care, 14*(6), 731–750.

Post, S. G. (2005). Altruism, happiness and health: It's good to be good. *International Journal of Behavioral Medicine, 12*(2), 66–77.

Ramirez, V. J., & Brown, A. U. (2003). Latinos' community involvement in HIV/AIDS: Organizational and individual perspectives on volunteering. *AIDS Education and Prevention, 15*(Suppl. 1), 90–104.

Ross, M. W., Greenfield, S. A., & Bennett, L. (1999). Predictors of dropout and burnout in AIDS volunteers: A longitudinal study. *AIDS Care, 11*(6), 723–731.

Schoen, K. (1998). Caring for ourselves: Understanding and minimizing the stresses of HIV caregiving. In B. J. Thompson & D. M. Aronstein (Eds.), *Psychosocial issues of HIV/AIDS* (pp. 527–536). Binghamton, NY: Harrington Park/Haworth.

Snyder, M., & Omoto, A. M. (1992). Volunteerism and society's response to the HIV epidemic. *Current Directions in Psychological Science, 1*(4), 113–116.

Soskolne, V., Acree, M., & Folkman, S. (2000). Social support and mood in gay caregivers of men with AIDS. *AIDS and Behavior, 4*(3), 220–232.

Thoits, P. A., Hohmann, A. A., Harvey, M. R., & Fletcher, B. (2000). Similar-other support for men undergoing coronary artery bypass surgery. *Health Psychology, 19,* 264–273.

Vitaliano, P. P., Zhang, J., & Scanlan, J. M. (2003). Is caregiving hazardous to one's physical health? A meta analysis. *Psychological Bulletin, 129*(6), 946–972.

Wight, R. G. (2000). Precursive depression among HIV infected AIDS caregivers over time. *Social Science and Medicine, 51*(5), 759–770.

Wight, R. G., Aneshensel, C. S., & Leblanc, A. J. (2003). Stress buffering effects of family support in AIDS caregiving. *AIDS Care, 15*(5), 595–613.

Wight, R. G., Leblanc, A. J., & Aneshensel, C. S. (1998). AIDS caregiving and health among midlife and older women. *Health Psychology, 17*(2), 130–137.

6 Self-Initiated Volunteering and Mental Health

Marc A. Musick
Miranda R. Waggoner

Historically, researchers have spent considerable effort conducting studies of paid work; although this research has proved to be important, a major portion of the work sector has remained largely ignored: volunteering. In recent years, however, researchers have addressed this deficiency by learning more about how and why people volunteer and how volunteering affects people's lives. For example, recent research has indicated that older adults who volunteer tend to live longer than older adults who do not engage in that activity (Musick, Herzog, & House, 1999; Oman, Thoresen, & McMahon, 1999; Shmotkin, Blumstein, & Modan, 2003). Other studies of older adults have shown benefits of the activity for physical functioning as well (e.g., Morrow-Howell et al., 2003). It is clear from emerging evidence that volunteering tends to benefit health, at least in older adult populations. Yet, we still do not fully understand why or how these linkages exist.

The purpose of this chapter is to further explore the association between volunteering and health by concentrating on a particular type of volunteering and its effects on mental health. More specifically, we will propose and test a theory focused on self-initiated volunteering, that is, volunteering which is done by someone who has not been asked to do the volunteering. As we discuss below, our belief is that persons who engage in this type of volunteering will reap greater mental health rewards from that activity than those who volunteer after being asked to do so.

In pursuit of this goal, the chapter proceeds as follows. In the first part, we review the literature on volunteering and mental health and then discuss how self-initiated volunteering should fit into this framework. Next, we test our expectations using a newly collected data set that contains extensive measures of volunteering and mental health. We conclude with a discussion of our findings and what future research might do to further our knowledge in this domain.

LITERATURE ON VOLUNTEERING AND MENTAL HEALTH

Generally speaking, it is believed that volunteering is beneficial for mental well-being. However, much of the evidence of this effect remains limited to older adults; indeed, there exists ample evidence that volunteering benefits older persons' psychological well-being (Jirovec & Hyduk, 1998; Morrow-Howell et al., 2003; Wheeler, Gorey, & Greenblatt, 1998). Likewise, at least two studies have found beneficial volunteering effects for older adults but not younger ones (Musick & Wilson, 2003; Van Willigen, 2000). In contrast, Thoits and Hewitt (2001) found that the psychological benefits of volunteering accrued to both younger and older adults. Although these findings generally overlap and are supportive of a beneficial effects hypothesis, the field must continue to look at the dynamics of the volunteering process and how that might play a role in the psychological consequences of the activity.

Previous research in this domain has discussed the meaning of roles, social interaction, and formal versus informal forms in understanding the salutary nature of volunteering. For example, Thoits and Hewitt (2001) argued that social causation and social selection operate concurrently, that is, there exists a positive cycle of people with greater well-being investing more in volunteering and volunteering itself producing a positive well-being in volunteers. Other researchers (Greenfield & Marks, 2004) have found that volunteering acts as a protective factor against a reduced sense of purpose in later life, indicating that role identities may play a major factor in the positive effects of volunteering on psychological well-being. Musick and Wilson (2003) have found suggestive evidence that formal but not informal social interaction improves mental health, and the fact that volunteering is associated with better mental health can be interpreted in terms of role salience. However, research has also pointed to the informal support of others as having a positive effect on well-being, although similar positive effects do not result from helping others within formal organizational contexts (Krause, Herzog, & Baker, 1992). In short, there is an understanding in the literature that volunteering is dynamic and multifaceted and must be fully considered when gauging its impact on well-being.

ALTRUISM, SELF-INITIATED VOLUNTEERING, AND HEALTH

Altruism and Self-Initiated Volunteering

A common perception holds that when people volunteer, they do so in altruistic ways. This may or may not be the case, but before discussing our conception of altruistic volunteering, we must first provide a working definition of altruism. Midlarsky and Kahana define *altruism* as a voluntary behavior that is "motivated by concern for the welfare of the other, rather than by the anticipation of rewards" (1994, p. 11); likewise, Dunkel-Schetter et al. (1992, p. 87) state that "altruistically motivated support attempts are those made without expectation of reward or personal gain." Smith (1982, p. 27) explains that altruism is a "net motivation of the individual actor who does not expect reciprocity." He further claims that a variable for absolute altruism does not exist and, furthermore, that the essence of volunteerism lies not in altruism but rather always in some form of selfishness. Although, as Smith claims, absolute altruism may not be possible, it should be feasible to classify some acts as more altruistic than others.

In terms of volunteering, it could be argued that those who volunteer without being asked to do so are more altruistic in the act than those who have been asked to volunteer. This contrast should be true because the process of being asked to volunteer implies an exchange-oriented or obligatory relationship. Along these lines, Midlarsky and Kahana (1994) actually outline a set of criteria for attributions of altruism. These include motives, whether the act is costly, the degree to which the act is voluntary, and whether alternative acts are available. They explain that if an act is required or expected, then it does not fit the criteria for an altruistic act. Thus, in accord with our own thinking, volunteering that is self-initiated proves to be more altruistic than that which is solicited, at least according to these criteria.

Self-Initiated Volunteering and Mental Health

Although no extensive research has been conducted on the health effects of self-initiated volunteering compared to the invited form, some research has explored the dynamics of the asking-volunteering process. Varese and Yaish (2000), in a study on the rescue of Jews in World War II Nazi Europe, single out "being asked" as the most significant factor in explaining altruistic assistance behavior. When Musick, Wilson, and Bynum (2000) examined the predictors of being asked to volunteer, they found that certain characteristics, including socioeconomic status, race, and social integration, played an important role in the likelihood of someone being sought out to volunteer. They also found, not surprisingly, that respondents who were asked to volunteer were much more likely to do so than those who had not been asked. However, it is certainly true that not all volunteers are asked to do so; rather, there likely exists a large pool of individuals who volunteer under their own initiative. Some researchers (e.g., Thoits & Hewitt, 2001) have raised the question of whether people take the initiative to seek out volunteer opportunities or whether organizations recruit volunteers. Yet, this subject has remained relatively unexplored.

Research on the health effects of self-initiated volunteering is also minimal. Some results have indicated that long-term volunteerism, while associated with higher levels of well-being, does not result in even higher levels of well-being when the individual initiates the activity (Pushkar, Reis, & Morros, 2002). It should be noted that "initiation" in this study was measured using a motivation scale involving categories such as altruism and personal rewards. In another study, Morrow-Howell et al. (2003) similarly found that volunteers' assessment of perceived benefits toward others did not affect well-being outcomes. In short, the evidence on this issue is scant, and what exists appears to support the idea that how volunteering is initiated or perceived has little effect on its health benefits.

Regardless of these findings, it is still possible to believe that volunteering which is self-initiated is better for mental health than volunteering which is invited. Generally speaking, researchers have argued that the positive mental health benefits that come from volunteering might flow from two sources: improvement of self-evaluations (e.g., enhanced self-esteem) and higher levels of social integration (Musick & Wilson, 2003). These benefits, when they exist, should adhere to both self-initiated and invited volunteers. Yet, one could argue that these benefits are likely greater for the self-initiated volunteers. For example, enhancements in self-evaluations due to volunteering often flow from the feeling that one is "doing good" or benefiting society when helping others. For self-initiating volunteers, these feelings of doing good are unclouded by the notion that the volunteering was conditioned on the invitation. In other words, there can be little doubt in the self-initiated volunteers' minds that their activity was of their own choosing and of their own accord; among those who were invited, this sense of mission is not as pure, though it is likely that they too will feel the positive self-appraisals that often come through helping others.

Likewise, although both self-initiated and invited volunteers may also benefit in terms of increased social integration, differences in this benefit are also likely. Many who initiate their volunteering will move into completely new social spheres, allowing them to construct completely new social networks. In contrast, invited volunteers are more likely to enter already established networks, albeit in new roles. As such, the social integration that flows from self-initiated volunteering is more likely to entail an expansion of networks, and the possibility for supportive network ties, than volunteering that is invited. In sum, although it should be the case that self-initiated and invited volunteering should both be beneficial for mental health, the additional benefits that flow from the former should generate stronger mental health benefits for that group.

DATA

To test this idea, we used data from the Survey of Texas Adults (SoTA; Musick, 2004). Conducted between November 2003 and January 2004, the SoTA is representative of community-dwelling adults residing in Texas and aged 18 and over. The data collection process yielded 1,504 completed telephone interviews (household-level cooperation rate: 37%; respondent-level cooperation rate: 89%; American Association for Public Opinion Research, 2004). Data were weighted on known population characteristics to match the sample to the population from which it was drawn.

Sampling was conducted using a modified Random Digit Dialing (RDD) design with a sampling frame constructed by Survey Sampling, Inc. (SSI). That is, SSI generated a list of working telephone exchanges throughout the state of Texas and then produced telephone numbers using four-digit randomization. Those phone numbers were then screened against yellow pages directories to find and eliminate phone numbers for businesses and thereby increase the likelihood of eligible phone numbers. Once a household was contacted, a list of eligible respondents was created and used to select the sample member from the household.

Data collection was conducted by the Office of Survey Research at the University of Texas at Austin. Each Computer Assisted Telephone Interviewing (CATI) survey lasted approximately 30–35 minutes and consisted of questions on a variety of topics, including but not limited to health, community participation, and religion. The instrument was also translated into Spanish and administered by Spanish-speaking interviewers for respondents who were more comfortable answering in that language. Of the 1,504 completed interviews, 137 (9.1%) were conducted in Spanish.

MEASUREMENT

Dependent Variable

The only dependent variable was psychological distress ($\pm$ = .81). The outcome is a six-item mean index which taps negative affect, somatic-retarded activity, and anxiety. For each item, respondents were asked how often over the past 30 days they had felt that way. Response categories ranged from 1 = "never" to 5 = "very often." The specific distress symptoms include feeling (a) so sad that nothing could cheer you up, (b) nervous, (c) restless or fidgety, (d) hopeless, (e) everything was an effort, and (f) worthless.

Independent Variables

Volunteering

Respondents were asked whether they had volunteered in any of 11 areas over the past 12 months. The areas were (a) health; (b) education; (c) religious groups; (d) human services; (e) environment/animal rescue; (f) public/society benefit; (g) recreation/coaching; (h) arts, culture, humanities; (i) work-related; (j) political; and (k) youth development. Respondents who said that they had done unpaid work in one or more of these areas were coded as having volunteered; otherwise, respondents were coded zero (0). A second set of three dichotomous variables was created, reflecting the number of areas in which respondents volunteered: (a) one or two areas, (b) three or four areas, and (c) five or more areas. The reference for all three variables was respondents who did not volunteer.

Asked to Volunteer

This item was a dichotomous variable coded one (1) for respondents who had been asked to volunteer at any time during the past 12 months and 0 otherwise.

Physical Health

Respondents were asked to rate their physical health at the present time. Responses ranged from 1 = "poor" to 5 = "excellent."

Religious Service Attendance

This variable was an indicator of how often respondents attended religious services. Responses included (1) never, (2) less than once a month, (3) 1–3 times a month, (4) once a week, and (5) several times a week.

Sociodemographic Controls

Other variables included in the analyses were gender (female: 1 = female, 0 = male), race (non-Hispanic Black: 1 = non-Hispanic Black, 0 = others; Hispanic: 1 = Hispanic, 0 = others), age (in years), education (five categories ranging from 1 = "none" to 5 = "graduate degree"), family income (six categories ranging from 1 = "less than $15,000" to 6 = "$85,000 or more per year"), and marital status (1 = married, 0 = others).

RESULTS

We begin a presentation of the results with a listing of descriptive statistics for study variables, as shown in Table 6.1. According to these findings, levels of psychological distress were relatively low, with a mean score of 1.98 on a 1–5 scale. Over the past year, about 44% of respondents mentioned that they had been asked to volunteer, and 61% of respondents mentioned that they had actually volunteered in one or more of the areas noted previously. Of those who volunteered, most (26%) volunteered in only one to two areas; however, a substantial portion of the sample (17%) did volunteer in five or more areas.

We have previously argued that, for many people, the gateway to volunteer exists in the form of a personal invitation. To shed more light on this issue, at the bottom of Table 6.1, we display the various patterns that exist between being asked to volunteer and actually doing so. The most common combina-

Table 6.1. Descriptive Statistics of Study Variables

	Range	Mean	Standard Deviation
Psychological Distress	1–5	1.98	.80
Volunteering Variables			
Asked to volunteer	0–1	.44	.50
Any volunteering	0–1	.61	.49
Volunteer in 1–2 areas	0–1	.26	.44
Volunteer in 3–4 areas	0–1	.18	.39
Volunteer in 5+ areas	0–1	.17	.38
Control Variables			
Female	0–1	.51	.51
Non-Hispanic Black	0–1	.11	.32
Hispanic	0–1	.37	.49
Age	18–94	41.46	17.29
Education	1–5	2.24	1.18
Family income	1–6	2.64	1.73
Physical health	1–5	3.39	1.12
Married	0–1	.53	.50
Religious services attendance	1–5	3.07	1.36
Being Asked × Volunteering			
Not asked–No volunteering	0–1	.34	.48
Not asked–Volunteering	0–1	.22	.42
Asked–No volunteering	0–1	.05	.21
Asked–Volunteering	0–1	.40	.49

tion of these variables represents people who are completely involved in the volunteering culture, that is, 40% of respondents reported that they were both asked to volunteer and did so during the past year. The second most common category shows the opposite pattern: people who were neither asked to volunteer nor did so. For the purposes of this chapter, the most interesting category represents people who were not asked to volunteer but did so. These are the self-initiated volunteers, who should profit the most from their volunteering. Although not as common as people who were asked and volunteered, they are still well represented in the sample at 22%. In contrast, a rare group in the sample, comprising only 5% thereof, is those respondents who were asked to volunteer but did not do so. Because being asked to volunteer implies a sort of social exchange, we would expect that respondents who are asked are very unlikely to decline; this small number is supportive of that expectation.

The ultimate goal of this chapter is to determine whether the documented (e.g., Musick & Wilson, 2003) mental health benefits of volunteering are stronger for those who were not asked to volunteer than for those who were asked to volunteer. There are several ways we could accomplish this objective. For example, we could regress psychological distress on the asked-volunteering typology shown in Table 6.1 to determine the effects of being in one category of that arrangement versus others. However, by using the dichotomous variables in the typology, we are unable to isolate the main effects of volunteering and being asked on psychological distress. Another approach, and the one we adopt here, is to create cross-product terms between being asked to volunteer and actually doing so. When regressing psychological distress on these terms, along with their component items, we can gauge both the main effects of volunteering and being asked to volunteer and how levels of one variable affect the relationships of the other. More specifically, we can determine the effects of volunteering among those who were asked and those who were not asked to volunteer and then make a contrast to determine whether the effects are significantly different. The analyses to explore the moderating effect of being asked on volunteering are shown in Table 6.2.

This table displays two panels of models. In the first model of panel 1, we regress psychological distress on any volunteering, being asked to volunteer, and other controls. According to the findings in this model, being asked to volunteer has no impact on distress; likewise, volunteering has a marginal effect on distress, albeit not in the direction we anticipated. According to the coefficient for volunteering ($b = .09$), having volunteered in the past year is associated with more psychological distress, though this effect is only marginally significant ($p < .10$). Turning to the controls in this model, we see results that are consistent with many other studies of mental health. For example, women report more distress; older adults report less distress; those with higher levels of education, income, and physical health all report less distress. Contrary to other studies (e.g., Ellison et al., 2001), our results indicate that religious services attendance

Table 6.2. Estimated Net Effects of Being Asked to Volunteer and Volunteering on Psychological Distress (OLS Regression Estimates)

	Panel 1		Panel 2	
	Model 1	Model 2	Model 1	Model 2
Volunteering Variables				
Asked to volunteer	.03	.29**	.04	.29**
Any volunteering	.09+	.16**	——	——
Volunteer in 1–2 areas	——	——	.11	.16*
Volunteer in 3–4 areas	——	——	.08	.22*
Volunteer in 5+ areas	——	——	.02	.07
Interaction Effects				
Asked × Any volunteering	——	−.34**	——	——
Asked × Volunteer 1–2	——	——	——	−.29*
Asked × Volunteer3–4	——	——	——	−.42**
Asked × Volunteer 5+	——	——	——	−.29+
Control Variables				
Female	.09*	.10*	.09*	.10*
Non-Hisanic Black	.07	.06	.07	.07
Hispanic	−.13**	−.13**	−.13**	−.13**
Age	−.01***	−.01***	−.01***	−.01***
Education	−.07***	−.06***	−.06**	−.06**
Family income	−.03*	−.03*	−.03*	−.02+
Physical health	−.19***	−.19***	−.19***	−.19***
Married	−.13**	−.13**	−.13**	−.14***
Religious services attendance	−.02	−.02	−.02	−.02
Intercept	3.32	3.28	3.31	3.28
Adjusted R^2	.14	.14	.14	.14

Note: $N = 1,496$. $+ p < .10$; $*p < .05$; $**p < .01$; $***p < .001$.

has no effect on distress. The results shown in this model for the control variables are consistent across all models in our study; therefore, we will not discuss them further.

The second model in the first panel is identical to the first model except that it adds a cross-product term between volunteering and being asked to volunteer. As shown in the table, the cross-product term is negative and significant ($b = −.34$, $p < .01$). In contrast to Model 1, the main effects for volunteering and being asked to volunteer are positive and significant in this model. To interpret these coefficients, one must first understand to what portions of the sample they apply. In the case of the main effects, the coefficients represent the effect of the variable in question among people who were coded 0 on the other variable in the cross-product term. For example, the coefficient of .16 for any volunteering indicates the effect size of that variable among people who were coded 0 on asked to volunteer, that is, those people who were not asked to volunteer. Likewise, the coefficient of .29 for asked to volunteer is the effect size of that variable for people who did not volunteer. The positive and significant nature of both of these variables indicates that either volunteering or being asked to volunteer in the *absence* of the other is associated with higher levels of psychological distress. To understand the effect of the cross-product term, one only has to add that coefficient to one of the main effect coefficients, depending on the contrast desired. For example, in this chapter, we are most concerned about the moderating effect of being asked on volunteering. We know the effect of volunteering among those not asked: It is .16, as shown in the table. To get the effect of volunteering among people who were asked, we add the cross-product term coefficient, which in this case is negative, so we subtract it. The resulting coefficient is –.18, indicating that the effect of volunteering among those who were asked is negative, that is, volunteering among those who were asked leads to lower levels of psychological distress. The significance of the cross-product term indicates that the effect of volunteering among those who were asked versus those who were not asked is significantly different.

In the second panel of Table 6.2, we display models similar to those in the first panel, but we substitute levels of volunteering for the any volunteering variable. We examine levels of volunteering because there is some evidence (e.g., Musick et al., 1999) to indicate that the amount or range of volunteering one does is an important part of understanding the health consequences of the activity in general. According to these models, we find effects very similar to those shown in the first panel. For example, in the first model, we find no effect of being asked to volunteer and only a modest effect of the lowest level of volunteering. As was the case for the original main effect of any volunteering, volunteering in one or two areas is associated with higher levels of psychological distress. Turning to the second model, we see more results that are consistent with the first panel. All three cross-product terms are significant, though the one for volunteering in five or more areas is only marginally so. All of the cross-product terms are negative, indicating that to get the effect of volunteering among those who were asked to volunteer, one must subtract the cross-product coefficients from the main effect ones for volunteering. This math yields effect sizes of –.13 for one or two areas, –.20 for three or four areas, and –.22 for five or more areas. The significance levels further indicate that the relationships between volunteering and distress are significantly different between respondents who were asked and those who were not. Finally, it should be noted that in both panels, there is virtually no change in the adjusted R^2 once the interactions are introduced. This lack of change indicates that the cross-product terms are not explaining new variances in distress; rather, they are simply reallocating what was already explained in the model.

We have made some effort in the text above to fully explain the meanings of the main effects and cross-product terms in the first set of models. To further elucidate the differences we observed in those models, we display a new set of models that regress psychological distress on volunteering. However, unlike the previous models, these new ones are sorted by being asked to volunteer, as shown in Table 6.3. According to the findings in the first panel, the effect of any volunteering among those who were not asked is positive and significant. In other words, among those who were not asked, volunteering is associated with more distress. In contrast, among those who were asked to volunteer, doing so was associated with less psychological distress. The same patterns emerge in the second panel, which contrasts the effects of the number of areas in which respondents volunteered. Among those not asked, volunteering in either one or two or in three or four areas was associated with more distress; however, among those who were asked, volunteering at all levels was associated with less distress, with more of the benefit accruing to the most involved volunteers. In short, these sorted models show results similar to those found in the models with cross-product terms. Moreover, in both cases, it is clear that our expectations were not supported. Recall that we expected that higher levels of volunteering would be associated with less distress and that this beneficial effect of volunteering would be strongest for respondents who had not been asked to volunteer. Our findings rebuffed these expectations in two ways. First, the main effects of volunteering either were not significant or behaved opposite to our expectations. Second, among those asked, volunteering was associated with less distress, but among those not asked, it was associated with more. Clearly, we found evidence that runs counter to our expected findings.

DISCUSSION

What might account for the disconnection between our findings and expectations? Several explanations are possible. First is the idea that we have not adequately measured the altruistic form of volunteering. We know that volunteers report a variety of reasons for engaging in that behavior. For example, some volunteers do so because they feel a strong need to help and be compassionate toward others. Other volunteers give reasons that are more focused on themselves, such as volunteering to help a career or because they had been helped in the past and wanted to repay the kindness. Given these various reasons, it is possible that altruistic volunteering is really volunteering done for certain reasons and is not based on being self-initiated, as we have speculated here. To adequately test the idea that altruistic volunteering, based on the motivations for volunteering, is beneficial for health, researchers would need measures of volunteering and reasons for the volunteering and health outcomes. As it happens, the Survey of Texas Adults contains some measures of volunteer motiva-

Table 6.3. Estimated Net Effects of Volunteering on Psychological
Distress by Being Asked to Volunteer (OLS Regression Estimates)

	Panel 1 (N = 676)		Panel 2 (N = 820)	
	Not Asked	Asked	Not Asked	Asked
Volunteering Variables				
Any volunteering	.17*	–.20*	——	——
Volunteer in 1–2 areas	——	——	.17*	–.16+
Volunteer in 3–4 areas	——	——	.25*	–.24**
Volunteer in 5+ areas	——	——	.03	–.25**
Control Variables				
Female	.09	.10*	.11	.10*
Non-Hispanic Black	.11	–.00	.11	.00
Hispanic	–.20 *	–.02	–.18*	–.02
Age	–.01***	–.01***	–.0***	–.01***
Education	–.07+	–.06**	–.06+	–.05*
Family income	–.04*	–.01	–.04+	–.01
Physical health	–.19***	–.18***	–.19***	–.18***
Married	–.10	–.15**	–.10	–.16**
Religious services attendance	–.02	–.01	–.04	–.01
Intercept	3.36	3.51	3.36	3.51
Adjusted R²	.12	.18	.12	.18

Note: + $p < .10$; *$p < .05$; **$p < .01$; ***$p < .001$.

tion, though they are very limited and are only representative of people who
had volunteered in the past year.

   To test the idea that volunteering motivated for more altruistic reasons is
beneficial for mental well-being, we chose to focus on two measures from the
SoTA. Each asked all volunteers how important each of the following reasons
was in their decision to volunteer: (a) "I feel compassion towards people in need";
and (b) "It's part of my religious belief or philosophy of life to give help." Because each of these reasons for volunteering is focused on helping others or on
a general philosophy of helping others, we feel they tap the ideals we envision
in altruistic volunteering. Based on each of these measures, we split the sample
into two groups: those who said a reason was "very important" in their decision
to volunteer versus all others. Because only volunteers were asked the questions,
we could not assess differences between volunteers and nonvolunteers in this
context. Instead, we regressed distress on volunteering in three or four areas and
in five or more areas, making the reference category those who volunteered in
only one or two areas. Net of other controls, we found that among people who
endorsed these reasons as very important, volunteers who volunteered in five

or more areas had significantly lower levels of psychological distress than volunteers who volunteered in only one or two areas (compassion indicator: $b = -.14$, $p < .05$; philosophy indicator: $b = -.12$, $p < .10$); there were no significant differences for the three or four areas group. In contrast, volunteering had no effect on distress for respondents who did not say that either of the reasons was very important. Finally, we created a new variable from these two measures, indicating whether respondents answered "very important" for *both* reasons. We again split the sample according to this variable and regressed distress on the two measures of volunteering. We found that among respondents in the altruistic category, volunteering in both three or four ($b = -.13$, $p < .10$) and five or more ($b = -.15$, $p < .10$) areas was associated with lower levels of distress compared to those volunteering in only one or two areas. For the other group, volunteering had no effect on depression. In sum, if we assume that altruistic volunteering can be defined in terms of motivation, then we do find evidence that volunteering in altruistic ways is more beneficial for mental health than volunteering in other ways. However, given the very limited nature of these measures and the way in which they were collected (only of volunteers), this analysis should be replicated with other data containing more extensive measurement.

A second possible explanation for our unexpected findings involves the dynamics of being asked to volunteer. The moment one is asked to volunteer, both the inviter and the invitee enter an exchange relationship. We have previously defined the person being asked in this exchange as being under an obligation to act given the extension of the offer. If the offer is refused, not only is the exchange imbalanced, but the person who refuses the offer may suffer some guilt given normative expectations of a willingness to help others. It is clear from our study that once people are asked to volunteer, they are very unlikely to not volunteer: In our data, only 5% of respondents fell into this category. However, it may be unwarranted to say that someone who volunteers out of the obligation entailed from the exchange should not still benefit from that exchange. Volunteers clearly benefit in very concrete ways, as Wilson (2000) has outlined in a recent review of the volunteering literature. In this article, he specifically addresses the psychological benefits of the activity when he writes, "A volunteer might feel good about doing the right thing, but she does not do it because it makes her feel good; rather it makes her feel good because she thinks she ought to have done it" (Wilson, 2000, p. 222). As Wilson states, part of the psychological benefit can derive from the act itself, but part can also depend on the normative expectations of voluntary action. If the expectation to volunteer exists in the form of personal philosophies or motivations, it can lead to psychological benefits, as we showed above. However, if the expectation is also derived from social forces, in this case being asked to volunteer, then performing the act should yield even more benefits given that it is done under the social expectation that it ought to be done.

In other words, when we think about the relationship between altruistic volunteering and mental health, we must keep in mind the fact that when people volunteer, they are usually observed in the activity, often by the person or organization doing the asking. By fulfilling these social expectations, volunteers who were invited are gaining those psychological benefits by living up to others' expectations. Additionally, they gain the benefit from knowing that, at a moral or philosophical level, the volunteering act is something that ought to be done. If this second explanation is closer to the truth, then we must revise our original thinking about altruistic volunteering. It should be the case that volunteering for the "right" reasons should lead to better mental health outcomes, and when this altruistic form of volunteering is coupled with a fulfillment of social expectations, it should be even more beneficial for mental health. Given our limited data, this idea would be a difficult one to test in a rigorous way. As such, we leave it to future investigators to determine whether this idea is worthwhile.

As previously noted, research on the relationship between volunteering and multiple forms of health has accumulated at a quick pace over the past few years. Investigators are still mostly focusing on the main effects of volunteering on mental and physical health outcomes. Although this basic research is important, investigators must also begin to spend more time looking at the subtleties of the relationship between volunteering and health. It is clear that volunteering comes in many forms, through different avenues, and for different reasons. It is possible that all volunteering, regardless of how and why it is done, has similar effects on health, but it is unlikely. Therefore, researchers must pay more heed to the vagaries of the process when examining this relationship. Our study is a small step in that direction.

The data used in this chapter were made available (in part) by the Population Research Center at the University of Texas at Austin and by funding provided by the RGK Center for Philanthropy and Community Service and the College of Liberal Arts at the University of Texas at Austin. These entities bear no responsibility for the analyses and interpretations presented here.

REFERENCES

American Association for Public Opinion Research. 2004. *Standard Definitions: Final Dispositions of Case Codes and Outcome Rates for Surveys.* 3rd ed. Lenexa, KS: AAPOR.

Dunkel-Schetter, C., Blasband, D. E., Feinstein, L. G., & Herbert, T. B. (1992). Elements of supportive interactions: When are attempts to help effective? In S. Spacapan & S. Oskamp (Eds.), *Helping and being helped* (pp. 83–114). Newbury Park, CA: Sage.

Ellison, C. G., Boardman, J. D., Williams, D. R., & Jackson, J. S. (2001). Religious involvement, stress, and mental health: Findings from the 1995 Detroit Area Study. *Social Forces, 80,* 215–249.

Greenfield, E. A., & Marks, N. F. (2004). Formal volunteering as a protective factor for older adults' psychological well-being. *Journal of Gerontology: Social Sciences, 59B*(5), S258–S264.

Jirovec, R. L., & Hyduk, C. A. (1998). Type of volunteer experience and health among older adult volunteers. *Journal of Gerontological Social Work, 30*(3–4), 29–42.

Krause, N., Herzog, A. R., & Baker, E. (1992). Providing support to others and well-being in later life. *Journal of Gerontology: Psychological Sciences, 47*(5), 300–311.

Midlarsky, E., & Kahana, E. (1994). *Altruism in later life.* Thousand Oaks, CA: Sage.

Morrow-Howell, N., Hinterlong, J., Rozario, P. A., & Tang, F. (2003). Effects of volunteering on the well-being of older adults. *Journal of Gerontology: Social Sciences, 58B*(3), S137–S145.

Musick, M. A. (2004). *Survey of Texas adults* [computer file]. Austin: University of Texas.

Musick, M. A., Herzog, A. R., & House, J. S. (1999). Volunteering and mortality among older adults: Findings from a national sample. *Journals of Gerontology: Psychological Sciences and Social Sciences, 54B*(3), S173–S180.

Musick, M. A., & Wilson, J. (2003). Volunteering and depression: The role of psychological and social resources in different age groups. *Social Science & Medicine, 56*(2), 259–269.

Musick, M. A., Wilson, J., & Bynum, W. B. (2000). Race and formal volunteering: The differential effects of class and religion. *Social Forces, 78*(4), 1539–1571.

Oman, D., Thoresen, C. E., & McMahon, K. (1999). Volunteerism and mortality among the community-dwelling elderly. *Journal of Health Psychology, 4*(3), 301–316.

Pushkar, D., Reis, M., & Morros, M. (2002). Motivation, personality and well-being in older volunteers. *International Journal of Aging and Human Development, 55*(2), 141–162.

Shmotkin, D., Blumstein T., & Modan, B. (2003). Beyond keeping active: Concomitants of being a volunteer in old-old age. *Psychology and Aging, 18*(3), 602–607.

Smith, D. H. (1982). Altruism, volunteers, and volunteerism. In J. D. Harman (Ed.), *Volunteerism in the eighties* (pp. 23–44). Lanham, MD: University Press of America.

Thoits, P. A., & Hewitt, L. N. (2001). Volunteer work and well-being. *Journal of Health and Social Behavior, 42*(2), 115–131.

Van Willigen, M. (2000). Differential benefits of volunteering across the life course. *Journals of Gerontology: Psychological Sciences and Social Sciences, 55B*(5), S308–S318.

Varese, F., & Yaish, M. (2000). The importance of being asked: The rescue of Jews in Nazi Europe. *Rationality and Society, 12*(3), 307–334.

Wheeler, J. A., Gorey, K. M., & Greenblatt, B. (1998). The beneficial effects of volunteering for older volunteers and the people they serve: A meta-analysis. *International Journal of Aging & Human Development, 47*(1), 69–79.

Wilson, J. (2000). Volunteering. *Annual Review of Sociology, 26*, 215–40.

7 Altruism and Health: Is There a Link During Adolescence?

Peter L. Benson
E. Gil Clary
Peter C. Scales

The links between prosocial action and health in adolescence have not been a central area of inquiry in the social sciences. Nevertheless, there is a growing body of literature that provides some hint about this intersection. This is partly due to the relatively recent national interest in volunteerism and the forms of it mandated or encouraged by school districts. These forms of service often travel under the banners of service learning and community service (Billig, 2004; Clary & Roehlkepartain, in press; Scales, & Benson, 2005; Scales & Roehlkepartain, 2004). And a voluminous body of research has documented the relationship of these programs to various indicators of adolescent well-being. Complementing this wave of research is an assortment of studies looking at other forms of adolescent engagement in actions variously labeled as prosocial behavior, generosity, or altruism. In exploring the linkages between these behaviors and health, this chapter (1) defines adolescent health, (2) synthesizes the published literature, (3) explores a large data set on 6th- to 12th-grade students to address additional empirical issues, and (4) recommends new lines of inquiry needed to advance knowledge about the altruism and health relationship.

DEFINING AND MEASURING ADOLESCENT HEALTH

The definition of health during adolescence tends to fall into three major categories. The first covers traditional domains of physical health, including nutrition, body weight, and exercise. The second looks at a range of health-compromising or risk behaviors. These behaviors are assumed to either compromise health status or place a person at risk for significant health issues. These behaviors include alcohol use, tobacco use, drug use, unsafe sexual activity, and violence. This constellation of risk behaviors has dominated studies of adolescence since the 1960s, and their prevention and treatment have been at the forefront of public policy funding and programming (Benson, 1997; Benson, Scales, Hamilton, & Sesma, 2006). A third line of inquiry has recently emerged and represents, in somewhat broader ways, another approach to adolescent health. This work yields such concepts as well-being and thriving with the intent of capturing behaviors which promote individual and/or societal good. Included in this domain are such concepts as academic success, connectedness, resilience, and civic engagement (Lerner, 2004; Scales, Benson, & Roehlkepartain, in press). Though these kinds of thriving concepts appear to be more in the realm of social-emotional health, there are strong theoretical reasons to posit that they constitute significant health promotion strategies (Benson, 1997).

A number of scholars argue that the definition of developmental success most deeply entrenched in public policy and practice conceives of health as the absence of disease or pathology. In recent decades, the dominant framework driving federal, state, and local interventions with youth has been that of risk behaviors, including alcohol use, tobacco use, other drug use, nonmarital pregnancy, suicide, antisocial behavior, violence, and school dropout (Benson, 1997; Eccles & Gootman, 2002; Hein, 2003; Takanishi, 1993). While positive youth development advocates readily accept that reductions in these health-compromising behaviors are important markers of developmental success, there is simultaneously a growing interest in defining the other side of the coin—that is, the attributes, skills, competencies, and potentials needed to succeed in the spheres of work, family, and civic life. This dichotomy is well captured in the youth development mantra "problem free is not fully prepared" (Pittman & Fleming, 1991). Accordingly, an important aspect of current positive youth development science is the conceptualization and measurement of dimensions of positive developmental success. Among these areas of work are efforts to define indicators of child well-being (K. A. Moore, 1997; K. A. Moore, Lippman, & Brown, 2004), thriving (Benson, 2003; Lerner, 2004; Scales & Benson, 2005; Theokas et al., 2005), and flourishing (Keyes, 2003). Within this inquiry on positive markers of success, an emerging issue has to do with expanding the conceptualization of developmental success to include not only what promotes individual well-being but also what promotes the social good (Benson & Leffert, 2001; Benson, Mannes, Pittman, & Ferber, 2004; Damon, 1997; Lerner, 2004).

The literature reviewed in this chapter explores the relationship of altruism to the prevention of risk behaviors. We argue that the enhancement of thriving success in these broader domains of health could well translate into lower rates of morbidity and mortality by either lowering risk or increasing relationships, supports, and opportunities known to promote physical health. And there is some theoretical reasoning that altruism can, by virtue of being one avenue by which persons exert control and influence, directly provide immunological protection against mortality and morbidity (Piliavin, 2003; Rodin & Langer, 1977).

THE RELATIONSHIP OF PROSOCIAL ORIENTATION TO RISK AND THRIVING MEASURES

As a first look at the relation of altruism and health in adolescents, we consider operationalizations of altruism that focus on internal states that reflect prosocial orientation and cross-sectional, correlational studies of American youth that examine the link between these forms of altruism and measures of developmental success. Scales, Benson, and Roehlkepartain (in press), based on a recent review of the literature, noted that prosocial values, attitudes, and behaviors have generally been found to be related to numerous indicators of well-being, including friendship-making ability (Vernberg, Ewell, Beery, & Abwender, 1994), perceived self-competence (Cauce, 1986), decreased loneliness (Inderbitzen-Pisaruk, Clark, & Solano, 1992), higher levels of helpfulness, sharing, and cooperation (Litvack-Miller, McDougall, & Romney, 1997), and lower levels of aggression and behavior problems (Hastings, Zahn-Walker, Robinson, Usher, & Bridges, 2000). With only a few exceptions (e.g., Rodkin, Farmer, Pearl, & Van Acker, 2000), the literature consistently shows that children with behavior problems tend to be more socially isolated and that children with prosocial orientations involving generosity, empathy, and being helpful are more popular, well adjusted, and connected (Rydell, Hagekull, & Bohlin, 1997).

Wentzel (1993) utilized peer ratings to assess both prosocial and antisocial behavior patterns among middle-school students and related these to academic performance. These peer ratings were thoroughly associated with both grade point average (GPA) and the Stanford Test of Basic Skills: Prosocial ratings were positively connected to both, and antisocial ratings were negatively correlated. Particularly important was the finding that prosocial orientation was a significant, independent predictor of both measures after controlling for gender, family structure, intelligence, and ethnicity.

Scales, Benson, and Roehlkepartain (in press) utilized similar multivariate analytical procedures to isolate the contribution of a prosocial orientation to multiple forms of risk behavior and thriving. A sample of 5,136 6th- to 12th-grade students in Colorado was assessed on a seven-item scale composed of four items measuring attitudes and values about helping others and three that tap behavioral intentions to help others. Zero-order correlations showed that prosocial orientation was positively linked to multiple forms of thriving (e.g., ability to overcome adversity, active engagement in promoting one's physical health, school success) and negatively to multiple forms of risk behavior (e.g., alcohol use, tobacco use, illicit drug use, violence, gambling, and antisocial behavior). To further clarify the predictive validity of the prosocial orientation construct, it was included in a stepwise regression analysis. Overall, prosocial orientation added a meaningful proportion of explained variance over and above demographic variables (e.g., grade, race/ethnicity, parental education levels). Among both genders, prosocial orientation helped to explain a positive orientation to school success, connectedness to school, valuing diversity, and active coping. Among girls, prosocial orientation explained 18% of the variance in sexual behavior risk. Among boys, it explained 14% of the variance in school problems.

THE RELATIONSHIP OF COMMUNITY SERVICE ACTIVITIES AND HEALTH

The work considered in the previous section was primarily concerned with measures of prosocial orientation, by which we mean the extent to which the adolescent possesses internal psychological states like attitudes, values, and emotional reactions (e.g., empathy) that value other people and especially others in need. This research points to a connection of altruism and indicators of well-being and risk tendencies. In this section, we examine studies that have operationalized altruism by involvement in prosocial activities and then correlated participation in these activities with health-related behaviors and outcomes in large samples (N's > 1,000) of adolescents.

Before turning to this work, we should first note that research on prosocial behavior includes a broad range of activities, from interventions into spontaneously arising emergencies to planned involvement in volunteer work. It is this latter type of prosocial activity that is often the focus in studies on the consequences—for the helper—of behaving prosocially, including the consequences for the helper's health. For several reasons, the planned helpfulness of volunteering seems to be most promising as a contributor to health-related outcomes. Among other features, volunteer activity often involves the helper (1) seeking out the opportunity to help, (2) deliberating about how and where to help, (3) helping regularly over a period of time, and (4) helping without remuneration (Clary & Snyder, 1999). In other words, volunteering contains features that are similar to such health practices as diet and exercise, including its deliberate and voluntary nature and the fact that the practice must often occur over time.

Volunteer work, as the name implies, is often voluntary; of course, not all volunteer work is voluntary, as when college students are required to participate in community service (see Stukas, Clary, & Snyder, 1999) or when offenders are ordered by the courts to engage in community service (Allen & Treger, 1990). Similarly, adolescents are faced with similar options, as volunteer work may be chosen as an extracurricular activity or may be a requirement for graduation (as in the case of the state of Maryland; National Youth Leadership Council, 2004) or to pass a course. In recent years, some research on volunteering among adolescents has explored this latter option, as many schools now offer service-learning courses where some kind of volunteer or community service is included as a significant component (see Raskoff & Sundeen, 2000).

Prosocial Activities Broadly Defined

Several studies have explored relations between involvement in prosocial activities and health-related behaviors and outcomes using diverse measures of each of the key constructs. In Eccles and Barber's (1999) investigation, the measure of prosocial activity was participation in volunteer work and/or church attendance, and the researchers studied the associations of these and four other categories of socially valued extracurricular activities with present and future risk behaviors. Analyses found that students indicating involvement in one of these prosocial activities in the 10th grade, versus those who did not, reported lower levels of alcohol and drug use concurrently and in a 2-year follow-up. Generally speaking, involvement in other types of extracurricular activities did not have these relations with risk behaviors, and those students involved in sports reported greater levels of alcohol use at the follow-up.

A somewhat similar finding with respect to the protective effects of prosocial activities was obtained by Jessor, Turbin, and Costa (1998). In this investigation, the measure of prosocial behavior was involvement in volunteer work, family activities, and school clubs other than sports, and this measure was conceptualized as one of several "conventionality-related (distal) protective factors" (p. 791). This analysis, which sought to predict health-enhancing behavior, found that, first, the set of conventionality-related factors contributed to the model beyond the contributions of the more proximal risk (e.g., parents smoking) and protective (e.g., parents modeling healthy behaviors) factors, and second, that prosocial activities, along with several other conventional behavior measures, was significantly related to the criterion. The key interpretation here, according to the authors, is that while factors that directly impact health-related behaviors have a stronger effect, activities like prosocial involvement—activities that do not have a direct impact on health-related behavior—also play an important role in health.

Prosocial Activities Defined as Volunteering

While the investigations by Eccles and Barber and Jessor et al. (1998) defined prosocial activities more broadly than volunteer work, other studies have assessed the associations of involvement in volunteer work and health-related behaviors and outcomes. Murphey, Lamonda, Carney, and Duncan (2004) examined the relations of volunteering, along with five other developmental assets (e.g., participation in other nonsports extracurricular activities, communication between students and their parents about school) and several risk behaviors (e.g., use of alcohol, cigarettes, and marijuana and physical fighting), and health-promoting behaviors (e.g., seat belt use, regular exercise) for almost 31,000 Vermont adolescents. While, overall, the total number of assets was negatively related to the risk behaviors and positively related to health-promoting behaviors, volunteer work was the single most important asset for exercise and was nonsignificantly related to risk behaviors concerning alcohol use, sexual activity, and contemplating suicide. In a longitudinal study, Uggen and Jenikula (1999) found that during the last 2 years of high school volunteers, relative to nonvolunteers, were less likely to report having been arrested in the young adult years. Finally, using the first waves of the same data set of Uggen and Jenikula (i.e., when students were still in high school), Johnson, Beebe, Mortimer, and Snyder (1998) found that after controlling for several bases of selection into volunteering, volunteer work was positively related to several outcomes (e.g., work-related values) but was unrelated to outcomes associated with health (well-being, depressive affect).

Prosocial Activities: Search Institute Data Set

As a final look at correlational approaches to the relation of prosocial activities to health-related behaviors and outcomes, we turn to analyses of a large aggregate data set collected through the work of Search Institute. Specifically, in the 1999–2000 academic year, a sample of more than 200,000 6th- through 12th-grade students in 318 communities throughout the United States responded to a 156-item survey. This instrument asked young people about their experiences in their homes, schools, neighborhoods, and communities; their relationships with others; their extracurricular activities; their characteristics; and backgrounds. Among the activities students were asked about were the number of hours of volunteer work they perform in an average week (0, 1, 2, 3–5, 6–10, 11 or more). The survey instrument has been primarily used to assess developmental assets as these have been conceptualized by Benson and his colleagues (Benson, 1997; Benson & Leffert, 2001; Benson, Leffert, Scales, & Blyth, 1998).

The survey also included items concerning well-being and risk behaviors. The measure of well-being included eight positive attitudes and behaviors that society regards as desired outcomes of socialization. These markers of developmental success or, more simply, indicators of thriving are school success (gets mostly A's), helping friends or neighbors, valuing diversity (places high importance on getting to know people of other ethnic groups), maintaining good health (good nutrition and exercise), exhibiting leadership (has served as a leader in an organization in the past year), resisting danger, delaying gratification (saves money for something special rather than spending it immediately), and overcoming adversity (does not give up when things get difficult). The measure of risk consists of 10 patterns of high-risk behaviors. The risk behaviors are alcohol problems (used alcohol three or more times in the past month or got drunk once or more in the past 2 weeks), tobacco use (smokes one or more cigarettes every day or frequently uses chewing tobacco), illicit drug use (three or more times in the past year), sexual intercourse (three or more times in lifetime), depression and suicide (frequently depressed and/or suicide attempt), antisocial behavior (three or more incidents of shoplifting, trouble with police, or vandalism in the past year), violence (three or more acts of fighting, hitting, injuring another, carrying/using a weapon, or threatening harm in the past year), school problems (skipped school two or more times in the past month and/or has below a C average), drinking and driving (self or ridden with another three or more times in the past year), and gambling (three or more times in the past year). These risk and thriving measures are discussed in more detail in Scales et al. (1998) and Leffert et al. (1998).

With this large aggregate data set, we have very simply calculated the zero-order correlations between involvement in volunteer work and each of these indicators of thriving and risk behaviors for the sample as a whole and for gender, ethnic groups, and a sampling of ages (early, mid-, and late adolescence); the correlations for thriving are presented in Table 7.1 and those for risk behaviors are in Table 7.2. Review of these correlations immediately reveals that (1) almost all of the associations for this very large sample are statistically significant; (2) the associations between volunteering and the thriving measures are positive and between volunteering and the risk behaviors are negative; (3) the correlations are modest at best (the exception involves the correlation of the more formal volunteer helping and the more informal helping of friends and neighbors); (4) the pattern observed for the sample as a whole tends to be replicated across the various groupings; and (5) volunteering tends to be more strongly associated with the indicators of thriving than with high-risk behaviors.

The correlations presented here provide perhaps the most basic look at the relation of prosocial behavior and health-related behaviors and outcomes, and do so with a large diverse sample (diverse in terms of communities, demographic variables, and indices related to health). And with this diversity, we see a persistent tendency for involvement in the prosocial activity of volunteering to be related, albeit modestly, to health indicators. At the same time, these relations are, at best, described as modest, and some attention to the failure to find strong relations is needed. While later sections of this chapter will explore other factors that may moderate or mediate the relation of prosocial behavior and health, we should at this point consider the role of the measure of prosocial behavior that this and other studies often employ. To be specific, the measure of volunteer activity may only provide a rough or approximate measure of actual volunteer

Table 7.1. Relations of Volunteering and Measures of Thriving for Demographic Groupings

Thriving Measures	Total	Gender		Ethnicity						Age		
	Sample	Female	Male	AmIn	Asian	AfAm	Hisp	Cau	Multi	13yrs	15yrs	17yrs
Danger resistance	.05	.04	.03	.07	.03	.03	.04	.05	.06	.04	.04	.05
Affirming diversity	.16	.14	.16	.15	.13	.14	.14	.17	.16	.17	.15	.15
Physical health	.14	.14	.15	.16	.12	.13	.14	.14	.13	.15	.13	.11
Impulse control	.10	.11	.11	.12	.08	.11	.11	.10	.12	.10	.10	.08
Informal helping	.40	.37	.42	.46	.42	.43	.38	.40	.42	.42	.40	.34
Leadership	.20	.20	.20	.15	.21	.20	.19	.20	.20	.19	.21	.22
Resiliency	.02	.05	.01	-.00*	.04	-.01	-.01	.04	.05	.02	.02	.05
School success	.04	.02	.04	.10	.06	.06	.08	.04	.04	.02	.05	.07

Notes: *The correlation did not exceed conventional levels of statistical significance.
AmIn = American Indian, AfAm = African American, Hisp = Hispanic, Cau = Caucasian, Multi = Multiracial.

Table 7.2. Relations of Volunteering and Measures of Risk Behaviors for Demographic Groupings

Risk Measures	Total	Gender		Ethnicity						Age		
	Sample	Female	Male	AmIn	Asian	AfAm	Hisp	Cau	Multi	13yrs	15yrs	17yrs
Alcohol	-.05	-.05	-.04	-.10	-.06	-.01	-.04	-.06	-.05	-.03	-.04	-.06
Antisocial behavior	-.05	-.04	-.03	-.06	-.06	.01*	-.02	-.06	-.06	-.03	-.04	-.06
Drinking-driving	-.04	-.04	-.03	-.05	-.03	-.01	-.03	-.05	-.03	.01*	-.03	-.08
Depression/suicide	-.03	.00	-.02	-.02*	.04	.07	.02	-.02	.02*	.04	.04	.02
Illicit drugs	-.07	-.06	-.06	-.07	-.05	-.04	-.06	-.07	-.09	-.03	-.06	-.09
Gambling	-.03	.01	-.02	-.05	-.02*	-.03	.00*	-.03	.00	-.01*	-.04	-.03
School problems	-.05	-.04	-.05	-.08	-.06	-.04	-.08	-.06	-.06	-.03	-.04	-.08
Sexual intercourse	-.03	-.04	-.01	-.07	-.01*	-.04	-.02	-.04	-.04	.01*	.00*	-.03
Tobacco use	-.03	-.05	-.04	-.05	-.05	-.03	-.04	-.06	-.05	-.02	-.04	-.08
Violence	-.06	-.05	-.05	-.06	-.03	-.03	-.02	-.03	-.01*	-.01*	-.01*	-.04

Notes: *The correlation did not exceed conventional levels of statistical significance.
AmIn = American Indian, AfAm = African American, Hisp = Hispanic, Cau = Caucasian, Multi = Multiracial.

work. In the context of a lengthy survey, a respondent is asked to first recall volunteer work with the prompt "helping other people without getting paid (such as helping out at a hospital, day care center, food bank, youth program, or community service agency, or doing other things) to make your city a better place for people to live" and then is asked to calculate the number of hours volunteered in an average week. Among other concerns, it may be that some activities may not come to mind as readily (e.g., volunteering that is episodic and not routine); that some volunteering is not voluntary; somewhat similar, that some volunteering may more clearly impact another person and thus is "more prosocial" than other activities; or that the benefits of helping vary with the way in which the help is given (e.g., alone versus with others). In other words, the measure of volunteering could be more precise, which then raises the question of whether the relation with health would vary if other aspects of the prosocial activity were taken into consideration.

Taking this and the correlational studies, which use large community samples of adolescents, as a whole, one often finds that involvement in prosocial activities is related to health-related behaviors and outcomes. At the same time, the findings are not always consistent with respect to specific health outcomes, in large part because different studies focus on different outcomes. Moreover, studies are also not consistent in their measures of prosocial activities, as some studies have focused exactly on volunteer work and others have combined participation in volunteer work with involvement in other activities; and those that focused on volunteering often used a single and in some cases dichotomous measure. Finally, it almost goes without saying that observed correlations of prosocial involvement and health outcomes may be due to other factors, although many of the studies discussed above did control for other possible influences and still found that prosocial activities contributed, if not directly, in some way to important health outcomes.

INTERVENTION STUDIES INVOLVING COMMUNITY SERVICE AND HEALTH

Many of the concerns that arise with the correlational studies reviewed thus far can be addressed with investigations that provide some students with a volunteering experience and compare them to those who do not have this experience, especially when students are randomly assigned to conditions. Allen and his colleagues (Allen & Philliber, 2001; Allen, Philliber, Herrling, & Kuperminc, 1997) have examined the impact of the community service program Teen Outreach on teen pregnancy and school problems, with assignment to the program or the control group being done randomly sometimes at the individual level, at others at the classroom level, and in Allen and Philliber (2001), the comparison group also included students who were nominated by program students or school staff. High school students participating in the Teen Outreach program perform at least 20 hours of supervised volunteer work, participate in classroom discussions about this experience, and engage in classroom activities related to the developmental tasks facing these adolescents. The key finding here is that students participating in the program were at less risk for teen pregnancy (and school problems), relative to the comparison group and after controlling for other relevant predictors.

An effect of involvement in a community service program was also obtained in an investigation by O'Donnell et al. (1999), in this case for violence. Specifically, classrooms of 7th- and 8th-grade students in the school where the intervention was developed were randomly assigned to a health instructional program or the same program combined with a weekly community service experience; a similar school was selected as the comparison group. Analyses found that while there were no program effects for the sample as a whole, 8th-grade students in the combined health and community service program reported less violence at the 6-month follow-up than the other two groups, after controlling for entry-level violence and biographical variables.

Somewhat similar effects were reported by Switzer, Simmons, Dew, Regalski, and Wang (1995), although in this case the health-related outcomes were depressive affect and problem behaviors in school. Here, 7th-grade students in a junior high school were assigned to classrooms in one of two subgroups, and students in one subgroup participated in some kind of helping activity during the academic year (some students engaged in a formal program that also included weekly discussion groups, while others participated in service work with community organizations), and those in the other served as the comparison group. While there was not an overall effect of the service program, boys in the service group did show improvement on depressive affect and problem behaviors, relative to boys in the comparison group and girls in either group.

EXPLAINING THE RELATIONSHIPS

The studies reviewed here, which included both correlational studies with relatively large community samples and intervention studies that compared a treatment group to a comparison group, suggest that involvement in prosocial activities plays a role in health-related behaviors and outcomes. It should be noted that at this point there is not clear evidence of a pure effect of prosocial action, as the measures used in several studies combined the sustained helpfulness of volunteering with other somewhat similar experiences, and the intervention studies generally packaged volunteer service with other experiences. Moreover, it should also be noted that studies often examined different types of health-related consequences, although the diversity of consequences does suggest that the impact of prosocial involvements may be a general one.

With these indications that participation in prosocial activities contributes to health-related outcomes, important questions about the mechanisms that may be responsible for this relation need to be considered. To begin with one broad perspective, the Carnegie Corporation of New York, in its 1992 report *A Matter of Time*, posited three potential benefits of constructive time use by adolescents, of which service and volunteering are one example. First, such engagement diverts time away from opportunities to engage in risk behaviors. Second, it can provide access to role models, supportive relationships, and social networks instrumental for health promotion. Finally, such engagement potentially nurtures social competencies and skills germane to health and well-being. It is to some of the more precise mechanisms that we now turn.

In the intervention studies, we noted that these investigations combined a community service experience with classroom-based activities where, presumably, students had the opportunity to discuss these experiences. This experience of explicitly considering the service in terms of educational objectives, commonly referred to as *reflection*, is regarded as a critical feature of good service-learning programs and appears to be necessary for a service experience to have an impact (Eyler, 2002). In other words, it appears that engaging in a prosocial activity in the absence of an opportunity where the young person can consider the meaning of the experience for him- or herself and the larger implications of the experience is less likely to produce the desired effects.

Much of the thinking about the impact of reflection with prosocial action has focused on the cognitive changes that take place, as young people who engage in this action-reflection experience develop new understandings of social problems, improve in their ability to analyze these matters in more abstract and complex ways, and enhance their ability to develop action-based solutions to problems (Eyler, 2002). Other investigations suggest that action-reflection experiences provide additional qualities for adolescents, especially surrounding identity development. More specifically, Youniss and Yates (1997, 1999) argue that students develop a moral identity through this experience (in their case, students worked in a soup kitchen as part of a social justice course), developing compassion and respect for the less fortunate and a sense of agency as a moral actor who has a responsibility to work for a better society. We should also note that the Eccles and Barber (1999) study discussed earlier also found support for the contributions of identity, although their conception of identity differed somewhat from that of Youniss and Yates (i.e., those engaging in prosocial activities had identities related to being an excellent student, tended to have peers who were similar, and tended to not engage in risky behaviors).

With the connection of prosocial action and identity and especially with the possibility that involvement in community service may promote certain specific features of identity, one might then begin to explore other aspects of personality that may be relevant here. One good candidate for inclusion is the trait of *conscientiousness*, defined generally as being careful, dutiful, and guided by one's conscience (see McCrae & Costa, 1987), which is one personality factor that research has tied to health outcomes (e.g., Friedman, Tucker, Schwartz, Tomlinson-Keasey, Martin, Wingard, & Criqui, 1995). In a recent meta-analysis, Boggs and Roberts (2004) found that, first, overall conscientiousness and health-related behaviors were correlated, and second, that several of the six facets of conscientiousness were more strongly related to health behaviors (in particular, responsibility, self-control, and traditionalism) than the others. Finally, we should note that Boggs and Roberts suggested that the traditionalism facet of conscientiousness appeared to be linked to the work of Jessor and his colleagues (1998) on conventionality, which we discussed earlier. Prosocial activities, as well as health practices, are all supported by social institutions, and certainly one important goal of socialization is that adolescents internalize norms of conventionality.

INTERCONNECTIONS

As we discussed in the previous section, a number of mechanisms may be at work in creating a connection between involvement in prosocial behavior and health-related behaviors and outcomes. In our discussion of these factors and processes, we have tried to emphasize the possibility that there may be important interconnections among the individual factors, which may be especially important as research explores the link between prosocial activities and health behavior for adolescents. In fact, interconnections of this sort are at the center of the work of Search Institute on developmental assets.

In the Search Institute framework, there are 40 environmental and psychological strengths that may be available to young people, which have been empirically connected to risk behaviors (negatively) and to indicators of thriving (positively) (Benson, Leffert, Scales, & Blyth, 1998; Leffert, Benson, Scales, Sharma, Drake, & Blyth, 1998; Scales, Benson, Leffert, & Blyth, 2000). These strengths consist of a mixture of external assets (e.g., positive relationships with parents, neighbors, and schools and constructive use of time) and internal assets (e.g., compassion, self-control, achievement motivation, and interpersonal competence). As suggested by these examples, involvement in prosocial activities is likely to enhance the development of one or more external assets in the life of a young person, and the mechanisms of identity, conscientiousness, and conventionality discussed earlier are viewed within this framework as internal assets.

In analyses of the responses of more than 200,000 adolescents from more than 300 communities to the Search Institute measure of the 40 developmental assets, relatively modest correlations have been obtained between reports of involvement in volunteer work and thriving indicators and a smaller but statistically significant negative relation has been obtained with a measure of risk behaviors. In a longitudinal study of almost 400 adolescents in one community, stronger associations were observed when several extracurricular activities were combined into an index of total civic involvement (in addition to volunteering, these include religious involvement, sports teams, school clubs, and nonschool nonsports clubs). This pattern, we should note, is similar to the Murphey et al. (2004) investigation where stronger relations were obtained when health outcomes were correlated with six assets than when each asset was examined individually.

The conceptual approach adopted by Search Institute, along with other current approaches to adolescent development (e.g., Lerner), and the findings that have examined these approaches raise several points. First, to begin with the more obvious observation, stronger effects are often obtained when combining separate influences than when looking at those influences individually; this, of course, can occur for both measurement and conceptual reasons. Second, from a more conceptual perspective, it is important to consider interconnections among features that are similar in nature. In the Search Institute framework of developmental assets, for example, external assets include involvement in traditional prosocial activities like volunteering and also participation in other activities that may not be "helping" in the traditional sense but that may certainly contribute to a community (e.g., sports and sense of community). Finally, it is important to consider the nature of the interconnections and particularly the likelihood that the key components of prosocial activities (broadly defined), psychological mechanisms, and health-related behaviors occur in a framework like Bandura's (1986) triadic reciprocity. That is, along with involvement in prosocial activities indirectly influencing health via the psychological mechanisms and, perhaps even more directly, the psychological mechanisms influencing prosocial involvements, health is also likely to impact both psychological states and prosocial activities. In other words, the relations among these components are dynamic.

ISSUES FOR FUTURE RESEARCH

The studies that have been conducted exploring a possible connection of involvement in prosocial activities and health-related behaviors and outcomes for adolescents suggest a relationship. At the same time, we should recognize, first, that only a relatively few studies have been conducted with adolescents, and second, that there is uncertainty about the precise nature of the connection. That being said, the relation of prosocial activities and health behaviors and outcomes does appear to be a promising area of research, both in terms of being a topic worthy of further exploration and in terms of having the potential to examine interesting questions and find important answers.

In one sense, there is a need to conduct more studies along the lines of those that have already been conducted. Additional correlational investigations with other and more diverse samples of adolescents and including a broader range of prosocial activities, psychological mechanisms, and health-related behaviors would be welcome; these studies, of course, would provide the opportunity to explore the interconnections among categories of variables (e.g., the categories of prosocial activities, psychological mechanisms, and health outcomes). Moreover, experiments and quasi experiments where some adolescents receive a prosocial experience and a comparison group does not are always desirable, and they offer opportunities to vary the experience itself and to assess several health-related behaviors and outcomes.

The most promising research strategy, however, and one consistent with the proposed dynamic and reciprocal quality of the relation of prosocial activities to health, is an investigation that incorporates elements of both the correlational and intervention approaches in a longitudinal format. Here, we envision a study where a pre-test includes, among others, measures of prosocial involvement, several psychological mechanisms, and health-related behaviors and outcomes. Adolescents then would be randomly assigned to a prosocial experience or a comparison group; relevant psychological mechanisms, along with other variables, then would be assessed over time to detect any changes; and health-related behaviors and outcomes would be assessed at a more distant point in time. This, it seems to us, represents one of the best possibilities for capturing the dynamic relations among prosocial activities, psychological mechanisms (e.g., moral or civic identity, conventionality, and conscientiousness), and health-related behaviors and outcomes, if these factors are actually related in this way.

REFERENCES

Allen, G. F., & Treger, H. (1990). Community service orders in federal probation: Perceptions of probationers and host agencies. *Federal Probation, 54,* 8–14.

Allen, J. P., & Philliber, S. (2001). Who benefits most from a broadly targeted prevention program? Differential efficacy across populations in the teen outreach program. *Journal of Community Psychology, 29,* 637–655.

Allen, J. P., Philliber, S. P., Herrling, S., & Kuperminc, G. P. (1997). Preventing teen pregnancy and academic failure: Experimental evaluation of a developmentally-based approach. *Child Development, 64,* 729–742.

Bandura, A. (1986). *Social foundations of thought and action: A social cognitive theory.* Englewood Cliffs, NJ: Prentice-Hall.

Benson, P. L. (1997). *All kids are our kids: What communities must do to raise caring and responsible children and adolescents.* San Francisco: Jossey-Bass.

Benson, P. L. (2003). Toward asset-building communities: How does change occur? In R. M. Lerner & P. L. Benson (Eds.), *Developmental assets and asset-building communities: Implications for research, policy, and practice* (pp. 213–221). New York: Kluwer Academic/Plenum.

Benson, P. L., & Leffert, N. (2001). Childhood and adolescence: Developmental assets. In N. J. Smelser & P. G. Baltes (Eds.), *International encyclopedia of the social and behavioral sciences* (pp. 1690–1697). Oxford: Pergamon.

Benson, P. L., Leffert, N., Scales, P. C., & Blyth, D. A. (1998). Beyond the "village" rhetoric: Creating healthy communities for children and adolescents. *Applied Developmental Science, 2*(3), 138–159.

Benson, P. L., Mannes, M., Pittman, K., & Ferber, T. (2004). Youth development, developmental assets, and public policy. In R. M. Lerner & L. Steinberg (Eds.), *Handbook of adolescent psychology* (2nd ed., pp. 781–814). New York: Wiley.

Benson, P. L., Scales, P. C., Hamilton, S. F., & Sesma, A., Jr. (2006). Positive youth development: Theory, research, and applications. In W. W. Damon & R. M. Lerner (Eds.), *Handbook of child psychology* (6th ed., Vol. 1, Theoretical models of human development) (pp. 894–941). New York: Wiley.

Billig, S. H. (1994). Heads, hearts, and hands: The research on K-12 service-learning. In National Youth Leadership Council, *Growing to greatness: The state of service-learning project* (pp. 12–25). St. Paul, MN: National Youth Leadership Council.

Billig, S. (2004). Heads, hearts, and hands: The research on K-12 service-learning. In *Growing to greatness: The state of service-learning report*. St. Paul, MN: National Youth Leadership Council.

Boggs, T., & Roberts, B. W. (2004). Conscientiousness and health-related behaviors: A meta-analysis of the leading behavioral contributors to mortality. *Psychological Bulletin, 130,* 887–919.

Carnegie Corporation of New York. (1992). *A matter of time: Risk and opportunity in the non-school hours.* Waldorf, MD: Carnegie Council on Adolescent Development.

Cauce, A. M. (1986). Social networks and social competence: Exploring the effects of early adolescent friendships. *American Journal of Community Psychology, 14,* 607–628.

Clary, E. G., & Roehlkepartain, E. C. (in press). Adding it up: Youth involvement in community life. *Search Institute Insights and Evidence.*

Clary, E. G., & Snyder, M. (1999). The motivations to volunteer: Theoretical and practical considerations. *Current Directions in Psychological Science, 8,* 156–159.

Damon, W. (1997). *The youth charter: How communities can work together to raise standards for all our children.* New York: Free Press.

Eccles, J. S., & Barber, B. L. (1999). Student council, volunteering, basketball, or marching band: What kind of extracurricular involvement matters? *Journal of Adolescent Research, 14*(1), 10–43.

Eccles, J. S., & Gootman, J. A. (2002). *Community programs to promote youth development.* Washington, DC: National Academy Press.

Eyler, J. (2002). Reflection: Linking service and learning—linking students and communities. *Journal of Social Issues, 58,* 517–534.

Friedman, H., Tucker, J., Schwartz, J., Tomlinson-Keasey, C., Martin, L., Wingard, D., & Criqui, M. (1995). Psychosocial and behavioral predictors of longevity: The aging and death of the "Termites." *American Psychologist, 50,* 69–78.

Hastings, P. D., Zahn-Walker, C., Robinson, J., Usher, B., & Bridges, D. (2000). The development of concern for others in children with behavior problems. *Developmental Psychology, 36,* 531–546.

Hein, K. (2003). Enhancing the assets for positive youth development: The vision, values, and action agenda of the W. T. Grant Foundation. In R. M. Lerner & P. L. Benson (Eds.), *Developmental assets and asset-building communities: Implications for research, policy, and practice* (pp. 97–117). New York: Kluwer Academic/Plenum.

Inderbitzen-Pisaruk, H., Clark, M. L., & Solano, C. H. (1992). Correlates of loneliness in midadolescence. *Journal of Youth and Adolescence, 21,* 151–167.

Jessor, R. (1984). Adolescent development and behavioral health. In J. D. Matarazzo, S. M. Weiss, J. A. Herd, N. E. Miller, & S. M. Weiss (Eds.), *Behavioral health: A handbook of health enhancement and disease prevention* (pp. 69–90). New York: Wiley.

Jessor, R., Donovan, J. E., & Costa, F. M. (1991). *Beyond adolescence: Problem behavior and young adult development.* New York: Cambridge University Press.

Jessor, R., Turbin, M. S., & Costa, F. M. (1998). Protective factors in adolescent health behavior. *Journal of Personality and Social Psychology, 75*(3), 788–800.

Johnson, M. K., Beebe, T., Mortimer, J. T., & Snyder, M. (1998). Volunteerism in adolescence: A process perspective. *Journal of Research on Adolescence, 8,* 309–332.

Keyes, C. L. M. (2003). Complete mental health: An agenda for the 21st century. In C. L. M. Keyes & J. Haidt (Eds.), *Flourishing: Positive psychology and the life well-lived.* Washington, DC: American Psychological Association.

Leffert, N., Benson, P. L., Scales, P. C., Sharma, A. R., Drake, D. R., & Blyth, D. A. (1998). Developmental assets: Measurement and prediction of risk behaviors among adolescents. *Applied Developmental Science, 2*(4), 209–230.

Lerner, R. M. (2004). *Liberty: Thriving and civic engagement among America's youth.* Thousand Oaks, CA: Sage.

Litvack-Miller, W., McDougall, D., & Romney, D. M. (1997). The structure of empathy during middle childhood and its relationship to prosocial behavior. *Genetic, Social, and General Psychology Monographs, 123,* 303–324.

McCrae, R. R., & Costa, P. T. (1987). Validation of the five-factor model of personality across instruments and observers. *Journal of Personality and Social Psychology, 52,* 81–90.

Moore, C. W., & Allen, J. P. (1996). The effects of volunteering on the young volunteer. *Journal of Primary Prevention, 17*(2), 231–258.

Moore, K. A. (1997). Criteria for indicators of child well-being. In R. M. Hauser, B. V. Brown, & W. R. Prosser (Eds.), *Indicators of children's well-being* (pp. 36–44). New York: Russell Sage Foundation.

Moore, K. A., Lippman, L., & Brown, B. (2004). Indicators of child well-being: The promise for positive youth development. *Annals of the American Academy of Political and Social Science, 591,* 125–145.

Murphey, D. A., Lamonda, K. H., Carney, J. K., & Duncan, P. (2004). Relationships of a brief measure of youth assets to health-promoting and risk behaviors. *Journal of Adolescent Health, 34,* 184–191.

National Youth Leadership Council. (2004). *Growing to greatness 2004: The state of service learning project.* St. Paul, MN: Author.

O'Donnell, L., Stueve, A., San Doval, A., Duran, R., Atnafou, R., Haber, D., Johnson, N., Murray, H., Grant, U., Juhn, G., Tang, J., Bass, J., & Piessens, P.

(1999). Violence prevention and young adolescents' participation in community youth service. *Journal of Adolescent Health, 24,* 28–37.

Piliavin, J. A. (2003). Doing well by doing good: Benefits for the benefactor. In C. L. M. Keyes & J. Haidt (Eds.), *Flourishing: The positive psychology and the life well lived* (pp. 227–247). Washington, DC: American Psychological Association.

Pittman, K. J., & Fleming, W. P. (1991). *A new vision: Promoting youth development: Written transcript of live testimony by Karen J. Pittman given before the House Select Committee on Children, Youth, and Families.* Washington, DC: Center for Youth Development and Policy Research.

Raskoff, S. A., & Sundeen, R. A. (2000). Community service programs in high school. *Law and Contemporary Problems, 62,* 73–111.

Rodin, J., & Langer, E. (1977). Long-term effects of a control-relevant intervention with the institutionalized aged. *Journal of Personality and Social Psychology, 35,* 897–902.

Rodkin, P. C., Farmer, T. W., Pearl, R., & Van Acker, R. (2000). Heterogeneity of popular boys: Antisocial and prosocial configuration. *Developmental Psychology, 36,* 14–24.

Rydell, A., Hagekull, B., & Bohlin, G. (1997). Measurement of two social competence aspects in middle childhood. *Developmental Psychology, 33,* 824–833.

Scales, P. C., Benson, P. L., Leffert, N., & Blyth, D. A. (2000). The contribution of developmental assets to the prediction of thriving outcomes among adolescents. *Applied Developmental Science, 4*(1), 27–46.

Scales, P. C. & Benson, P. L. (2005). Prosocial orientation and community service. In K. A. Moore & L. Lippman (Eds.), *What do children need to flourish?* (pp. 339–356). New York: Kluwer Academic/Plenum.

Scales, P. C., & Leffert, N. (2004). *Developmental assets: A synthesis of the scientific research on adolescent development* (2nd ed.). Minneapolis, MN: Search Institute.

Scales, P. C., & Roehlkepartain, E. C. (2004). *Community service and service-learning in U.S. public schools, 2004: Findings from a national survey.* St. Paul, MN: National Youth Leadership Council.

Scales, P. C., Sesma, A., & Bolstrom, B. (2004). *Coming into their own: How developmental assets promote positive growth in middle childhood.* Minneapolis, MN: Search Institute.

Stukas, A., Clary, E. G., & Snyder, M. (1999). The effects of "mandatory volunteerism": Satisfaction, intentions, and motivations to volunteer. *Psychological Science, 10,* 59–64.

Switzer, G. E., Simmons, R. G., Dew, M. A., Regalski, J. M., & Wang, C. (1995). The effects of a school-based helper program on adolescent self-image, attitudes, and behavior. *Journal of Early Adolescence, 15,* 429–455.

Takanishi, R. (1993). An agenda for the integration of research and policy during early adolescence. In R. M. Lerner (Ed.), *Early adolescence: Perspectives on research, policy, and intervention* (pp. 457–469). Hillsdale, NJ: Erlbaum.

Theokas, C., Almerigi, J., Lerner, R. M., Dowling, E. M., Benson, P. L., Scales, P. C., & von Eye, A. (2005). Conceptualizing and modeling individual and ecological asset components of thriving in early adolescence. *Journal of Early Adolescence, 25*(1), 113–143.

Uggen, C., & Jenikula, J. (1999). Volunteerism and arrest in the transition to adulthood. *Social Forces, 78,* 331–362.

Vernberg, E. M., Ewell, K. K., Beery, S. H. & Abwender, D. A. (1994). Sophistication of adolescents' interpersonal negotiation strategies and friendship formation after relocation: A naturally occurring experiment. *Journal of Research on Adolescence, 4,* 5–19.

Wentzel, K. R. (1993). Motivation and achievement in early adolescence: The role of multiple classroom goals. *Journal of Early Adolescence, 13,* 4–20.

Youniss, J., McLellan, J. A., Su, Y. & Yates, M. (1999). The role of community service in identity development: Normative, unconventional, and deviant orientations. *Journal of Adolescent Research, 14,* 248–261.

Youniss, J., & Yates, M. (1997). *Community service and social responsibility in youth.* Chicago: University of Chicago.

Youniss, J., & Yates, M. (1999). Youth service and moral-civic identity: A case for everyday morality. *Educational Psychology Review, 11,* 361–376.

8   Rx: Volunteer: A Prescription for Healthy Aging

Adam S. Hirschfelder
with Sabrina L. Reilly

In a recent *San Francisco Chronicle* article (Rosen, 2004), Joyce, a widower, discusses her experiences in helping Johnay, an 11-year-old son of Nicaraguan immigrants, become a better reader. The experience, she says, gives her "tremendous satisfaction." Similarly, a recent *New York Times* article (Olson, 2004) describes how David, a retired 67-year-old, has been affected by volunteering with elementary school students in Baltimore. "I feel good. . . . I look forward to getting up in the morning and doing this. . . . I'm a lot more active now. I'm walking more, I'm standing more." Meanwhile, in the *Wall Street Journal* (Zaslow, 2003), Paul, a 95-year-old retired salesman, mentions one of the benefits of his volunteer work with his local police department: "When I got here, my contemporaries sat in the clubhouse and twiddled their lives away. Now they're all gone."

When researchers describe the health benefits of volunteering, particularly for older adults, they are often referring to citizens like Joyce, David, and Paul, whose mental and physical health improved by helping others (outside of friends, neighbors, or relatives) with no expectation of pay or other material benefit (Yum & Lightfoot, 2005, pp. 38–39). An implication from much of the research in the area, including several of the articles referenced in this volume, is that these acts of volunteerism are beneficial, of course, and that there would be a dual benefit to society from having greater numbers of older adults engaged in activities such as tutoring children and providing support for local safety efforts. Given the inherent limitations of many of these studies, however, little attention has been given to the practical public health implications of these findings.

If research shows that because of their volunteer work, older adults are more optimistic, physically active, socially engaged, and less likely to die within 10 years, what, if anything, does this mean for the public's health? And if it does mean something positive (and it does), what can be done to translate the research on the health benefits of volunteerism into real-world interventions, programs, and initiatives that can be implemented, evaluated, and replicated so that society achieves a greater number of healthier, happier older citizens engaged in meaningful activities with potentially lower health costs? In short, how can we increase the number of volunteers like Joyce, David, and Paul?

This chapter attempts to provide one answer to this question by outlining one potentially useful yet, to date, virtually unexamined practical public health application of the research on the health benefits of volunteerism—the involvement of primary care physicians as volunteerism advocates. It also serves as a call to action for more integrated research that explicitly links volunteering with clinical medical practice—two fields that operate mostly in isolation from each other. Given the confluence of large and noted trends in the aging, civic engagement, and health care fields, the time has come for the important research on the health benefits of volunteerism (and altruism) to be part of the broader discussion of health care for older adults and for volunteering to be viewed as a real public health issue.

THE AGING REVOLUTION

The fact that the United States is facing an unprecedented demographic shift—the graying of America—toward an aging population that promises to transform all aspects of society is hardly news. Still, the numbers are worth briefly recounting since they provide the impetus for much of the research in this chapter. According to the Federal Interagency Forum on Aging-Related Statistics (2004, p. 2), in 2003, nearly 36 million people aged 65+ lived in the United States, accounting for just over 12% of the total population. During the 20th century, the older population grew from 3 million to 35 million and is projected to grow to almost 87 million by 2050. A major factor, of course, for the surge is the approximately 77 million babies born during the "boom years" of 1946–1964. Due to the baby boom, the older population in 2030 is projected to be *twice* as large as its counterpart in 2000, growing to 71.5 million and representing nearly 20% of the total U.S. population.

Just as important to society as the sheer number of older adults is the increased longevity these citizens can expect to experience. According to the National Center for Health Statistics (2004, p. 77), thanks to a broad range of advances in medical care, boomers who reach age 65 can expect to live, on average, at least another 18.1 years compared to an average life expectancy of 47 for those born in 1900. America now possesses the largest and fastest-growing population of older adults in history. As the Centers for Disease Control and Prevention Web site notes (2004a), "America is on the brink of a longevity revolution."

Until recently, much of the attention, particularly among policy makers and the media, on the impact of aging on America has focused on the negative impact that massive numbers of older citizens will have on public programs, such as Social Security and Medicare (Freedman, 1999, pp. 14–15; Magee, 2004, p. 1). However, a growing number of researchers (Freedman, 1999), academic institutions (Center for Health Communication, 2004), think tanks (Civic Ventures, 2002; Magee, 2004), and nonprofit organizations (Gerontological Society of America, 2004; Independent Sector, 2000; National Council on Aging, 2003) have begun focusing instead on what Freedman (1999) terms the "aging opportunity" (pp. 19–23).

Rather than look at the vast new generation of older adults as a burden, this new approach focuses on the potentially transformative *positive* impact that this cohort can have on society through increased and sustained civic engagement. Adler (2002) notes that "the older population is not simply a bundle of costs, but represents an untapped social asset" (p. 2). Independent Sector (2000, p. 1) finds that adults 55+ give a staggering total of 5 billion hours in volunteer time annually. Civic Ventures (2002) points out that, if society can find ways to "motivate [retiring boomers] to apply a portion of their newfound time and accumulated experience toward public service—helping to fill some of the most urgent needs in our society—the result will be a windfall for American civic life" (p. 2).

What makes the coming generation of older Americans such a source of interest is that it is composed of citizens who are better educated, healthier, wealthier, and more active than any previous generation of elders (Freedman, 1999, p. 16). Just as important, this cohort expects volunteerism to play a significant role in its retirement, a decision in part spurred by the September 11, 2001, terrorist attacks (Peter D. Hart Research Associates, 2002). According to Freedman and Gomperts (2004), research shows that 54% of boomers say that doing work that helps others is very important to them, and 78% of Americans say that they expect volunteer work to be an important part of their retirement. Further, from a community needs standpoint, seniors are especially valuable since charities and congregations find that one of their greatest challenges is recruiting volunteers during the workday, a flexible time for many retirees (Urban Institute, 2004, p. 5). Older adults may be "our nation's only growing natural resource" (Freedman, 1999, p. 16).

To be sure, a major theme of many of the new civic engagement efforts is that there is no guarantee that the coming generation of older citizens will produce millions of new volunteers. There is evidence (Putnam, 2000) that boomers are less civically engaged than previous generations of Americans. Further, as Prisuta (2004) notes, boomers are noteworthy for their "independence, self-reliance and self-indulgence, factors not typically associated with a propensity to volunteer" (p. 85). Also, research indicates that rates of volunteering traditionally drop in retirement and decline as people age (Center for Health Communication, 2004, p. 4). Because of these trends, many of the new initiatives call for new programs and recruitment efforts to harness the civic potential of older adults.

HEALTHY AGING

One major challenge facing older adults who may want to volunteer more is, naturally, their own health. Because of advances in medicine, many older Americans now survive diseases that used to be fatal and live many years with chronic diseases—thus reducing volunteer ability (Magee, 2004, p. 5). Similarly, Prisuta (2004) finds that health status plays a critical role in determining if seniors volunteer and, if so, where and how often they do so. Given the United States' aging population, it should be no surprise that health-related factors should impact volunteer rates. Indeed, the issue of how to improve the quality and years of healthy life for older adults is at the top of the nation's health care agenda (Centers for Disease Control and Prevention, 2003a; U.S. Department of Health and Human Services, 2000). As the Centers for Disease Control and Prevention (CDC) finds, "[T]he aging of the population is one of the public-health challenges of the 21st Century" (American Society on Aging, 2003, p. 1).

According to the CDC (2003a, p. 2), almost one third of total U.S. health care expenditures is for older adults, and spending will increase by 25% simply because the population will be older. Medicare spending, meanwhile, has grown sevenfold in the past two decades from $33.9 billion in 1980 to $252.2 billion in 2002 and is projected to double again by 2012. According to the Centers for Medicare and Medicaid Services (International Council on Active Aging, 2003a, p. 2), poor health cost the United States $1.42 trillion in 2001 and is forecasted to cost $2.8 trillion by 2011. In addition to fiscal costs, chronic diseases (80% of seniors have at least one) exact a societal toll since they contribute to disability, diminished quality of life, and increased demands on caregivers (Centers for Disease Control and Prevention, 2004b).

Needless to say, given the unprecedented impact (financial and otherwise) that the health of older adults will have on society in the coming decades, finding ways to encourage and promote "healthy aging" has captured the interest of government agencies, researchers, policy makers, foundations, and health maintenance organizations (HMOs). This increased interest is due, in part, to influential reports (e.g., Rowe & Kahn, 1998) that suggest that poor health is not a natural consequence of aging and that vast numbers of older citizens—contrary to stereotypes—are very capable of living healthy and fulfilling lives, including volunteer work. Furthering interest in the issue, research indicates that many chronic diseases can be prevented or managed with behavior changes (see Centers for Disease Control and Prevention, 2003a; Institute of Medicine Committee on Assuring the Health of the Public in the 21st Century, 2002; Smedley & Syme, 2000, pp. 1–36).

Fiscal issues, of course, are also boosting attention to healthy aging issues since research shows that preventing (or minimizing) health problems is one of the few proven ways to stem rising health care costs (Centers for Disease Control and Prevention, 2003b). According to the Institute of Medicine (2001, p. 7), as much as 95% of health care spending goes to medical care and biomedical research though lifestyle behaviors are responsible for more than 70% of avoidable mortality. Healthy lifestyles are as influential, if not more so, than genetic factors in helping older people to avoid aging-related deterioration (see Centers for Disease Control and Prevention, 2003a; Merck Institute of Aging & Health, 2002). These findings build on "compression of morbidity" research (Fries, 1980, 2003) which posits that disability in old age can be delayed and medical utilization reduced through behavioral changes and health promotion efforts.

The recent medical focus on the importance of prevention and health promotion for older adults is mirrored in the social gerontology field where the issue of healthy aging is described in broader theoretical concepts. For example, Hinterlong et al. (2001) refer to "productive aging" as a term that "draws our attention away from a narrow biological treatment of aging and toward the contributions made by older adults" (p. 4). Morrow-Howell et al. (2001) propose that "productive aging" should be further defined as "productivity in later life," which "suggests that productivity is among many possible pursuits of later life [and] . . . more about social institutions, policies and programs than about individuals" (pp. 285–306). Whatever the definition, the authors make clear that older citizens and society alike benefit when older adults are engaged in meaningful activities such as volunteering.

From a more individualistic perspective, Rowe and Kahn (1998) use the term "successful aging." They define it as "the ability to maintain three key behaviors or characteristics: low risk of disease and disease-related disability; high mental and physical function; and active engagement with life" (p. 38). The authors make clear that it is a combination of all three that represents the concept of successful aging, yet they also stress that "successful aging goes beyond potential; it involves activity." Of particular interest are activities such as volunteering (pp. 169–174). Similarly, Schneider and Miles (2003) refer to "ageless" habits that older adults can adopt "to live longer with more zest and vitality" (p. 2). Included among these ageless habits (pp. 192–195) are social engagement activities such as volunteer work. In fact, some older adults themselves believe that volunteering is essential to healthy aging (Canadian Ethnocultural Council, 2002).

Whether it is referred to as "healthy aging," "productive aging," "productivity in later life," "successful aging," "active aging," or "ageless," it is clear that there are many behavior changes that older adults can make to increase their chances of having a healthier, longer life. Of these, increased physical activity has received, perhaps, the most attention from the health and aging fields. A brief look at the research in this area and some of the initiatives that have been created in response provides the context for a practical application of the research on the health benefits of volunteerism.

A large body of research indicates that being physically active is beneficial for the prevention, management, and treatment of the chronic conditions and illnesses most prevalent in older adults and that increased physical activity increases the quality and years of healthy life (e.g., Balde et al., 2003; Damush et al., 1999, U.S. Department of Health and Human Services, 1996). For example, regular physical activity reduces several health-risk factors which are associated with cardiovascular disease, the leading cause of death among the old (Merck Institute of Aging & Health, 2004a, p. 11). Equally important, exercise reduces mortality and disability from mental health disorders (U.S. Department of Health and Human Services, 2002).

Yet despite the overwhelming evidence that physical activity offers one of the best ways to extend the years of active independent life, reduce disability, and improve quality of life, only a relatively small number of older adults exercise regularly (Damush et al., 1999, p. M423). According to the U.S. Department of Health and Human Services (2002, p. 2), approximately one third of persons aged 65+ lead a sedentary lifestyle. Up to three fourths of the older population doesn't exercise at recommended levels (Nied & Franklin, 2002, p. 419). Naturally, this lack of physical activity has a substantial economic impact on the U.S. health care system. The Medicare and Medicaid programs spend an estimated $84 billion in direct costs annually on chronic conditions that could be improved by increased exercise (U.S. Department of Health and Human Services, 2002, pp. 4–5). In response to the low rates of exercise among older adults, many large public and private initiatives have been launched. Of particular note, in 2001, a group of more than 40 large organizations in the health and aging fields came together to launch a massive effort to get more seniors to exercise: the National Blueprint: Increasing Physical Activity Among Adults Age 50 and Older (Robert Wood Johnson Foundation, 2001). To meet its lofty goals, the National Blueprint identifies several sectors of society that need to be engaged, including communities, families, employers, medical systems, policy makers, researchers, and the media (Robert Wood Johnson Foundation, 2001, p. 7). Similarly, several HMOs have also launched new efforts to get older adults to exercise (see Fitzner et al., 2002, pp. 29–41; HMO Workgroup on Care Management, 2002, pp. 5–13; Martinson et al., 2003; Partnership for Prevention, 2002).

THE HEALTH BENEFITS OF VOLUNTEERISM
FOR OLDER ADULTS

For more than 30 years, researchers, including many in this volume, have looked at the relationship between volunteering and well-being in later life. Much of this research has found that volunteerism, like exercise, is associated with a broad range of physical and mental health benefits for older adults. Nevertheless, the impact of some of these studies was limited somewhat by researchers' inability to determine the selection effect on health outcomes and by a lack of control groups and objective outcome measures (Yum & Lightfoot, 2005, p. 32). However, a more recent body of research conducted with improved methodologies (control variables, longitudinal data, etc.) has further documented a link between volunteering and improved physical and mental health for older adults (see Greenfield & Marks, 2004; Morrow-Howell et al., 2003; Parker-Pope, 2004; Yum & Lightfoot, 2005).

Among the newer studies, of particular interest is a recent evaluation (Fried et al., 2004) of Experience Corps (EC), an innovative intergenerational program which places older adult volunteers in schools to improve the academic outcomes of low-income children. In addition to its educational mission, EC is explicitly designed to yield health improvements by providing older volunteers with a rigorous, structured, and engaging experience that includes—through teams of volunteers at the same school—opportunities for ongoing peer interaction. The study notes that EC has been specifically developed "to increase volunteers' physical, social and cognitive activity simultaneously, hypothesizing that improvement in any of these pathways would have health benefits" (p. 65). In this study, older adults committed to at least 15 hours of EC service per week over a full school year to ensure a high "health promotion dose" (p. 65). In a randomized trial of volunteers assigned to either the EC program or a comparison group, EC participants saw substantial improvements in physical activity and strength (including reduced cane use and falls) and cognitive activity when compared to controls. Further, more than 80% of the participants expect to volunteer longer than one school year, extending the health benefits.

This EC study adds to the growing body of research that indicates that there is something about volunteering itself—whether through lowering stress hormones, improving outlook, adding social roles, increasing interpersonal contact, improving self-image, boosting physical activity, or some combination thereof—that promotes better health and reduces mortality. As King (1996) notes, "Volunteering is unique in its integration of a broad range of benefits for its participants. It offers productive roles in a variety of settings that can provide older adults with feelings of usefulness, mental challenge, and social integration" (p. 4). Similarly, Musick et al. (1999) find that "[v]olunteer work can . . . protect the older person from the hazards of retirement, physical decline and inactivity" (pp. S173–S180). One study (Oman et al., 1999) found that the reduction in mortality associated with volunteering is larger than the reduction associated with physical activity.

VOLUNTEERISM AND OLDER ADULTS:
A PUBLIC HEALTH ISSUE

From a public health perspective, what this growing body of research suggests is that volunteering appears to be the type of social and behavioral approach to health improvement that offers great promise to reduce morbidity and mortality (Smedley & Syme, 2000). The EC study (Fried et al., 2004, pp. 103–104) notes that the tutoring program should be considered as a type of multilevel health intervention—combining individual, organizational, and community components—that offers benefits that other health efforts do not. More bluntly, the director of the Center for Health Communication at the Harvard School of Public Health claims that "civic engagement in retirement is the next health club in terms of fitness, good health and longevity" (Powell, 2004).

In addition to being similar to physical activity in its association with a range of health (and community) benefits, volunteerism shares another similarity to exercise: Participation rates by older adults are relatively low. While finding an exact measure of the percentage of older adults who volunteer is difficult to determine (due to religion, sampling procedures, question wording, etc.), the rates of volunteering by older adults is smaller compared to other age cohorts, with rates increasing in age, peaking in midlife, then declining for adults 65+ (Prisuta, 2004, pp. 60–61). In its official estimate, the Bureau of Labor Statistics (2004, p. 1) finds that only 23% of older adults volunteer. Other research has found a somewhat higher rate. For example, Prisuta (2004, p. 61) estimates that, based on studies from the American Association of Retired Persons (AARP), Independent Sector, and the Points of Light Foundation, approximately half of American adults are currently or were recently involved in some type of volunteering, with much of the efforts episodic and rates dropping at older ages. What this means is that, like exercise, there is a clear opportunity to increase volunteerism rates among older adults. The major challenge is: how?

RECRUITING OLDER ADULTS TO SERVE

Since 1961, when the first White House Conference on Aging brought national attention to the importance of engaging older adults in useful activities (Gartland, 2001, p. 15), a range of public and private efforts to get older adults to volunteer has been launched. In 1965, the U.S. government began creating the Retired Seniors and Volunteer Program (RSVP), which was designed to provide opportunities for retired persons aged 60+ to participate more fully in the life of their communities through volunteerism (Lindbloom, 2001, p. 8). Today, RSVP along with the Foster Grandparent Program and the Senior Companion Program comprise the National Senior Service Corps (Senior Corps). Through the network of Senior Corps programs (74,000 nonprofits, community-based organizations, and faith-based institutions), approximately a half million older adult volunteers annually provide services in the areas of health, economic development, education, housing, disaster relief, and homeland security (Corporation for National and Community Service, 2004a, p. 140).

The call for more seniors to volunteer continues to be a national priority. In his 2002 State of the Union speech—4 months after the 9/11 terrorist attacks—President George W. Bush launched USA Freedom Corps, a White House effort to engage more citizens, particularly older adults, in volunteer work (Bridgeland et al., 2003). Evidence indicates that older adults responded positively to this renewed national attention, with two in five older Americans saying that the attacks made them more likely to volunteer (Peter D. Hart Research Associates, 2002, p. 2). The Corporation for National and Community Service finds that those aged 55+ accounted for nearly a third of the 4 million increase in volunteers from 2002 to 2003 and that volunteering by members of that group, who traditionally give the most hours per year, rose from 25.1% of the total number of volunteers to 25.6% (Corporation for National and Community Service, 2004a).

As mentioned earlier, despite this positive news, there is no guarantee that society will continue to see increased rates of volunteerism among older adults. Recognizing this challenge, a broad range of organizations has launched major initiatives to boost civic engagement among older adults. Similar in scope to exercise initiatives such as the National Blueprint, these new efforts seek to engage many sectors of society. For example, the new Harvard School of Public Health–MetLife Foundation Initiative on Retirement and Civic Engagement (Center for Health Communication, 2004) calls for including policy makers, nonprofit organizations, employers, local governments, educational institutions, and faith-based institutions in the process. Perhaps the most noteworthy element of this effort is a call (p. 4) for a major mass media campaign, based on successful social marketing initiatives, such as the "designated driver" campaign of the 1980s, to inspire greater numbers of older adults to volunteer.

Similarly, the National Council on Aging (2003) has launched RespectAbility, a new initiative "to help community organizations and decision makers identify and advance methods to enhance [the] civic and professional participation of older Americans." Among the elements of this multiyear effort are research to deepen the understanding of structural, policy, and programmatic barriers to engaging older adults in volunteer positions; media advocacy; town hall meetings; and new community assessment tools. Meanwhile, the Gerontological Society of America (2004) has created Civic Engagement in Older America, a campaign to "produce and promote research that will contribute to the development of more effective social institutions, programs, and policies that will increase civic participation by older adults." Other recent efforts have called for a new federally supported "boomer corps" with stipends and scholarships for older volunteers (Magee, 2004). Meanwhile, Senior Corps (2003) has launched a new Internet-based recruitment site.

THE MISSING ELEMENT: PHYSICIANS

As shown by these varied new civic engagement efforts, there are broad similarities between the efforts to increase volunteerism among older adults and those designed to boost physical activity. Some commonalities include government leadership, national organization involvement, foundation support, new promotional campaigns, media advocacy, policy development, and challenges to local governments and community-based organizations to restructure. Yet there is one major difference between the two types of efforts. While nearly all of the new civic engagement efforts highlight the health benefits of volunteerism for older adults, *none* include outreach to the medical community as an explicit component. In contrast, the roles of physicians and the "medical system" are major parts of nearly all of the exercise initiatives, particularly the National Blueprint (Centers for Disease Control and Prevention, 2002a, p. 2). Given the important role that the health care system, particularly doctors, plays in the lives of older adults, this is clearly a missed opportunity and one worthy of more attention.

With increased attention on engaging older adults in preventive health activities and the growing recognition that volunteering is a behavior essential to healthy aging, it is a strategically important time to include the medical system in the larger conversation on increasing civic engagement among older adults. Not only can physicians be effective advocates for behavior change—in this case, increased volunteerism—but the health care system, particularly through the health insurance industry, can provide a cost-benefit framework that may provide, as it has for physical activity (e.g., Martinson et al., 2003), a fiscal rationale for the type of increased investment in recruitment efforts, organizational restructuring, and community planning called for by the new civic engagement initiatives. A brief look at the role of physicians in promoting exercise (and other healthy behaviors) provides further context for a new effort that engages doctors in the endeavor to increase volunteerism among older adults.

A broad range of research shows that while many sources of information about physical activity exist, including health associations, government agencies, community organizations, and health and fitness clubs, health care providers are essential to reach and motivate older adults to become and remain active (Active for Life, 2002, p. 7). One study (Ades et al., 1992) found that the strength of a primary physician's recommendation is the most powerful predictor of exercise initiation for older patients. Research on the positive impact of physician recommendations on adults' physical activity levels (see Andersen et al., 1997; Balde et al., 2003; Bull & Jamrozik, 1998; Estabrooks et al., 2003; Nied & Franklin, 2002; O'Connor, Rush, Prochaska, Pronk, & Boyle, 2001; Pinto, Goldstein, & Marcus, 1998) has led to several calls to action for physicians to "prescribe" physical activity to patients (e.g., International Council on Active Aging, 2003b, p. 2; Manson & Greenland, 2004). The issue has reached the popular press as well (Associated Press, 2004).

There are several reasons that doctors, particularly primary care physicians (PCPs), can play an influential role in promoting healthy behaviors to older adults. First, Americans over age 65 represent 13% of the population, but account for half of physician visits (Merck Institute of Aging & Health, 2004a, p. 27). Annually, 31% of adults age 65+ have between 1 and 3 doctor visits; 36% have between 4 and 9; and 24% have 10 or more (National Center for Health Statistics, 2004, p. 247). The CDC (Cherry et al., 2003, p. 18) finds that patients aged 65+ make an average of 6 office visits per year. Thus, doctors have multiple opportunities to encourage patients to adopt healthier lifestyles (Andersen et al., 1997, p. 2). Also, regular care offers opportunities for physicians to track progress and provide feedback on healthy behavior adoption and adherence (Whitlock et al., 2002, p. 269).

Boosting the impact of multiple office visits, patients are receptive to receiving health information from their physicians. For example, patients report that PCPs are expected sources of preventive health recommendations (Whitlock et al., 2002, p. 269). A Center for the Advancement of Health (2001) study on the integration of health behavior counseling into routine medical care concludes that "[w]hen individuals seek medical care, they are unusually open to accepting guidance from an authority in whom they have trusted their well-being" (p. 4). Balde et al. (2003) note that the CDC and the American College of Sports Medicine recommend that physicians counsel patients to exercise because "patients respect their physician's advice [and] . . . are more likely to change their exercise behaviors as a result" (p. 91).

Older adults, in particular, are attentive to recommendations from their doctors. For example, "physicians and other health care professionals have a considerable influence over the health behaviors of mid-life and older patients, and a tremendous opportunity exists to influence adult health and health behaviors through clinical practice" (Active for Life, 2002, p. 19). Part of what makes physicians so influential in the lives of older adults is that while older adults believe that taking care of their health is very important, barely more than a third feel they are knowledgeable about how to prepare for a healthy old age (Cutler et al., 2002, p. 51). Supporting this finding, the Merck Institute of Aging & Health finds that over 40% of older adults would eat healthier and exercise more if their doctors told them how (Merck Institute of Aging & Health, 2004b, p. 2).

To be sure, there is extensive evidence that indicates that engaging physicians in preventive health counseling with older patients is difficult. For example, although doctors generally have positive attitudes toward preventive care, the Centers for Disease Control and Prevention (2002b, p. 2) find that only 52% of older adults reported being asked during routine check-ups about physical activity. Other studies have found similar results (see Balde et al., 2003, p. 93; Damush et al., 1999). Meanwhile, one large study finds that only 40% of physicians recalled having discussed physical activity with their patients (Morey & Sullivan, 2003, p. 206). Further, evidence indicates that high-risk patients are more often asked about exercise than are healthy ones (Pinto, Goldstein, & Marcus, 1998, p. 507), thus limiting the impact to a smaller cohort as opposed to the entire population.

A range of studies (e.g., Ainsworth & Youmans, 2002; Estabrooks et al., 2003; Manson & Greenland, 2004; Pinto, Goldstein, & Marcus, 1998) attributes the low rates of physical activity counseling to several factors, including lack of physician training and counseling skills, lack of time, lack of relevant materials, lack of organizational support, little or no reimbursement from insurance companies, and perceived ineffectiveness. On a more positive note, evidence indicates that despite the challenges of integrating behavioral counseling into office visits, health care providers generally accept and value their role in promoting disease prevention to patients (Whitlock et al., 2002, p. 269). Further, counseling interventions that include well-structured physician (and staff) training produce positive results (Ainsworth & Youmans, 2002; Albright et al., 2000; Eakin et al., 2004; Marcus et al., 1997; Pinto, Goldstein, & Marcus, 1998).

VOLUNTEERISM AS A BEHAVIORAL INTERVENTION

Given the health care system's increased focus on prevention, those interested in promoting volunteering by older adults may find allies within the medical system—if volunteerism is positioned as an easy-to-implement preventive health behavior. Ironically, one of the strongest arguments for doctors to embrace volunteerism as a health intervention is that many older adults are resistant to participating in exercise programs. As Nied and Franklin (2002) note, "[E]lderly patients face an array of personal, socioeconomic and environmental barriers to exercise" (p. 424). These include fear of injury, discomfort, and disability. Because of this, patients successfully recruited into exercise interventions are highly motivated and healthier, but even then adherence to recommendations drops off substantially after 6 months (Fried et al., 2004, p. 65). Further, other evidence indicates that some physicians have lingering concerns about a lack of solid evidence regarding exercise specifically tailored to older adults (Morey & Sullivan, 2003, pp. 204–207).

Also providing an opening for including volunteerism in medical care is the fact that many older urban adults live in unsafe neighborhoods. Because of this, many are reluctant to walk (or exercise) outside regularly (Fried et al., 2004, p. 65; HMO Workgroup on Care Management, 2002, p. 9). Thus, involving older patients in volunteer programs may be an attractive alternative for physicians. In fact, a program such as the aforementioned Experience Corps has been designed to "offer a community-based approach to health promotion that could attract diverse older adults, including many not likely to participate in more traditional health promotion activities" (Fried et al., 2004, p. 74). While EC's highly structured model is unique and only operating (as of December 2004) in 13 cities, national programs such as Senior Corps offer thousands of local volunteer opportunities nationwide, making it a widely accessible activity (King, 1996).

From a medical standpoint, there is also research to suggest that discussing volunteerism within a preventive health context might contribute to the patient-physician relationship. For example, patients prefer doctors who use a "patient-centered" approach that focuses on communication, partnership, and health promotion (Little et al., 2001, p. 468). Other research (Fincham & Wertheimer, 1986, p. 5) indicates that patient satisfaction in an HMO is influenced by physicians' discussion of preventive health activities. Whitlock et al. (2002, p. 272) note that clinician advice is associated with increased satisfaction with medical care. Other data (Schauffler et al., 1996) indicate that physicians may achieve higher levels of patient satisfaction if lifestyle and behaviors are discussed in a prevention context. Further, a high proportion of patients are willing to engage in two-way communication with physicians to improve their health (O'Connor et al., 1996). What better way to improve patient-physician communication than to discuss opportunities for local community involvement and volunteerism?

Undeniably, the notion of asking physicians to add another preventive measure to discuss with patients will not be fully embraced by the medical community. There is already broad concern among doctors about not having enough time to cover many of even the smallest preventive services recommended by the U.S. Preventive Services Task Force (Yarnall et al., 2003, p. 635). Further, if some physicians are reluctant to prescribe exercise to older adults because of a lack of evidence-based activities suitable for these patients, recommending volunteerism may be even more problematic since there is disagreement in the volunteerism research itself about how much and how often an older adult needs to volunteer to achieve the associated health benefits (Yum & Lightfoot, 2005, pp. 35–36).

Still, it is clear that older adults benefit from even small amounts of volunteer activity (e.g., Morrow-Howell et al., 2003). And rather than look at volunteerism as a well-defined "prescription" with specific hours and activities, just having physicians ask patients whether they volunteer and emphasizing that it is important to do so may be enough to increase volunteer rates. Research (Strange et al., 2002) indicates that preventive health counseling does not need to be long or extensive to make a difference. Further, advice from a physician may "prime patients to become more aware of and attentive to health information, programs, and services" (Kreuter et al., 2000, pp. 428–429), and an office visit may "plant a seed that will sprout later" (Manson & Greenland, 2004, p. 256). Taking this into account, medical offices can easily facilitate volunteerism by patients. For example, based on other prevention efforts (e.g., Elley et al., 2003; Kreuter et al., 2000; Pinto, Goldstein, & Marcus, 1998), medical staff can be

provided with patient handouts that contain information on local service opportunities. Also, self-help volunteer guides can be distributed in office waiting
rooms.

Once older patients leave an office visit where volunteerism is emphasized
(primed), the hope is that they will seek out service opportunities or be more
likely to volunteer if asked by a friend, family member, community leader, or
faith-based institution or via some other recruitment method. Similar to exercise interventions, between office visits, medical staff can also play a simple but
important role in reinforcing the volunteerism message (Whitlock et al., 2002).
This could include sending patients material about new local volunteer opportunities, making regular calls to patients to see if they have volunteered, and
coordinating patient activities with local community groups. In short, there is
no reason that volunteerism can't be readily integrated into the regular medical
care of older adults.

Before discussing a new initiative that integrates volunteerism into medical care, it should be noted that introducing an activity like volunteering into
primary care raises many important questions. First, medicalizing social issues
raises concerns regarding personal versus societal responsibility for health problems (Callahan & McHorney, 2003, p. 390). Second, volunteering is a personal
decision, and some older adults may not be comfortable with physician involvement in that area of their lives, particularly since many older adults volunteer
through faith-based institutions (Independent Sector, 2000). Thus, integrating
volunteerism into medical care may unintentionally introduce religion into
medical practice, a controversial issue (see Miller & Thoresen, 2003; Sloan et al.,
2000). It is interesting to note, however, that some research indicates that discussion of religion, like health behavior counseling, can improve the patient-
physician relationship (Sloan & Bagatelle, 2000, pp. 1915–1916).[1] Finally, it is
worth noting again that there is no consensus in the gerontology field on whether
older adults can achieve health benefits from relatively small amounts of volunteering or whether engagement needs to be a sustained, committed effort to
produce an impact (Yum & Lightfoot, 2005).

VOLUNTEERISM AS A HEALTH
PROMOTION STRATEGY?

Throughout this chapter, questions have been raised about the integration of
volunteerism into medical care. One of the reasons that there is so little clarity
on the issue is that very little formal research exists on whether it is feasible (or
desirable) for civic engagement to be a primary care physician–recommended
activity. We don't how doctors (or staff) would feel about recommending it and,
most important, what impact (if any) a recommendation, or prescription, to
volunteer would have. What is clear, however, is that the act of volunteering—

for whatever reason—clearly produces health benefits. In a time when prevention is increasingly the norm (or goal) in medical care, when health care costs are rapidly increasing, and with a demographic wave soon to hit, interventions that translate basic research into low-cost practical health interventions must be tested. As Syme (2003) notes:

> Our medical care system might be strained now, but it will be overwhelmed within the next 40 years. . . . It is therefore essential that we vigorously explore opportunities to prevent disease and promote health and not simply wait for medical care to solve problems after the fact. To do that, we will need to be more creative and effective in developing intervention programs to encourage successful aging. (p. 402)

Recognizing, like others (e.g., Fries, 2002, p. 3165), that there are many potentially valuable preventive health measures that have not been implemented, the California-based Public Health Institute (PHI) in 2003 launched an initiative to evaluate the feasibility of volunteerism as a medical intervention. Entitled Rx: Volunteer: A California Initiative to Promote Service and Healthy Aging, the project is based on similar studies (e.g., Bull & Jamrozik, 1998; Elley et al., 2003; Goodwin et al., 2001; Marcus et al., 1997; Pinto, Goldstein, DePue, & Milan, 1998) that evaluate physician adoption of a specific behavioral health intervention, adherence to the intervention protocol, and impact on patient behavior.

California provides a unique setting for the effort since legislators have identified volunteerism as critical to the state's plans for its aging population (California Integrated Elder Care and Involvement Act, 2002; California Strategic Plan on Aging Advisory Committee, 2004). In fact, California's Health and Human Services Agency's "Staying Well" vision (2003, pp. 46–48) identifies volunteering as a preventive health activity for seniors on a par with activities such as exercise (with *no* mention of physicians). Further, studies show a low number of older California residents involved in service (Ramakrishman & Baldassre, 2004, p. 2), though many express interest in doing so (Governor's Office on Service and Volunteerism, 2001).

Physicians and patients in the Rx: Volunteer study will be recruited from the Medicare practice of a large HMO in Northern California. The 18-month research effort (ending in 2006) includes:

- A survey of Bay Area physicians who treat large numbers of older adults (65+) regarding their knowledge about the health benefits of volunteerism; whether they have ever recommended or discussed volunteer service with patients; and, if not, whether they would ever do so and what types of training and materials they would need.
- A survey of patients regarding their knowledge about the health benefits of volunteerism; current or past volunteer experiences; whether they recall

ever discussing volunteering with their physician; how they would feel if their doctor recommended it to them; and what impact it might make.

- A survey of office staff to measure their knowledge about the health benefits of volunteerism; whether they have ever recommended or discussed volunteer service with patients; what type of community resources they currently use for patients; and how comfortable they would be with referring a patient to volunteer programs.

- A small intervention study involving 5–10 physician offices, including doctors and staff, to evaluate whether it is feasible to include volunteering counseling as part of regular office care and what impact, if any, it has on a patient's intentions to volunteer, actual volunteer rates, and adherence to volunteer activity.

- To encourage patients to volunteer, physicians will make mention of it in the office visit. To reinforce the prescription, the physician, office staff, health educators, and social workers in the HMO will reinforce the importance of volunteerism by contacting patients by phone and mail as well as in health education classes offered by the HMO.

- To facilitate the placement of older patients in engaging volunteer opportunities, a dedicated referral service has been created that will handle patient interviews to gauge areas of interest and to make placements in community organizations.

If the initial small Rx: Volunteer study is successful and if physicians, staff, and patients accept the idea of physician-directed volunteer counseling, whether or not volunteer rates increase, a much larger study, involving a control group, will be conducted with the HMO to measure the specific impact of receiving a volunteerism prescription within a medical context.

ENGAGING THE MEDICAL SYSTEM: THE MISSING LINK?

Recommending that those interested in promoting volunteerism among older adults engage the medical community by no means suggests, of course, that physician outreach should in any way replace new efforts to restructure nonprofits, provide incentives, use the mass media, and remove other barriers to community service. Nor does it imply, in any way, that volunteerism should replace existing behavioral health counseling efforts. Rather, it should be considered as another effective medical tool available to physicians to improve patients' health.

Finally, this call to action is made with full recognition that older adults consider many motives and other time commitments when deciding to volunteer (see Choi, 2003; Rouse & Clawson, 1992) and that even the most effective physician-based behavioral health interventions have only modest behavior

change impacts, with just 5–15% of patients making clinically significant behavior changes (Whitlock et al., 2002, p. 272). Still, if a similar impact could
be found on volunteer rates, the implications, spread across the population, could
be tremendous (Manson & Greenland, 2004, p. 256). As Morrow-Howell et al.
(2003) note, "[F]rom a public health perspective . . . programs that bring older
adults into volunteer roles, even at modest amounts of commitment, will be
beneficial" (p. 142).

Quite simply, linking civic engagement to larger trends in medicine and public
health, such as prevention and healthy aging, opens up a range of untapped chan-
nels to promote volunteerism. For example, beginning in 2005, all new Medicare
beneficiaries now receive a "welcome to Medicare physical." This new benefit,
authorized by the Medicare Modernization Act of 2003, is the result of the U.S.
government's increased focus on prevention-oriented health care and will focus
on providing education and counseling to older patients to increase the adoption
of healthy behaviors (U.S. Department of Health and Human Services, 2004).
Thus, physicians will have an unprecedented opportunity to affect the preventive health behaviors of millions of older adults. If volunteerism were included in
just a small number of these visits, the results could be remarkable.

To make this vision a reality, what is needed now are expanded partner-
ships between volunteer advocates and physicians. In fact, many medical providers already have links with community organizations. For example, one large
California HMO partners with social service agencies to assist with the care of
the elderly (Wilber et al., 2003). Yet in this partnership (like others), elders are
the *recipients* of services, including in-home care, nutrition/exercise advice, and
transportation. From the framework of volunteerism as a health intervention,
physicians could just as easily identify patients who could be volunteer *providers* of these services as well. Also, many health insurers promote volunteerism
as part of healthy aging on their Web sites (e.g., www.mylifepath.com). Physicians could easily direct patients to these and other electronic resources.

Comparable to recommendations outlined in the National Blueprint to
promote physical activity among older adults, similar steps are needed to integrate volunteerism into medical care:

1. Disseminate information on the health benefits of volunteerism to the
   medical community, including HMOs, medical societies, advocacy organizations, and public health agencies.
2. Include civic engagement experts when developing preventive health
   intervention recommendations for physicians.
3. Create profiles of the older adults most likely to benefit from involvement in community service so that screening and assessment tools can
   be developed and distributed to physicians.
4. Identify—via research—which volunteer activities produce the most
   health benefits for older adults, so evidence-based recommendations can
   be provided to physicians.

5. Include study of the health benefits of volunteerism in medical schools.
6. Provide funding for studies that evaluate volunteerism as a doctor-recommended activity.

The convergence of several interrelated trends in the aging, volunteerism, and health care fields provides a unique opportunity to establish volunteerism by older adults as a public health issue. Engaging physicians is an essential step of this process. A broad range of research shows that the most effective way to get older adults to volunteer is merely to ask them. Imagine the impact of physicians "asking" with a prescription that reads: "Volunteer for 2 hours and call me in the morning."

NOTE

1. Encouraging the general promotion of volunteerism within medical care might be a compromise strategy to harness the potential health benefits of religiosity (since many patients would volunteer at a house of worship) while preserving physician neutrality and avoiding interreligious conflict.

REFERENCES

Active for Life. (2002). *The role of midlife and older consumers in promoting physical activity through health care settings.* Retrieved October 20, 2004, from www.activeforlife.info/resources/reports_papers.html.

Ades, P. A., Waldmann, M. L., McCann, W. J., & Weaver, S. O. (1992). Predictors of cardiac rehabilitation participation in older coronary patients. *Archives of Internal Medicine 152*(5), 1033–1035.

Adler, R. (2002). *Engaging older volunteers in after-school programs.* San Francisco: Civic Ventures.

Ainsworth, B. E., & Youmans, C. P. (2002). Tools for physical activity counseling in medical practice. *Obesity Research, 10,* 69S–75S.

Albright, C. L., Cohen, S., Gibbons, L., Miller, S., Marcus, B., Sallis, J., Imai, K., Jernick, J., & Simmons-Morton, D. G. (2000). Incorporating physical activity into primary care: Physician-delivered advice within the activity counseling trial. *American Journal of Preventive Medicine, 18*(3), 225–234.

American Society on Aging. (2003). *CDC backgrounder: Crucial issues in elder health: What the CDC is doing to prevent and protect.* Retrieved May 30, 2003, from http://www.asaging.org/media/pressrelease.cfm?id=36.

Andersen, R. E., Blair, S. N., Cheskin, L. J., & Bartlett, S. J. (1997). Encouraging patients to become physically active. *Annals of Internal Medicine, 127*(5), 395–400.

Associated Press. (2004, February 10). Doctors urged to discuss fitness with their patients. Retrieved February 15, 2004, from http://www.usatoday.com/news/health/2004-02-10-doctors-fitness_x.htm.

Balde, A., Figueras, J., Hawkins, D. A., & Miller, J. R. (2003). Physician advice to the elderly about physical activity. *Journal of Aging and Physical Activity, 11*(1), 90–97.

Bridgeland, J. M., Goldsmith, S., & Lenkowsky, L. (2003). Service and the Bush administration's civic agenda. In E. J. Dionne, K. M. Drogosz, & R. E. Litan (Eds.), *United we serve: National service and the future of citizenship* (pp. 52–59). Washington, DC: Brookings Institution Press.

Bull, F. C., & Jamrozik, K. (1998). Advice on exercise from a family physician can help sedentary patients to become active. *American Journal of Preventive Medicine, 15*(2), 85–94.

Bureau of Labor Statistics. (2004). *Volunteering in the United States, 2004.* Retrieved December 17, 2004, from http://www.bls.gov/news.release/volun.nr0.htm.

California Health and Human Services Agency. (2003). *Strategic plan for an aging California population.* Retrieved May 20, 2004, from http://www.chhs.ca.gov/SB910/SB910.html.

California Integrated Elder Care and Involvement Act. (2002). SB 953. Retrieved May 20, 2004, from http://info.sen.ca.gov/pub/01–02/bill/sen/sb_0951–1000/sb_953_bill_20020915_chaptered.html.

California Strategic Plan on Aging Advisory Committee. (2004). *Planning for an aging California population: Preparing for the "aging baby boomers."* Retrieved June 1, 2004, from http://www.calaging.org/works/work_preparing.html.

Callahan C. M., & McHorney, C. A. (2003). Successful aging and the humility of perspective. *Annals of Internal Medicine, 139*(5, Pt. 2), 389–390.

Canadian Ethnocultural Council. (2002). *Ethnic seniors and healthy aging: Perceptions, practices, and needs.* Retrieved November 1, 2004, from http://www.ethnicaging.ca/Healthyaging/01.asp.

Center for the Advancement of Health. (2001). *Integration of health behavior counseling in routine medical care.* Retrieved January 2, 2001, from http://www.prescriptionforhealth.org/dowloads/integration2001.pdf.

Center for Health Communication, Harvard School of Public Health. (2004). *Reinventing aging: Baby boomers and civic engagement.* Boston: Author.

Centers for Disease Control and Prevention. (2002a). *Promoting active lifestyles among older adults.* Retrieved June 20, 2003, from http://www.cdc.gov/nccdphp/dnpa/physical/pdf/lifestyles.pdf.

Centers for Disease Control and Prevention. (2002b). Prevalence of health-care providers asking older adults about their physical activity levels: United States, 1998. *Morbidity and Mortality Weekly Report, 51*(19), 412–414.

Centers for Disease Control and Prevention. (2003a). Public health and aging. *Morbidity and Mortality Weekly Report, 52*(6), 101–106.

Centers for Disease Control and Prevention. (2003b). *The power of prevention: Reducing the health and economic burden of chronic disease.* Atlanta, GA: Department of Health and Human Services, Centers for Disease Control and Prevention.

Centers for Disease Control and Prevention. (2004a). *Healthy aging.* Retrieved November 18, 2004, from http://www.cdc.gov/aging.

Centers for Disease Control and Prevention. (2004b). *Healthy aging: Preventing dis-*

ease and improving quality of life Among older Americans. Retrieved December 1, 2004, from http://www.cdc.gov/nccdphp/aag/aag_aging.htm.

Cherry, D. K., Burt, C. W., & Woodwell, D. A. (2003). *National ambulatory Medicare care survey: 2001 summary: Advance data from vital and health statistics.* Hyattsville, MD: National Center for Health Statistics.

Choi, L. H. (2003). Factors affecting volunteerism among older adults. *Journal of Applied Gerontology, 22*(2), pp. 179–196.

Civic Ventures. (2002). *Recasting retirement: New perspectives on aging and civic engagement.* San Francisco: Author.

Corporation for National and Community Service. (2004a). *Testimony before the House Appropriations Subcommittee on Labor, Health and Human Services, Education, and Related Agencies, March 17, 2004.* Retrieved July 12, 2004, from http://www.nationalservice.org/news/davideisner/031704.html.

Corporation for National and Community Service. (2004b). *Corporation for national and community service FY 2004 performance and accountability report, Washington, D.C.* Retrieved December 1, 2004, from http://www.nationalservice.org/pdf/about/reports/par2004.pdf.

Cutler, N. E., Whitelaw, N. A., & Beattie, B. L. (2002). *American perceptions of aging in the 21st century.* Washington, DC: National Council on Aging.

Damush, T. M., Stewart, A. L., Mills, K. M., ing, A. C., & Ritter, P. L. (1999). Prevalence and correlates of physician recommendations to exercise among older adults. *Journal of Gerontology: Medical Sciences, 54A,* M423–M427.

Eakin, E. G., Brown, W. J., Marshall, A. L., Mummery, K., & Larsen, L. (2004). Physical activity promotion in primary care: Bridging the gap between research and practice. *American Journal of Preventive Medicine, 2004, 27*(4), 297–303.

Elley, C. R., Kerse, N., Arroll, B., & Robinson, E. (2003). Effectiveness of counseling patients on physical activity in general practice: Cluster randomized controlled trial. *British Medical Journal, 326,* 793–798.

Estabrooks, P. A., Glasgow, R. E., & Dzewaltowski, D. A. (2003). Physical activity promotion through primary care. *Journal of the American Medical Association, 289*(22), 2913–2916.

Federal Interagency Forum on Aging-Related Statistics. (2004). *Older Americans 2004: Key indicators of well-being: Federal interagency forum on aging-related statistics.* Washington, DC: U.S. Government Printing Office.

Fincham, J. E., & Wertheimer, A. L. (1986). Predictors of patient satisfaction in a health maintenance organization. *Journal of Health Care Marketing, 6*(3), 5–11.

Fitzner, K., Madison, M., Caputo, N., Brown, E., French, M., Bondi, M., & Jennings, C. (2002). Promoting physical activity: A profile of health plan programs and initiatives. *Managed Care Interface, 15*(12), 29–41.

Freedman, M. (1999). *Prime time: How baby boomers will reinvent retirement and revolutionize America.* New York: Public Affairs.

Freedman, M., & Gomperts, J. (2004, October 6). When I'm 64: Beatles refrain doesn't age well. *USA Today.* Retrieved from http://www.usatoday.com/news/opinion/editorials/2004-10-06-freedman-gomperts_x.htm.

Fried, L. P., Carlson, M. C., Freedman, M., Frick, K. D., Glass, T. A., Hill, J., McGill,

S., Rebok, G. W., Seeman, T., Tielsch, J., Wasik, B. A., & Zeger, S. (2004). A social model for health promotion for an aging population: Initial evidence on the Experience Corps model. *Journal of Urban Health: Bulletin of the New York Academy of Medicine, 81*(1), 64–78.

Fries, J. F. (1980). Aging, natural death and the compression of morbidity. *New England Journal of Medicine, 303,* 130–136.

Fries, J. F. (2002). Reducing disability in older age. *Journal of the American Medical Association, 288,* 3164–3166.

Fries, J. F. (2003). Measuring and monitoring success in compressing morbidity. *Annals of Internal Medicine, 139,* 455–459.

Gartland, J. P. (2001). *Senior Corps volunteer participation: An effective means to improve life satisfaction.* Retrieved November 1, 2003, from www.nationalserviceresources .org/filemanager/download/459/gartland.pdf.

Gerontological Society of America. (2004). *The Gerontological Society of America announces initiative on civic engagement in an older America.* Retrieved November 30, 2004, from http://www.geron.org/press/engagement.htm.

Goodwin, M. A., Zyzanski, S. J., Zronek, S., Ruhe, M., Weyer, S. M., Konrad, N., Esola, D., & Stange, K. C. (2001). A clinical trial of tailored office systems for preventive service delivery: The Study to Enhance Prevention by Understanding Practice (STEP-UP). *American Journal of Preventive Medicine, 21*(1), 20–28.

Governor's Office on Service and Volunteerism. (2001). *The giving years: Engaging the time, talent, and experience of older Californians in intergenerational service.* Retrieved May 20, 2004, from http://www.csc.ca.gov/aboutgs/reports.asp.

Greenfield, E. A., & Marks, N. F. (2004). Formal volunteering as a protective factor for older adults' psychological well-being. *Journal of Gerontology: Social Sciences, 59,* S258–S264.

Hinterlong, J., Morrow-Howell, N., & Sherraden, M. (2001). Productive aging: Principles and perspectives. In N. Howell, J. Hinterlong, & M. Sherraden (Eds.), *Productive aging: Concepts and challenges* (pp. 3–18). Baltimore: Johns Hopkins University Press.

HMO Workgroup on Care Management. (2002). Improving the care of older adults with common geriatric conditions. Washington, DC: AAHPF Foundation.

Independent Sector. (2000). *America's senior volunteers.* Washington, DC: Author.

Institute of Medicine Committee on Assuring the Health of the Public in the 21st Century, Board on Health Promotion and Disease Prevention. (2002). *The future of the public's health in the 21st century.* Washington, DC: National Academies Press.

International Council on Active Aging. (2003a). *Health trend makes physical and fiscal sense.* Retrieved January 10, 2004, from http://www.icaa.cc/PressInfo/ healthtrends.htm.

International Council on Active Aging. (2003b). *Organizations call on healthcare providers to help older Americans live healthier, more active lives.* Retrieved January 10, 2004, from http://www.icaa.cc/PressInfo/calltoaction.htm.

King, R. (1996). Volunteerism by the elderly as an intervention for promoting successful aging. In R. G. Stone (Ed.), *Gerontology manual.* Retrieved June 29, 2003, from http://otpt.ups.edu/Gerontological_Resources/Gerontology_Manual/King-R.html.

Kreuter, M. W., Shobhina, S. G., & Bull, F. C. (2000). How does physician advice influence patient behavior? Evidence for a priming effect. *Archives of Family Medicine, 9*, 426–433.

Lindbloom, D. (2001). *Baby boomers and the new age of volunteerism.* Retrieved January 15, 2004, from www.nationalserviceresources.org/filemanager/download/465/lindblom.pdf.

Little, P., Everitt, H., Williamson, I., Warner, G., Moore, M., Gould, C., Ferrier, K., & Payne, S. (2001). Preferences of patients for patient-centered approach to consultation in primary care: Observational study. *British Medical Journal, 322*(7284), 468–472.

Magee, M. (2004). Boomer corps: Activating seniors for national service. *Progressive Policy Institute.* Retrieved January 30, 2004, from www.ppionline.org/documents/Boomer_Corps_0104.pdf.

Manson, J. E., & Greenland, P. (2004). The escalating pandemics of obesity and sedentary lifestyle. *Archives of Internal Medicine, 164*, 249–258.

Marcus, B. H., Goldstein, M. G., Jette, A., Simkin-Silverman, L., Pinto, B. M., Milan, F., Washburn, R., Smith, K., Rakowski, W., & Dube, C. E. (1997). Training physicians to conduct physical activity counseling. *Preventive Medicine, 26*, 382–388.

Martinson, B. C., Crain, L., Pronk, N. P., O'Connor, P. J., & Maciosek, M. V. (2003). Changes in physical activity and short-term changes in health care charges: A prospective cohort study of older adults. *Preventive Medicine, 37*(4), 319–326.

Merck Institute of Aging & Health. (2002). *The state of aging and health in America.* Retrieved January 21, 2003, from http://www.miahonline.org/resources/reports.

Merck Institute of Aging & Health. (2004a). *The state of aging and health in America.* Retrieved November 30, 2004, from http://www.miahonline.org/resources/reports.

Merck Institute of Aging & Health. (2004b). *Survey by Merck Institute of Aging & Health shows doctors don't always provide older adults with adequate information on diet and exercise.* Retrieved May 4, 2004, from http://www.miahonline.org/press/content/4_24_04_survey.html.

Miller, W. M., & Thoresen, C. E. (2003). Spirituality, religion, and health: An emerging research field. *American Psychologist, 58*(1), 24–35.

Morey, M. C., & Sullivan, R. J., Jr. (2003). Medical assessment for health advocacy and practical strategies for exercise initiation. *American Journal of Preventive Medicine, 25*(3, Suppl. 2), 204–208.

Morrow-Howell, N., Hinterlong, J., Rozario, P. A., & Tang, F. (2003). Effects of volunteering on the well-being of older adults. *Journal of Gerontology: Social Sciences, 58B*(3), S137–S145.

Morrow-Howell, N., Hinterlong, J., Sherraden, M., & Rozario, P. (2001). Advancing research on productivity in later life. In N. Howell, J. Hinterlong, & M. Sherraden (Eds.), *Productive aging: Concepts and challenges* (pp. 285–311). Baltimore: Johns Hopkins University Press.

Musick, M., Herzog, A. R., & House, J. S. (1999). Volunteering and mortality among older adults: Findings from a national sample. *Journal of Gerontology: Social Sciences, 54B*, S173–S180.

National Center for Health Statistics. (2004). *Health, United States: With chartbook on trends in the health of Americans.* Hyattsville, MD: Author.

National Council on Aging. (2003). *NCOA launches RespectAbility.* Retrieved June 15, 2004, from http://www.respectability.org/whatshappening/news.html.

Nied, R. J., & Franklin, B. (2002). Promoting and prescribing exercise for the elderly. *American Family Physician, 65*(3), 419–426.

O'Connor, P. J., Rush, W. A., Prochaska, J. O., Pronk, N. P., & Boyle, R. G. (2001). Professional advice and readiness to change behavioral risk factors among members of a managed care organization? *American Journal of Managed Care, 7,* 125–130.

O'Connor, P. J., Rush, W. A., Rardin, K. A., & Isham, G. (1996). Are HMO members willing to engage in two-way communications to improve health? *HMO Practice, 10*, 17–19.

Olson, E. (2004, April 13). Medicine: Testing the idea that helping out is healthy. *New York Times.*

Oman, D., Thoresen, C. A., & McMahon, K. (1999). Volunteerism and mortality among the community-dwelling elderly. *Journal of Health Psychology, 4*, 301–316.

Parker-Pope, T. (2004, June 28). Work may hold one key to a longer life. *Wall Street Journal.*

Partnership for Prevention. (2002). *Promoting physical activities in communities: Forward-looking options from an executive roundtable.* Washington, DC: Author.

Peter D. Hart Research Associates. (2002). *Making commitment to community service: Older Americans set a new priority for retirement.* San Francisco: Civic Ventures.

Pinto, B. M., Goldstein, M. G., DePue, J. D., & Milan, F. B. (1998). Acceptability and feasibility of physician-based counseling: The PAL project. *American Journal of Preventive Medicine, 15*(2), 95–102.

Pinto, B. M., Goldstein, M. G., & Marcus, B. H. (1998). Activity counseling by primary care physicians. *Preventive Medicine, 27*, 506–513.

Powell, S. M. (2004, June 16). Boomers' key to long life? Volunteering, study says. *Seattle Post-Intelligencer.* Retrieved October 20, 2004, from http://seattlepi.nwsource.com/health/177958_volunteer16.html.

Prisuta, R. (2004). Enhancing volunteerism among aging boomers. In *Reinventing aging: Baby boomers and civic engagement* (pp. 47–89). Boston: Harvard School of Public Health, Center for Health Communication.

Putnam, R. (2000). *Bowling alone: The collapse and revival of American community.* New York: Simon and Schuster.

Ramakrishnan, S. K., & Baldassare, M. (2004). *The ties that bind: Changing demographics and civic engagement in California.* San Franciso: Public Policy Institute of California.

Robert Wood Johnson Foundation. (2001). *National blueprint: Increasing physical activity among adults age 50 and over.* Princeton, NJ: Author.

Rosen, R. (2004, May 24). Share your experience. *San Francisco Chronicle.*

Rouse, S., & Clawson, B. (1992). Motives and incentives of older adult volunteers. *Journal of Extension On-line, 30*(3). Retrieved March 15, 2004, from http://www.joe.org/joe/1992fall/a1.html.

Rowe, J. W., & Kahn, R. L. (1998). *Successful aging.* New York: Pantheon.

Schauffler, H. H., Rodriguez, T., & Milstein, A. (1996). Health education and patient satisfaction. *Journal of Family Practice, 42*(1), 62–68.

Schneider, E. L., & Miles, E. (2003). *AgeLess: Take control of your age and stay youthful for life.* Emmaus, PA: Rodale.

Seniors Corps. (2003). *Senior Corps seeks 100,000 volunteers for America's communities.* Retrieved September 20, 2003, from http://www.volunteerfriends.org/pressroom.asp.

Sloan, R. P., Bagiella, E., VandeCreek, L., Hover, M., Casalone, C., Jinpu Hirsch, T., Hasan, Y., Kreger, R., & Poulos, P. (2000). Should physicians prescribe religious activities? *New England Journal of Medicine, 342,* 1913–1916.

Smedley, B. D., & Syme, L. S. (2000). *Promoting health: Intervention strategies from social and behavioral research.* Washington, DC: National Academy Press.

Strange, K. C., Woolf, S. H., & Gjeltema, K. (2002). One minute for prevention: The power of leveraging to fulfill the promise of health behavior counseling. *American Journal of Preventive Medicine, 22*(4), 320–323.

Syme, S. L. (2003). Psychosocial interventions to improve successful aging. *Annals of Internal Medicine, 139*(5, Pt. 2), 400–402.

Urban Institute. (2004). *Volunteer management capacity in America's charities and congregations: A briefing report.* Washington, DC: Author.

U.S. Department of Health and Human Services. (1996). Physical Activity and Health: A report of the Surgeon General. Atlanta, GA: Centers for Disease Control.

U.S. Department of Health and Human Services. (2000). *Healthy people 2010: Understanding and improving health* (2nd ed.). Washington, DC: U.S. Government Printing Office.

U.S. Department of Health and Human Services. (2002). *Physical activity fundamental to preventing disease.* Retrieved June 30, 2003, from http://aspe.hhs.gov/health/reports/physicalactivity/index.shtml.

U.S. Department of Health and Human Services. (2004). *Medicare preventive benefits begin January 2005 with a goal of healthier seniors.* Retrieved November 10, 2004, from http://www.hhs.gov/news/press/2004pres/20041109.html.

Whitlock, E. P., Orleans, C. T., Pender, N., & Allan, J. (2002). Evaluating primary care behavioral counseling interventions: An evidence-based approach. *American Journal of Preventive Medicine, 22*(4), 267–384.

Wilber, K. H., Allen, D., Shannon, G. R., & Alongi, S. (2003). Partnering managed care and community-based services for frail elders: The Care Advocate Program. *Journal of the American Geriatrics Society, 51,* 807–812.

Wilson, J., & Musick, M. (1999). The effects of volunteering on the volunteer. *Law and Contemporary Problems, 62*(4), 141–168. Retrieved July 1, 2003, from http://www.law.duke.edu/journals/lcp/articles/lcp62dAutumn1999p141.htm.

Yarnall, K. S. H., Pollak, K. I., Ostbye, T., Kause, K. M., & Michener, J. L. (2003).

Primary care: Is there enough time for prevention? *American Journal of Public Health, 93*(4), 635–641.

Yum, T. Y., & Lightfoot, E. (2005). The effects of volunteering on the physical and mental health of older people. *Research on Aging, 27*(1), 31–55.

Zaslow, J. (2003, February 3). The granny patrol: Florida cops recruit elderly volunteers. *Wall Street Journal.*

PART II

The Contribution of Altruistic
Emotions to Health

Introduction

Stephen G. Post
Brie Zeltner

Based on the presentations in the previous part, it appears plausible to assert (with various caveats) that an association exists between volunteerism, on the one hand, and well-being, health, and possibly longevity, on the other. In this part, the focus shifts away from altruistic actions per se to interpretations of benevolent emotions in relation to happiness and health. Here, then, attention shifts to the positive psychology of altruistic emotions, including various models of how such emotions connect with health.

In "The Biology of Positive Emotions and Health," Andrea H. Marques and Esther M. Sternberg provide a summary of the existing literature on the biological pathways and mechanisms involved in social interactions and positive emotions and their potential relationship to enhanced health. In the first three sections of their chapter, the authors focus on the substantial body of research on the neural pathways of affiliative behavior, maternal-infant bonding, pair bonding, parental care, and some sexual behavior. The neurobiology of these systems has been largely worked out, and they may also play a role in the neurobiology of positive emotions and behaviors like altruism, spirituality (prayer and meditation), and exercise, where research has only just begun. Neurotransmitters and hormones, such as dopamine, oxytocin, prolactin, vasopressin, and glucocorticoids, will most likely play important roles in the biology of these processes and will help to explain a health connection in that all have implications for the immune system and stress response. The authors note that there will undoubtedly be a mix of genetic and environmental influences on the neurobiology underlying positive emotions and behavior, and their connections to health will interact differently in each individual. In the last section of their chapter, the authors explain the biology of the placebo effect and hypothesize that the powerful effects of classical conditioning (learning to associate a certain outcome with a stimulus) may be an intermediate link between positive emotions or behavior and enhanced health.

Jeff Levin, in "Integrating Positive Psychology Into Epidemiologic Theory: Reflections on Love, Salutogenesis, and Determinants of Population Health," provides a tour de force overview of what we know. The author's goal in this chapter is to advocate the integration of positive psychology into the field of epidemiology to promote the study of the health effects of virtues, such as love, hope, gratitude, forgiveness, and optimism. Traditional epidemiological methods can be applied to this pursuit, but the historical pathogenic focus of the field as well as confusion about population-level versus individual-level analyses have prevented any significant progress in the area. To remedy this, Levin advances the concept of salutogenesis, introduced by Antonovsky in the 1980s, as the framework for the study of the impact of positive emotions and prosocial tendencies on health. Resetting epidemiology's focus to salutogenesis and coherence (a global sense of the meaning of events and behaviors in a person's life) forces researchers to develop a theory of coping and to address not how people become ill (pathogenesis), but how they become well again. It is important to note that health is not simply the absence of disease, and salutogenesis is not simply the opposite of pathogenesis. The study of positive psychosocial constructs may necessitate an entirely different level of analysis and a different direction through the natural history of disease, as well as measurement of a different class of variables. In the second half of the chapter, the author reviews five different theoretical perspectives in psychosocial epidemiology and how the study of love fits within their frameworks. Each of the five theories addresses the influence of the psyche on human health, and the effects of loving kindness or prosocial behavior fit naturally into their study, particularly in the areas of mind-body medicine and the stress paradigm. In conclusion, the author believes that positive psychology can be successfully integrated into epidemiologic theory and will allow for the study of the potentially salutogenic effect of positive psychosocial "exposures," like love or altruism, on a population level.

George E. Vaillant, in "Generativity: A Form of Unconditional Love," uses the Study of Adult Development, Harvard Medical School's 60-year prospective study of the lives of college and inner-city men, to answer two questions about generativity. First, should the Eriksonian concept of generativity be distinguished from the human capacity for warm relationships, and second, does generativity lead to improved physical health in later life? The author begins by defining generativity not only as assuming responsibility for the growth and well-being of others, but also as community building and mentoring to the next generation, and he points out that generative relationships often require much greater maturity than does simple loving attachment. The author uses the examples of two men from the study's inner-city cohort to show that generativity is not dependent upon social privilege and that generative individuals do not always live long, healthy lives. The Study of Adult Development began in 1940 and followed 268 Harvard sophomores and 456 disadvantaged Boston teens until age 75, prospectively gathering information on their health and ability to work and love across the lifespan. The participants were rated on generativity (defined as a stable career identity and stable intimate relationship coupled with taking responsibility for the next generation), their capacity for warm relationships, and their life-coping skills (such as altruism, suppression, anticipation, humor). The author found evidence that volunteering increases longevity, but the effect was erased when alcoholism was taken into account. Generativity was strongly associated with mental health and the capacity for warm relationships, which were in turn associated with physical health. Yet, generativity itself was not associated with objective physical health. To explain the complicated relationships among generativity, altruism, and health, Vaillant concludes that generativity may be crucial to "aging well" but may not reduce mortality because it is more closely connected to maturity, which has little to do with physical health.

Bita Ghafoori and Robert Hierholzer, in "The Roles of Love, Attachment, and Altruism in the Adjustment to Military Trauma," summarize current research on the associations among love, attachment, altruism, and posttraumatic stress disorder (PTSD). PTSD occurs in some people after exposure to severe trauma and results in a persistent reexperiencing of the trauma, numbing of responsiveness, increased arousal, and avoidance behavior. PTSD invariably leads to relationship dysfunction because of a restricted range of affect and the sense of detachment of the sufferer from those around him. There is some evidence that both attachment style and altruistic intent are related to the development of PTSD. Attachment refers to the basic universal bond between child and caregiver that is formed in the earliest days of life and can either lead to a sense of security and confidence (secure attachment) or feelings of mistrust, rejection, and unease (insecure attachment), depending on the quality of the initial bond formed. Secure attachment enhances health and subjective well-being, and insecure attachment has been linked to stress response syndromes and higher levels of anxiety and depression. Positive, secure loving attachments enhance self-confidence and confidence in one's social network to provide support in times of stress. In their own work and in other recent studies, the authors have found evidence that securely attached people are less susceptible to PTSD and that, while childhood attachment styles tend to be persistent across the lifespan, they can be disrupted by severe trauma, making current attachments to a spouse or loved ones more relevant to PTSD. In terms of altruistic intent, the authors believe that secure attachment styles may be a prerequisite for the ability to act altruistically and to care for and empathize with others. This could explain why some studies have shown that those with higher levels of altruistic intent are less susceptible to PTSD, and further research in the area may find a place for volunteer-style intervention programs designed to strengthen a person's natural resistance to trauma.

Deborah D. Danner, Wallace V. Friesen, and Adah N. Carter, in "Helping Behavior and Longevity: An Emotion Model," present a possible mechanism—positive emotions—to account for the positive health outcomes of helping behavior. They believe that future-oriented positive emotions (like hope and optimism) form the basis of attitudes that lead to certain repeated choices in one's use of time and energy throughout life. These choices, which mostly involve choosing to spend one's time in pursuits that increase positive affect, are accompanied by physiological and cardiovascular responses that can extend life and improve health. The basis for this hypothesis came from the authors' review of the Nun Study, in which they found that sisters who expressed more positive emotions in their youth lived longer than those who expressed less. The authors have chosen to focus on older adults because there are more studies of helping behavior in this population; older adults have more time to devote to helping behavior; and research has shown that older adults increasingly choose to participate in activities that produce positive emotions (Carstensen, 1992). The authors believe that positive emotions must be of lasting duration to have an effect on health and that the particular positive emotions associated with helping behavior are those of motivation. Further, they argue that appraisal is one of the biggest challenges facing research on helping behavior because appraisal of need, the capacity to help, the recipient's willingness to receive, and the effectiveness of the relationship are critical to the emotional experience of helping. Despite the fact that there is significant research documenting the health impacts of positive emotions, research on helping behavior has generally focused on the decision to help, or not, and the motives behind helping behavior. Researchers must pay more attention to the emotions involved in all stages of the helping process as well as the helper's appraisal of her experience in order to better understand the health impacts of helping behavior. Because of the interrelatedness of positive emotion and helping behavior, integration of their study will no doubt lead to the better understanding of both.

Charlotte V. O. Witvliet and Michael E. McCullough, in "Forgiveness and Health: A Review and Theoretical Exploration of Emotion Pathways," address altruism in the manifestation of forgiveness. In this chapter, the authors address the possible positive health effects of forgiveness, which they define as an unusual expression of altruistic love that can only occur after a person has first suffered harm from an offender. Forgiveness is an act of gift giving to the undeserving offender that attempts to overcome injustice with goodness and potentially to edge out negative feelings associated with the transgression with prosocial emotions like empathy, compassion, and love. Based on emotion theory, they identify forgiveness as a positively valent low-arousal emotion (like peace and calm) and the opposite, "unforgiveness," as a negatively valent high-arousal emotion (like fear and anger). Using the dynamical systems neurovisceral integration model, we can view the emotional process of forgiveness as one of inhibition, a healthy interruption of the negative response of rumination or grudge bearing in response to transgression. The authors see forgiveness as an antidote to negative responses to transgression, and they present research on the negative health effects of hostility, stress, rumination, and suppression along with ways in which forgiveness can counter these effects. By promoting reappraisal of the offense, forgiveness encourages a response shift that decreases the original offense's emotional impact and inhibits the negative effects of preoccupation with self by promoting other-regarding love. Research on forgiveness has shown beneficial effects on mental health (better self-reported health, more positive emotions, more life satisfaction, reduced anxiety and depression, higher self-esteem) and physical health (lower cardiovascular reactivity and stress levels) of forgiving attitudes as compared to rumination and grudge bearing. Although extant research in the area of forgiveness and physical health can only speak to an immediate response (captured in the laboratory setting), the authors believe that because forgiveness reduces unforgiveness and because unforgiveness has been linked to sustained physiological activation (increased stress), it is reasonable to expect that forgiveness also has sustained health effects.

Marivic Dizon, Lisa D. Butler, and Cheryl Koopman, in "Befriending Man's Best Friends: Does Altruism Toward Animals Promote Psychological and Physical Health?" recommend that we care for pets. The authors discuss animal-directed altruism and the growing body of literature documenting psychosocial and physical health benefits of the human-animal relationship. The human-animal bond, a dynamic relationship between people and animals, most likely stems from a wider sense of kinship with nature and has led to our befriending and adoption of animals first as beasts of burden and then as pets. In the mental health area, studies have shown that pets act as social support to their owners, enhance social contact by facilitating communication and contact with other people, and may help to foster a sense of empathy and compassion for other animals, nature, and human beings. All of these services may contribute to improved mental health in human beings. Further, companion animals have been used in many settings as psychosocial interventions that improve the quality of life for the sick and socially isolated in nursing homes and that provide a sense of direction and meaning in life to inmates in prisons. There is also ample evidence that pet presence and interaction can lower stress, promote relaxation, and lower blood pressure. Further study is needed, however, to document and test any possible long-term effects of pet ownership on mortality. In conclusion, the authors identify several research questions that merit further study, including the influence of species on the benefits of the human-animal relationship, the impact of negative animal treatment on the perpetrator, and human-animal affinity as people's attempt to recognize their interdependence with nature in an age of increasing isolation from our environment.

9   The Biology of Positive
    Emotions and Health

Andrea H. Marques
Esther M. Sternberg

Among the ancient Greeks, the concept that mind and emotions could affect the course of illness was not only accepted, but assumed. Throughout the centuries, this assumption has waxed and waned, in relation to available scientific theories and technologies. In recent decades, the biological pathways underpinning emotions and disease have been explained due to advances in molecular and cellular biology, genetics, neuroscience, and brain imaging. These have revealed the many bidirectional connections between the neural and neuroendocrine systems and the immune system (Dantzer, 2003; Sternberg, 2000b). Many studies also have shown that a variety of physical and psychosocial stressors can alter immune responsiveness, which may lead to increased susceptibility to disease (Herbert & Cohen, 1993a, 1993b; Marques-Deak, Cizza, et al., 2005; Zorrilla, Luborsky, et al., 2001). Most recently, severe emotional stress has also been shown to precipitate reversible "stress cardiomyopathy" in patients without coronary disease (Brandspiegel, Marinchak, et al., 1998; Pavin, Le Breton, et al., 1997; Wittstein, Thiemann, et al., 2005). This syndrome consists of myocardial stunning precipitated by acute stress, which is associated with an exaggerated sympathetic adrenergic response (Wittstein, Thiemann, et al., 2005).

Much recent research in this field has focused on psychobiological models of resilience to stress and the influence of positive emotions on health (Charney, 2004; Miller & Wood, 1997). Interestingly, resilience studies have revealed a consistent pattern of individual characteristics associated with successful adaptation to stress. These include the effective self-regulation of emotion and attachment behaviors, a positive self-concept, optimism, altruism, good intellectual function, a capacity to convert traumatic helplessness into learned helpfulness, and an active coping style in confronting a stressor (Masten & Coatsworth, 1998; Richardson & Waite, 2002). Moreover, a diversity of social factors, such as religiousness, spirituality, social support, sociability, and altruistic behavior, has been shown both to help patients to cope with illness and also to be related to better health outcomes (Cohen, Doyle, et al., 2003;; House, Landis, et al., 1988; Irwin, 2002; Koenig, George, et al., 2004a; Koenig, George, et al., 2004b; Schwartz, Meisenhelder, et al., 2003).

Epidemiological studies have shown that religiousness and spirituality are associated with fewer depressive symptoms (Koenig, George, et al., 2004b), and longitudinal studies have described that religiousness predicts faster remission from depression in elderly patients (Idler & Kasl, 1997; Koenig, George, et al., 1998). Moreover, depressive symptoms have been shown to predict worse health outcomes in a sample of elderly medical in-patients (Koenig, Shelp, et al., 1989). In the last few decades, depression has been associated with alterations in the neuroendocrine system and immune function (Herbert & Cohen, 1993a; Zorrilla, Luborsky, et al., 2001). Although decreased immune system activity has been found in patients with depression, the clinical implications of these findings are still controversial in diseases such as cancer and infection (Irwin, 2002).

Religiousness and spirituality have also been associated with greater social support, better psychological health, and better health status in a large sample of older hospitalized patients (Koenig, George, et al., 2004a). The authors suggested that this may be related to the fact that religious beliefs help patients to accept and understand their medical conditions, which in turn may help them to integrate health changes into their lives. Moreover, religious practices can help patients to relax and to deal with loneliness and isolation during hospitalization (Koenig, George, et al., 2004a).

Social support is another factor that has been associated with a better health status and well-being (House, Landis, et al., 1988). Increased sociability has been shown to be associated with a decreased probability of developing viral rhinitis (the common cold) in a group of healthy subjects (Cohen, Doyle, et al., 2003), independent of baseline immunity, stress hormones, and health practices. One possible explanation is that sociability could be determined by genes that contribute to both sociability and biological processes that lead to greater ability to fight infections (Cohen, Doyle, et al., 2003). Sociability could also lead to a better health status as it could increase positive and decrease negative affect, promote healthier practices, and provide more social support (Uchino, Cacioppo, et al., 1996). Also, one of the personality traits found in people with increased sociability is extraversion, which reflects an individual's preferences for social settings. This personality dimension has been associated with low resting levels of electrocortical and sympathetic nervous system (SNS) activity (Geen, 1997). This correlation could explain why subjects with extraversion traits had reduced susceptibility to common cold viruses (Broadbent, Broadbent, et al., 1984; Cohen, Doyle, et al., 1997; Totman, Kiff, et al., 1980) (see the section below on SNS and immune response).

Psychosocial factors have also been related with better outcomes in diseases such as cancer (House, Landis, et al., 1988) and asthma (Miller & Wood, 1997). Emotional support has been associated with longer survival after a diagnosis of cancer, while patients with hopelessness and depression showed rapid morbidity and mortality (Spiegel, 2002). Stress responses can suppress some aspects of antitumor immunity (Antoni, 2003; Cohen & Rabin, 1998; Kiecolt-Glaser, Robles, et al., 2002), and emotional support may decrease the stress of having a cancer diagnosis. Conversely, chronic stress and depression have been linked to dysregulation of circadian rhythms (Chrousos, 1998; Deuschle, Schweiger, et al., 1997), which have also been associated with early mortality in patients with breast cancer (Chrousos, 1998; Deuschle, Schweiger, et al., 1997; Sephton, Sapolsky, et al., 2000; Sephton & Spiegel, 2003).

Positive emotional responses have also been associated with better pulmonary function in children (Miller & Wood, 1997) and adults (Kubzansky, Wright, et al., 2002), while negative emotional responses are associated with decreased pulmonary function (Miller & Wood, 1994). Emotional factors may influence the course of asthma by activating physiologic pathways (cholinergic system) implicated in the pathophysiology of the asthmatic process (airway reactivity) (Miller & Wood, 1994, 1997).

Finally, altruistic behaviors, such as engaging in helping others, have also been associated with higher levels of mental health (Schwartz, Meisenhelder, et al., 2003). Imaging studies have revealed that both altruistic cooperation and altruistic punishment are associated with activation of the reward neural pathways, which are mediated by dopamine (de Quervain, Fischbacher, et al., 2004; Fehr & Rockenbach, 2004; O'Doherty, 2004). Interestingly, genetic studies have found an association between altruistic behavior and polymorphisms in the dopaminergic receptor genes (DRD4 and DRD5 genes) (Bachner-Melman, Gritsenko, et al., 2005). Conversely, a different variant in the same gene (DDR4) has also been found in patients with attention deficit hyperactivity disorder, often comorbid with antisocial behavior (Faraone, Doyle, et al., 2001). These studies suggest that the balance between DDR4 gene variants may contribute to diverse behavioral phenotypes in the human population from altruistic behavior to more aggressive or perhaps antisocial types (Bachner-Melman, Gritsenko, et al., 2005).

In this chapter, we will summarize some possible biological pathways related to social interactions and positive emotions, and we will examine how those factors are associated with the improvement of health.

NEURAL AND NEUROENDOCRINE PATHWAYS OF AFFILIATIVE BEHAVIOR, SOCIAL INTERACTION, AND MATERNAL BEHAVIOR: DOPAMINE, OXYTOCIN, VASOPRESSIN, AND PROLACTIN

Evolutionary biology studies in brain behavior have hypothesized that the emergence of the thalamocingulate limbic system in the brain of mammals was associated with a new pattern of behavior related to social interactions (MacLean, 1990). In his work, MacLean speculated that drug addiction was an attempt to replace endogenous factors normally provided by social attachments, such as maternal behavior and pair bonding. Therefore, both conditions could share a common neurobiological pathway (MacLean, 1990). The neurobiology of reward has been largely elucidated from studies of addiction or substance abuse, and several lines of evidence implicate the mesocorticolimbic dopamine in addiction processes (Insel, 2003). The mesocorticolimbic pathway includes the ventral tegmental area (VTA), the nucleus accumbens, the ventral pallidum, and the thalamus. Thalamic projections activate the prefrontal and cingulate cortex, which in turn provide feedback to the VTA (Everitt & Wolf, 2002). (See Figures 9.1 and 9.2.) Dopamine is one of the main neurotransmitters modulat-

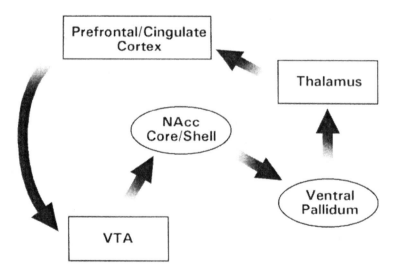

Figure 9.1. Putative reward circuit. Cartoon shows basic reward pathways from midbrain dopamine cell bodies in the ventral t tegmental area (VTA) to the nucleus accumbens (NAcc) which project via the ventral pallidum to the thalamus. There is a broad thalamic projection to the prefrontal and cingulate cortex which complete this loop with projections to the VTA. The VTA projects directly to cortex and amygdala in addition to the NAcc (not shown). Reprinted with permission from Physiology & Behavior.

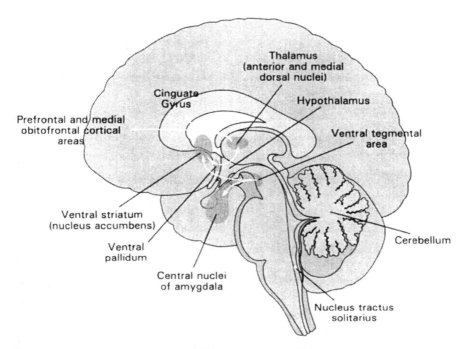

Figure 9.2. Anatomical locations of brain regions underpinning positive emotional behaviors: hypothalamus and mesocorticolimbic area. The following regions compromise the mesocorticolimbic area: ventral tegmental area, nucleus accumbens, ventral pallidum, thalamus, prefrontal cortex and cingulate cortex.

ing activity in this circuit (Nestler, 2001), and oxytocin (OT) and vasopressin (AVP) are the main neurohormones that activate this circuit.

Many studies have shown that dopamine mesocorticolimbic pathways mediate mother-infant interactions in rats (Hansen & Ferreira, 1986; Lee & Voogt, 1999; Lonstein, Simmons, et al., 1998; Stack, Balakrishnan, et al., 2002) and pair bonding in voles (Gingrich, Liu, et al., 2000; Wang, Yu, et al., 1999). Moreover, studies have suggested that OT and AVP play important roles in behaviors associated with monogamy, affiliation, paternal care, and pair bonding (Cho, DeVries, et al., 1999; Gingrich, Liu, et al., 2000; Insel, Winslow, et al., 1995; Wang, Yu, et al., 1999; Winslow, Hastings, et al., 1993; Young, Toloczko, et al., 1999). Sex steroid hormones have also been shown to control mating-behavior circuits through binding to nuclear receptors in ventromedial hypothalamic neurons that invoke regulation of gene expression (Mong & Pfaff, 2004; Pfaff 1999). Other hormones, neuropeptides, and neurotransmitters have also been implicated in the modulation of affiliative behaviors; they include prolactin, serotonin, endogenous opioids, and norepinephrine (Altemus, 1995; Keverne, Martensz, et al., 1989; Lightman & Young, 1989; Moskowitz, Pinard, et al.,

2003; Nelson & Panksepp, 1998; Stern, Goldman, et al., 1973). These will not be discussed here, but are reviewed extensively elsewhere (Graves, Wallen, et al., 2002; Insel & Winslow, 1998; Mong & Pfaff, 2003, 2004; Moskowitz, Pinard, et al., 2001; Moskowitz, Pinard, et al., 2003; Nelson & Panksepp, 1998; Ogawa, Robbins, et al., 1996; Pfaff 1999).

Animal and Human Studies of OT and AVP

OT and AVP are produced in the hypothalamus, among other sites, and stored in the pituitary. Peripherally, OT mediates the milk ejection during lactation and uterine contraction during parturition (Carter & Altemus, 1997), while AVP promotes reabsorption of water in the kidney. AVP is released after osmotic alteration, and both OT and AVP are released after vaginocervical stimulation (Gainer & Wray, 1994).

OT release is associated with different stimuli, including nipple stimulation, parturition, estrogen, progesterone, and certain social interactions, such as genital stimulation and sexual activity in some species (Carter, 1992; Mitchell & Schmid, 2001). In mammals, OT is described as being involved in the sexual behaviors of voles (Mahalati, Okanoya, et al., 1991), the onset of maternal care in rats (Insel, Young, et al., 1997), bonding between mother and infant in sheep (Kendrick, Da Costa, et al., 1997), social affiliations in rats (Witt, Winslow, et al., 1992), and pair bonding in voles (Insel, Winslow, et al., 1995), and OT has an inhibitory effect on aggressive behavior in rats (Giovenardi, Padoin, et al., 1997).

AVP acts within the central nervous system modulating various behaviors, including learning, memory, and social behaviors (Engelmann, Wotjak, et al., 1996; Le Moal, Dantzer, et al., 1987; Pitkow, Sharer, et al., 2001; Winslow, Hastings, et al., 1993; Young, Toloczko, et al., 1999). The influence of the AVP and OT system on social behavior in animals has been shown in studies comparing two rodent species: montane voles, which are nonmonogamous and show low social contact and only maternal care, as compared to prairie voles, which are monogamous, with high social contact and biparental care (Young, Wang, et al., 1998). Affiliative and attachment behavior are increased only in male prairie voles after the central administration of AVP, but not in montane voles after administration of AVP and OT (Winslow, Hastings, et al., 1993). Interestingly, the prairie vole exhibits a higher density of AVP (ventral pallidum) and OT receptors (nucleus accumbens and prelimbic cortex) in reward pathways than does the montane vole (Young, Toloczko, et al., 1999). In female prairie voles, the central infusion of OT facilitates the development of partner preference in the absence of mating (Insel, Winslow, et al., 1995), and infusion of a selective antagonist before mating blocks the formation of partner preference without interfering with mating (Insel, Winslow, et al., 1995). Thus, in male prairie voles, AVP is critical for partner preference formation, while in

Table 9.1. Behavior and Brain Functions That Comprise Different Elements of Positive Emotional and Social Interactions, Including Different Aspects of Love, Altruistic Behavior, and Empathy. Brain Pathways and Neurotransmitters Underpinning These Behaviors Are Also Listed. Illnesses Associated with Dysregulations in These Behaviors, Brain Pathways, or Neurotransmitters Are Also Shown.

Behavior/Function	Brain Pathways	Neurotransmitter/ Neurohormone	Illness	References
Reward Figures 9.1 and 9.2	Mesocorticolimbic area (VTA, NA, VP, thalamus, pre-frontal and cingulate cortex)	Dopamine	Addiction	Insel et al., 2003
Affiliation/attachment Pair bonding Figures 9.1 and 9.2	Hypothalamus Mesocorticolimbic area	OT (F), AVP (M) Dopamine	Autism (V1aR)	Insel et al., 1992 Carter & Altemus, 1997 Wassink et al., 2004
Maternal behavior Figures 9.1 and 9.2	Mesocorticolimbic	OT, prolactin	OCD	Altemus et al., 1992 Leckman et al., 1994 Pfaff, 1999
Sexual behavior Figure 9.3	Hypothalamus (ventromedial nucleus)	E, P, T		Mong et al., 2003 Mong &Pfaff, 2004
Empathy	Limbic system, cerebellum, frontal and temporal regions	Dopamine Serotonin Glutamate	Autism	Kemper & Bauman, 1993 Farrow et al., 2001 Preston, 2002 Harris, 2003
Initative behavior Empathy	"Mirror neurons" (humans) Parietal, premotor cortex, Broca's area, superior temporal sulcus		Echolalia/echopraxia Autism	Grafton et al., 1996 Rizzolatti et al., 1996 Fogassi et al., 1998 Iacoboni et al., 1999
Sickness behavior (social isolation) Figures 9.2 and 9.3	Choroid plexus, NTS, MPA, SN, amygdala	Interleukins	Depression	Young et al., 1998 Dantzer, 2003

Note: Ventral tegmental area (VTA); nucleus accumbens (NA); ventral pallidum (VP); oxytocin (OT); vasopressin (AVP); female (F); male (M); AVP receptor 1aR (V1aR); obsessive-compulsive disorder (OCD); estrogen (E); progesterone (P); testosterone (T); nucleus tractus solitarius (NTS); medial preoptic area (MPA); supraoptic nucleus (SN).

females, OT is responsible for affiliative behavior (Insel, 2003). OT has also been described to be involved in passive stress-coping strategies in rats during acute stress, by inhibiting the action of excitatory amino acids (glutamate and aspartate) released during stress (Ebner, Bosch, et al., 2005).

AVP acts through three receptor subtypes (V1a, V1b, and V2), each of which is associated with different actions (Bielsky, Hu, et al., 2004). The V1a receptor has been described to be critical in social recognition (Bielsky, Hu, et al., 2004; Dantzer, Bluthe, et al., 1987; Everts & Koolhaas, 1999) and anxiety-like behavior, such as repetitive grooming (Bielsky, Hu, et al., 2004; Landgraf, Gerstberger, et al., 1995; Meisenberg, 1988). AVP has been associated with increased aggressive behavior, increased attention, arousal, and sympathetic functions (Carter & Altemus, 1997), although it has also been related to anxiolytic effects (Appenrodt, Schnabel, et al., 1998; Landgraf, Gerstberger, et al., 1995).

Animal and Human Studies of Prolactin

Prolactin has been implicated in maternal behavior. Prolactin is a powerful antistress hormonal, and it is important in maternal milk production (Bridges & Ronsheim, 1990). It is produced by the pituitary gland and is regulated by hypothalamic factors and also by the stimulus of suckling (Carter & Altemus, 1997). Animal and human studies of females in the lactation state have shown a reduction in the production of stress hormones after exposure to stress (Altemus, Deuster, et al., 1995; Lightman & Young, 1989; Stern, Goldman, et al., 1973), reduction of heart rate and galvanic skin response (Weisenfeld, Malatesta, et al., 1985), and reduction in behavioral responses to stress (Hansen & Ferreira, 1986). Both prolactin and oxytocin have also been related, in animal studies, to anxiolytic effects (Neumann, Kromer, et al., 2000), enhanced social interactions (Witt, Winslow, et al., 1992), and suppressed stress hormonal responses in a stress situation (Neumann, Kromer, et al., 2000). There are some possible physiological mechanisms mediating the decreased stress response in lactating women, including GABA (gamma-aminobutyric acid, which is known to inhibit the stress response) and estrogen (which increases the stress response) (Handa, Nunley, et al., 1994; Qureshi, Hansen, et al., 1987). Interestingly, stress inhibits lactation (Newton & Newton, 1948), while lactation reduces the stress response. Therefore, during lactation, lowering the stress response may be an effective way of conserving energy needed for milk production. Moreover, it can minimize the psychological arousal or anxiety associated with the demands of the newborn (Altemus, 1995). Indeed, it has been demonstrated that anxiety symptoms are reduced during lactation in women with anxiety disorder (Klein, 1994). Furthermore, lowering the stress response can also enhance immune function, as an overactive stress response can suppress the immune system.

GENETIC AND ENVIRONMENTAL FACTORS

Maternal-Offspring Interactions in Early Development

Animal models have yielded important information regarding the relative contribution of genetics and environment on maternal behavior and pup responses in adult life (Gomez-Serrano, Tonelli, et al., 2001; Levine, 2001; Schmidt, Oitzl, et al., 2002; Winslow, Noble, et al., 2003). Mother-offspring interactions early in life have been shown to influence social behavior and endocrine stress responses in rats and monkeys. These have also been shown in humans (Gomez-Serrano, Tonelli, et al., 2001; Levine, 2001; Rutter, Andersen-Wood, et al., 1999; Weaver, Cervoni, et al., 2004; Winslow, Noble, et al., 2003; Zhang, Parent, et al., 2004).

Differential maternal behavior has been shown in inbred Lewis (LEW/N) and Fisher (F344N) rats, which also exhibit differential hypothalamic-pituitary-adrenal (HPA) axis responses and related differential inflammatory susceptibility and resistance (Sternberg, Hill, et al., 1989; Sternberg, Young, et al., 1989). In cross-fostering studies using these strains, some behavioral and neuroendocrine responses to stress have been shown to be mediated by both genetic and nongenetic factors, including differential rearing conditions (Gomez-Serrano, Tonelli, et al., 2001). In this model, pup gender also plays a role in determining the set point of the adult neuroendocrine stress response.

Another model of maternal effects in early development that has been extensively studied is based on a normal range of maternal licking and grooming. In these studies, the rate of maternal licking and grooming has been associated with the development of individual differences in behavioral and HPA responses to stress (Caldji, Diorio, et al., 2003; Francis, Diorio, et al., 1999; Zhang, Parent, et al., 2004). The offspring of high licking and grooming (LG) mothers show reduced activation of the stress response (HPA axis), increased expression of cortisol receptors, enhanced cortisol negative feedback sensitivity (Liu, Diorio, et al., 1997), decreased startle responses, increased open field exploration (Francis, Diorio, et al., 1999), increased density of central benzodiazepine receptors in the brain areas associated with fear (Caldji, Diorio, et al., 2003), increased sensitivity to benzodiazepines, and less fearfulness (Fries, Moragues, et al., 2004). Cross-fostering studies have shown that offspring of low-LG mothers reared by mothers with high-LG behavior resemble the offspring of high-LG mothers, and vice versa (Francis, Diorio, et al., 1999). These findings suggest that variations in maternal behavior can influence gene expression. In fact, maternal behavior has been described as altering a regulatory region of the glucocorticoid (GC) receptor gene by inducing methylation—one stable mechanism that suppresses gene expression (Weaver, Cervoni, et al., 2004). Pups that were neglected at birth also show increased levels of methylation in the promoter region of the receptor gene. This potentiates the suppression of the GC receptor gene, leading to fewer GC receptors and decreased HPA axis sensitivity to cortisol negative feedback (Weaver, Cervoni, et al., 2004). Cross-fostering studies in rats have also shown that the same pattern of GC receptor methylation was associated with the rearing mother pattern and not with the biological mother pattern (Francis, Diorio, et al., 1999).

Taken together, these data suggest that rearing conditions are associated with altered stress responsiveness and social behavior in adult life. Variations in maternal behavior have shown that environmental factors early in life can modulate genetic expression and individual stress reactivity.

Studies in primates have also demonstrated the influence of maternal interactions and offspring behavior. Male rhesus monkeys reared in a nursery away from the mother showed reduced social behavior, increased aggressive and solitary behavior, and high levels of stereotypy. Moreover, those offspring also had lower levels of oxytocin in their cerebrospinal fluid compared to mother-reared monkeys (Winslow, Noble, et al., 2003). An interaction of genetic background and early rearing conditions has also been shown in primates with polymorphisms in the serotonin transporter gene regulatory region (5-HTTLPR) (Champoux, Bennett, et al., 2002). Both mother-reared and nursery-reared rhesus macaque monkeys with hererozygous phenotypes of 5-HTTLPR(l/s) showed increased distress compared to homozygotes (l/l), indicating a genetic effect. Conversely, lower orientation scores were observed only in nursery-reared infants with the hererozygous phenotype of 5-HTTLPR(l/s). Finally, human studies have show that polymorphisms in the 5-HTTLPR are also associated with different levels of serotonin transporter expression and serotonin-mediated behavior and personality traits (Lesch & Mossner, 1998). Furthermore, human infants raised in extremely socially deprived environments have also been described as exhibiting decreased social interactions and some of the features of autism (Rutter, Andersen-Wood, et al., 1999).

Human Disorders Associated With Impaired Social Behavior

These data from animal studies have provided important information for understanding similar disorders in humans in which social behavior is impaired, such as autism and anxiety-related disorders, including obsessive-compulsive disorder (OCD). Autism is a developmental disorder characterized by deficits in communication, impaired social interactions, and repetitive, stereotyped motor and behavioral activity. Recent studies have found a polymorphism (Kim, Young, et al., 2002) and evidence of linkage disequilibrium (Wassink, Piven, et al., 2004) in the AVP receptor gene (V1aR) in autistic patients. Although it is not clear whether these alterations contribute to causing the disease, the AVP system remains a candidate for exploration in autistic disorder.

Another neurobiological characteristic observed in autism is related to difficulties in copying actions and imitation-like phenomena, such as echolalia (imitation of words or phrases) and echopraxia (imitation of actions). The dysregulated activation of mirror neurons has been proposed to explain these behaviors in patients with autism (Williams, Whiten, et al., 2001). Mirror neurons are a group of neurons that show activity in relation to both observed and executed actions (Harris, 2003). This concept was first described in monkeys, in which neurons from the prefrontal cortex area were activated not only when the monkey performed a certain action, but also when the monkey was watching the same action being performed by another individual (Williams, Whiten, et al., 2001). It is thought that other brain regions, such as the orbitofrontal cortex (Stevens, Fonlupt, et al., 2000) and motor pathways (Rizzolatti & Arbib, 1998), may operate to inhibit the action. It has also been speculated that mirror neurons may play a role in the imitation of the social interactions that characterize empathy and that early developmental alterations in such mirror neurons may be responsible for the impairment in social abilities and the lack of empathy (Williams, Whiten, et al., 2001) seen in autism. Anatomic studies in patients with autism have also shown alterations in the limbic system and cerebellum, which may be related to impaired social abilities, including lack of empathy (Kemper & Bauman, 1998).

Alterations in the AVP and OT system have also been associated with other psychiatric disorders, such as obsessive-compulsive disorder (Scantamburlo, Ansseau, et al., 2001). Some studies have found elevated AVP (Altemus, Pigott, et al., 1992) and oxytocin (Leckman, Goodman, et al., 1994) in the cerebrospinal fluid of patients with OCD. One study of patients with OCD also reported that the AVP-OT ratio was negatively correlated with symptom severity (Swedo, Leonard, et al., 1992), although normal oxytocin levels have also been reported (Altemus, Jacobson, et al., 1999). Thus, the AVP system may provide novel therapeutic targets for those disorders associated with social impairment and anxiety, although further investigation in humans is required (Bielsky, Hu, et al., 2004).

BIOLOGICAL PATHWAYS LINKING POSITIVE EMOTIONS AND AFFILIATIVE BEHAVIORS WITH BETTER HEALTH OUTCOMES

As is clear from the previous section of this chapter, the neurobiology of affiliative behaviors has been well worked out, including the neural pathways, brain regions, and neurohormones and neurotransmitters involved. In addition, it is clear

from epidemiological and clinical studies that positive emotions, affiliative behaviors, and salubrious activities (such as prayer, meditation, exercise, and happy
memories) are associated with better health outcomes. However, the biological pathways linking these positive emotions and behaviors with improved immune responses and health are less clear. This section will outline several neural
and neuroendocrine pathways that mediate the effects of positive emotions and
affiliative behaviors on immune responses and health. These include the activation of neural and neuroendocrine pathways that modulate and attenuate the
negative effects of stress responses on immunity, including acetylcholine, endogenous opioids, OT, prolactin, and GABA, as well as the release of endogenous
mediators that may directly positively affect immune responses (endogenous
opioids, dopamine, OT, AVP, and prolactin).

Finally, this section will describe the biology of the placebo effect, the process of active learning and association that allows positive actions and behaviors, and the mediators released to modify immune system responses and health.

Neural and Neuroendocrine Pathways of Positive Emotions and Affiliative Behaviors That Modulate the Stress Response and the Immune Response

The Biology of the Stress Response

The stress response results in the release of neurotransmitters and hormones that
serve as the brain's messengers for regulation of the immune and other systems.
The consequences of this response are generally adaptive in the short run, but
can be damaging when stress is chronic (Dhabhar & McEwen, 2001).

The primary neuroendocrine and neural components of the stress response
are the HPA axis and the sympathetic nervous system (see Figure 9.3). The main
anatomical components of the HPA axis are the paraventricular nucleus of the
hypothalamus, the anterior pituitary gland located at the base of the skull, and
the cortex of the adrenal gland. After exposure to stressful stimuli, the paraventricular nucleus of the hypothalamus produces and secretes the hormones
corticotrophin releasing hormone (CRH) and arginine vasopressin (AVP). In the
anterior pituitary gland, CRH, along with AVP, stimulates the expression and release of adrenocorticotropic hormone (ACTH), enkephalins, and endorphins.
ACTH then induces the adrenal glands to synthesize and release GCs (Tyrell, Finding, et al., 1994). Stress and CRH also activate the locus coeruleus-noradrenergic
center in the brainstem, which releases norepinephrine in noradrenergic brain
regions and in peripheral tissues through the SNS. Stress also stimulates the
production and release of catecholamines (epinephrine, norepinephrine, and
dopamine) from the adrenal medulla, a highly specialized part of the sympathetic nervous system. Studies have shown that there is a bidirectional positive
feedback loop between these systems. Thus, CRH and AVP activate the sym-

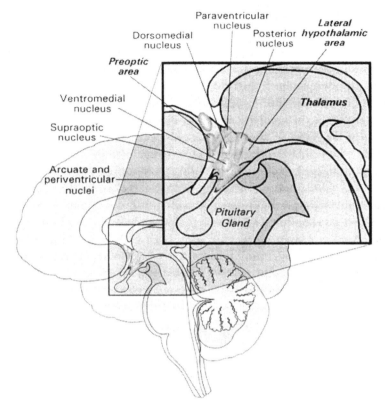

Figure 9.3. Hypothalamic nuclei involved in positive emotional behaviors.

pathetic nervous system and, conversely, norepinephrine stimulates the release of CRH (for reviews, see Gold, Goodwin, et al., 1988; Reiche, Nunes, et al., 2004; Sternberg, Chrousos, et al., 1992; Wilder, 1995).

The release of GCs from the adrenal cortex, catecholamines from the adrenal medulla, and norepinephrine from sympathetic nerve terminals prepares the individual to cope with the demands of metabolic, physical, and psychological stressors and serves as the brain's messengers for regulation of the immune and other systems (Elenkov, Wilder, et al., 2000). Generally, GCs inhibit the immune system, stimulating the immune cells to produce anti-inflammatory factors (anti-inflammatory cytokines) and inhibiting the production of pro-inflammatory factors (pro-inflammatory cytokines) (Chrousos, 2000; Madden, Sanders, et al., 1995; van der Poll, Coyle, et al., 1996). Cytokines are peptides synthesized by the immune system that play a crucial role in mediating inflammatory and immune responses, and they also serve as mediators between the immune and neuroendocrine systems.

Conversely, in the periphery, the immune system can be activated by pathogens and other injurious stimuli that enhance the production of pro-inflammatory cytokines. This leads to an acute inflammatory response that is normally limited by regulatory mechanisms, including the production of anti-inflammatory cytokines and stimulation of the HPA axis. Pro-inflammatory cytokines can cross the blood-brain barrier (BBB) at leaky points, such as at the organum vasculosum lamina terminalis, or median eminence, or they may be transported across the BBB (Banks, Satin, et al., 1995). Cytokines can also influence the brain by activation of secondary messengers, such as nitric oxide and prostaglandins (Elmquist, Scammell, et al., 1997). Finally, cytokines can also activate the HPA axis, through the cholinergic anti-inflammatory pathway, by stimulation of the vagus nerve, which is part of the parasympathetic nervous system (Tracey, 2002). Studies have also identified a common molecular basis for this central nervous system–immune system communication, with cells from the immune system producing and expressing receptors for hormones, neuropeptides, and neurotransmitters (Blalock, 1989; Cunningham, Wada, et al., 1992; Wong, Bongiorno, et al., 1995), and cells from the nervous system producing cytokines and expressing receptors for these molecules (Besedovsky, del Rey, et al., 1983; Goehler, Gaykema, et al., 2000; Goehler, Relton, et al., 1997; Watkins & Maier, 2005).

Thus, systemically, the immune response, through activation of the stress system, stimulates an important negative feedback mechanism that regulates susceptibility and resistance to autoimmune, inflammatory, infectious, and allergic diseases.

Neuronal and Hormonal Pathways Activated During Positive Emotions and Affiliative Behaviors: Direct and Indirect Effects on Immune Responses

Neurohormones, neuropeptides, and neurotransmitters released during positive emotional states can improve health by directly enhancing immune responses and/or by blocking or reducing the negative effects of stress responses on immunity. Molecules that suppress the stress responses (HPA axis) can enhance the immune response. Generally, this prepares the body to fight infections and injuries. However, if activation of the immune system is excessive, it can enhance susceptibility to autoimmune diseases and inflammatory diseases, such as arthritis, systemic lupus erythematosus, allergic asthma, and atopic dermatitis. Conversely, excessive activation of the HPA axis may predispose the host to more infection due to relative immunosuppression (Webster, Tonelli, et al., 2002).

Cortisol and catecholamines, which are released during activation of the HPA axis and SNS, respectively, normally inhibit the immune system. Although cortisol has generally been considered immunosuppressive (Fauci, 1979; Marx,

1995), recent studies have also shown that physiological concentrations of GCs exert immuno-modulating and immuno-enhancing effects (Wilckens, 1995). This dual dose-related effect of GCs has been shown in several assays of immune function, including delayed-type hypersensitivity (DTH) reactions (Dhabhar & McEwen, 1999); antibody production (Levo, Harbeck, et al., 1985); thymocyte proliferation and apoptosis (Whitfield, MacManus et al. 1970); T-cell mitogenesis (Wiegers, Reul, et al., 1994); macrophage phagocytosis (Forner, Barriga, et al., 1995); and cytokine production and receptor expression (Wiegers & Reul, 1998).

Effects of the Cholinergic Pathway on Immune Responses

While positive emotions may in part enhance health through inhibition of the negative effects of the stress response, they may also directly affect immunity through the cholinergic nervous system (parasympathetic system), which is activated during positive emotions (Miller & Wood, 1997). The parasympathetic nervous system and the sympathetic nervous system are the two branches of the autonomic nervous system. Acetylcholine is the principal parasympathetic neurotransmitter, while norepinephrine is the principal sympathetic neurotransmitter. Together, they continuously control many essential functions, often acting in opposition to mediate many physiological responses, although in some situations the two systems function synergistically (Tracey, 2002). While stimulation of the parasympathetic system is associated with slowing heart rate, induction of gastric mobility, dilation of arterioles, and constriction of pupils, activation of the SNS is associated with increased heart rate, constriction of arterioles, and dilation of pupils. In contrast, the effect of both systems on the immune response seems to be synergistic, resulting in an anti-inflammatory effect (Tracey, 2002). Moreover, activation of the sympathetic system during stress also stimulates the output of the parasympathetic system (Tracey, 2002).

The SNS innervates all lymphoid organs and through the action of catecholamines (norepinephrine and epinephrine) modulates several immune parameters. The adrenal medulla is a highly specialized part of the SNS that also releases epinephrine and norepinephrine (in a lower proportion) (Goldfien, 1994).

Catecholamines normally inhibit the production of pro-inflammatory cytokines and enhance the production of anti-inflammatory cytokines; however, under certain conditions, they may stimulate immune responses (Elenkov, Webster, et al., 1999; Elenkov, Wilder, et al., 2000; Sanders, Baker, et al., 1997). Denervation of lymph node noradrenergic fibers is associated with the exacerbation of inflammation (Lorton, Bellinger, et al., 1996; Lorton, Lubahn, et al., 1999), whereas systemic sympathectomy or denervation of joints is associated with a decreased severity of inflammation (Lorton, Lubahn, et al., 1999). Almost all immune cells express norepinephrine receptors (Sanders, Kasprowicz, et al., 2001; Sanders & Kohm, 2002). Stimulation of these receptors has been shown to maintain adequate levels of antibody production, decreased T-lymphocyte proliferation, and decreased release of pro-inflammatory cytokines by macrophages (for reviews, see Kohm & Sanders, 2001; Sanders & Kohm, 2002; van der Poll, Coyle, et al., 1996).

The activation of the parasympathetic nervous system via the cholinergic nerve fibers of the efferent vagus nerve results in the release of acetylcholine. In peripheral organs (spleen, heart, liver), acetylcholine attenuates the release of pro-inflammatory cytokines, but not anti-inflammatory cytokines (Borovikova, Ivanova, et al., 2000). Together with the afferent stimulation of the central nervous system via the sensory nerve fibers of the vagus nerve, this loop forms the "inflammatory reflex" (Czura & Tracey, 2005). Through this mechanism, inflammatory signals in the periphery (e.g., pro-inflammatory cytokines) rapidly activate the brain's anti-inflammatory cholinergic response. This mechanism can also activate the HPA axis, further enhancing the anti-inflammatory response via the production of cortisol (Pavlov & Tracey, 2004; Tracey & Warren, 2004). In summary, the actions of the parasympathetic and sympathetic systems in the immune response seem to be synergistic, leading to an anti-inflammatory effect.

Effects of Endorphins and Endogenous Opioids on Immune Responses

Another mechanism by which positive emotions may directly affect immunity is through the endogenous opiate system. Several studies have established a link between the positive emotional responses that occur following exercise and increased endogenous opiate production (Carr, Bullen, et al., 1981; Harte, Eifert, et al., 1995). An increase in endogenous opiates, OT, prolactin, and dopamine has been described in both humans and dogs during a positive human-dog interaction (Odendaal & Meintjes, 2003). Endogenous opioids have also been associated with analgesia, euphoria states, thermoregulation, blood pressure regulation, and modulation of fear (Bodnar & Klein, 2004; Osaki, Castellan-Baldan, et al., 2003).

Endorphins or endogenous opiates are neuropeptides synthesized in the anterior pituitary and in the periphery. The antinociceptive effects of opioids are mediated by opioid receptors in the brain and in the periphery (Vallejo, de Leon-Casasola, et al., 2004). The b-endorphins play a role in pain perception and are increased by stress and suppressed by GCs (Tyrell, Aron, et al., 1994). Opioid receptors are also expressed in immune cells (Carr, DeCosta, et al., 1989; Chuang, Killam, et al., 1995; Makman, 1994).

While exogenous opioids are associated with immunosuppression, endogenous opioids have been described as enhancing the immune response (Vallejo, de Leon-Casasola, et al., 2004). The acute and chronic administration of exogenous opioids is associated with altered antibody production (Bussiere, Adler, et al., 1992; Johnson, Smith, et al., 1982; Taub, Eisenstein, et al., 1991), suppressed delay-type hypersensitivity (Bryant & Roudebush, 1990; Molitor, Morilla, et al., 1992), suppressed antimicrobial resistance (Tubaro, Borelli, et al., 1983), increased pro-inflammatory cytokine (IL-6) production (Houghtling & Bayer, 2002), reduced leukocyte activities (Rogers, Steele, et al., 2000), and reduced "natural killer" (NK) cell activity (Shavit, Depaulis, et al., 1986). Conversely, endogenous opiates have been shown to enhance NK cell activity (Hsueh, Chen, et al., 1995). NK cells are important in viral infections and immunosurveillance. Opioids have also been shown to indirectly affect immune response by activation of the SNS (acute administration) and activation of the HPA axis (chronic administration) (Houghtling & Bayer, 2002; Vallejo, de Leon-Casasola, et al., 2004). In summary, exogenous opiates are associated with immunosuppression, while endogenous opioids enhance immunity.

Effects of Dopamine on Immune Responses

As described earlier in this chapter, dopaminergic pathways play a central role in mediating positive emotional responses. Numerous studies have also shown that dopamine has a direct role in the regulation of immune function (Basu & Dasgupta, 2000; Devoino, Alperina, et al., 1988; Neveu, 1993; Nistico, Caroleo, et al., 1994), and dopamine receptors are expressed in immune cells (Amenta, Bronzetti, et al., 1999; McKenna, McLaughlin, et al., 2002; Ricci, Veglio, et al., 1995). Direct effects of dopamine on immune cells have been described as having both suppressive and stimulatory effects (for review, see Basu & Dasgupta, 2000). Pharmacological and physiological doses of dopamine have been associated with the inhibition of pro-inflammatory cytokine production (IL-2, IL-4, IFN[3]) in *in vitro* studies (Ghosh, Mondal, et al., 2003), inhibition of T-lymphocyte proliferation (Cook-Mills, Cohen, et al., 1995; Ghosh, Mondal, et al., 2003; Morikawa, Oseko, et al., 1994; Saha, Mondal, et al., 2001), and induction of programmed cell death of T-lymphocytes (Bergquist, Tarkowski, et al., 1998; Offen, Ziv, et al., 1995). Moreover, dopamine injection into the brain, particularly into the caudate nucleus, has been associated with a reduced antibody response (Nanda, Pal, et al., 2005). Conversely, dopamine has also been described as enhancing many immune functions, including lymphocyte proliferation (Tsao, Lin, et al., 1997), enhancement of impaired cytokine production (IL-2) in patients with Parkinson's disease (Wandinger, Hagenah, et al., 1999), macrophage activation (Dasgupta & Lahiri, 1987; Sternberg, Wedner, et al., 1987), and stimulation of

NK cell activity (Deleplanque, Vitiello, et al., 1994; Won, Chuang, et al., 1995). It has also been shown to have a modulatory dose-related effect on apopotosis (Blandini, Cosentino, et al., 2004; Colombo, Cosentino, et al., 2003). Other immunological functions of dopamine include a selective inhibition of angiogenesis in stomach tumors, suggesting that dopamine could play a role in gastric cancer (Chakroborty, Sarkar, et al., 2004).

Hypo-dopaminergic activity of the central nervous system has been reported in patients with Parkinson's disease, while hyper-dopaminergic activity has been reported in patients with schizophrenia. Studies in patients with Parkinson's disease have shown a reduction in many immune parameters (Bokor, Farago, et al., 1992; Marttila, Eskola, et al., 1984). In contrast, immune activation is seen in patients with schizophrenia (Ganguli, Brar, et al., 1995; Maes, Bosmans, et al., 1995; Rabin, Ganguli, et al., 1988), although these findings have not been replicated in all studies (Arolt, Weitzsch, et al., 1997; Sperner-Unterweger, Barnas, et al., 1992). Interestingly, the use of haloperidol, a dopamine receptor antagonist in rats and mice, and the destruction of the caudate nucleus (an area rich in dopamine) in the rat brain are associated with the suppression of immune function (Devoino, Cheido, et al., 2003; Devoino, Idova, et al., 1994). In summary, dopamine has been shown to directly modulate many immune responses, and manipulation of dopaminergic brain pathways is also associated with changes in immune function.

Effects of OT, AVP, Prolactin, and Nitric Oxide on Immune Responses

As previously noted, OT and AVP mediate monogamy, affiliation, paternal care, and pair-bonding behaviors (Cho, DeVries, et al., 1999; Insel, Winslow, et al., 1995; Winslow, Hastings, et al., 1993; Young, Toloczko, et al., 1999), and prolactin plays a role in maternal behavior (Altemus, 1995; Lightman & Young, 1989; Stern, Goldman, et al., 1973). One way in which these neurohormones might affect immunity is through modulation of the stress response.

The release of OT in response to physical and psychological stress, peripherally and in certain brain areas, has been described (Ebner, Wotjak, et al., 2000; Engelmann, Ebner, et al., 1999; Gibbs, Vale, et al., 1984; Lang, Heil, et al., 1983; Wotjak, Ganster, et al., 1998). OT has been shown to suppress stress-induced HPA activity in male (Ebner, Bosch, et al., 2005; Neumann, Kromer, et al., 2000) and female (Neumann, 2001; Windle, Kershaw, et al., 2004; Windle, Shanks, et al., 1997) rats. OT release during stress could thus modulate the negative effects of stress responses on immunity. Few studies have described a direct action of OT on the immune system, but recently OT has been associated with cell survival in immature immune cells (Hansenne, Rasier, et al., 2004).

For many years, AVP was associated with activation of the HPA axis (Aubry, Turnbull, et al., 1997; Engelmann, Landgraf, et al., 2004; Sasaki, Watanobe, et al., 1995; Scott & Dinan, 1998). However, the role of AVP in the activation of the HPA axis has been recently debated in the literature (Engelmann, Landgraf, et al., 2004; Makara, Mergl, et al., 2004). Thus, an inhibitory effect of AVP has been shown, depending on its site of action and the type of stressor (for review, see Engelmann, Landgraf, et al., 2004), and in some studies AVP does not appear to activate the HPA axis in certain stress situations (for review, see Makara, Mergl, et al., 2004). AVP has also been implicated in activation of the sympathetic system (Antoni, 1993; Carter & Altemus, 1997; Engelmann, Landgraf, et al., 2004; Janiak, Kasson, et al., 1989). AVP may thus indirectly modulate the immune system via its effects on the HPA axis and sympathetic system.

AVP has been detected in immune tissues, where it exerts an immunomodulatory role (Baker, Richards, et al., 2003; Chowdrey, Lightman, et al., 1994; Geenen, Defresne, et al., 1988; Moll, Lane, et al., 1988). AVP has also been found in human lymphocytes (Ekman, Gobom, et al., 2001), and CRH and AVP have been shown to be coexpressed in the same subpopulation of immune cells (Baker, Richards, et al., 2003). Furthermore, AVP receptors have been found in a variety of immune cells (Bell, Adler, et al., 1992; Dardenne & Savino, 1994; Johnson & Torres, 1985). Thus, immune cells have the machinery to produce AVP and respond to it.

AVP derived from immune cells has been shown to act as a pro-inflammatory peptide in rats (Patchev, Mastorakos, et al., 1993), and it has also been implicated in lymphocyte activation (Bell, Adler, et al., 1992) and in the enhancement of pro-inflammatory cytokine production (INFg) (Johnson & Torres, 1985). Conversely, it has also been related to stress-induced immune suppression (Shibasaki, Hotta, et al., 1998) and is an indirect negative regulator of antibody production (Hu, Zhao, et al., 2003). Moreover, AVP and CRH have been shown to directly induce the production of ACTH (Reder, 1992) and endorphins (Kavelaars, Ballieux, et al., 1989) in lymphocytes.

Similarly to OT and AVP, prolactin has also indirect and direct effects on the immune system. Indirectly, it influences the HPA axis and the OT system (Carter & Lightman, 1987; Torner, Toschi, et al., 2002). Directly, it alters immune cell function through binding to receptors in these cells (Vera-Lastra, Jara, et al., 2002). Recently, an inhibitory role of prolactin on HPA axis responses to stress has been shown in male and nonlactating female rats (Torner, Toschi, et al., 2002), and in lactating rats (Torner, Toschi, et al., 2002). Prolactin has also been associated with decreased OT reactivity in response to stress (Torner, Toschi, et al., 2002). A direct effect of prolactin on immune function has also been described. In fact, immune cells synthesize and express receptors for prolactin (Bole-Feysot, Goffin, et al., 1998; Hiestand, Mekler, et al., 1986; Pellegrini, Lebrun, et al., 1992; Sabharwal, Glaser, et al., 1992; Yu-Lee, 2001). Prolactin has been associated with enhanced autoantibody production in mice (McMurray,

2001) and may play a role in the pathogenesis of some autoimmune diseases, such as systemic lupus erythematosus (SLE) (Peeva, Venkatesh, et al., 2004). Moreover, in vitro studies have shown that prolactin enhances lymphocyte proliferation (Hartmann, Holaday, et al., 1989), increases production of pro-inflammatory cytokines (INF g) (Cesario, Yousefi, et al., 1994), and increases production of nitric oxide and pro-inflammatory cytokines (IL-1) in macrophages (Kumar, Singh, et al., 1997). Nitric oxide (NO) is an oxygen radical produced by cells, which is associated with many important physiological and immunological effects. Recently, NO has been associated with antibacterial and antiviral action (for review, see Benz, Cadet, et al., 2002). Moreover, NO has been described as suppressing the activation of mast cells by antigens (Davis, Flanagan, et al., 2004). NO has also been shown to suppress the production of cytokines by mast cells and thus may play a role in the resolution of allergic processes (Davis, Flanagan, et al., 2004). An inhibitory role of NO in HPA axis activity has also been shown, and it is mediated by CRH, AVP, histamine, and the adrenergic and cholinergic systems (for reviews see Bugajski, Gadek-Michalska, et al., 2004; McCann, Kimura, et al., 2000). In summary, AVP, OT and prolactin modulate the immune system indirectly and directly. OT and prolactin both have inhibitory influences on the HPA axis and also directly activate immune cells.

Biology of the Placebo Effect: The Effects of Conditioning and Active Learning on Immune Responses

The process that links positive emotions to a positive effect on the immune system and thus to a positive health outcome is called the placebo effect. This effect involves learning. Positive emotional states can be triggered by different kinds of events and actions, including positive memories, prayer, social interactions, meditation, and even taking a pill. People learn to associate events, actions, and feelings. This form of learning, called classical conditioning, can become automatic (Ader, 1985; Ader & Cohen, 1993; Sternberg, 2000b). Both positive and negative associations can be learned. The effect of such conditioned responses on healing is termed the placebo effect. This effect is ubiquitous and occurs in relation to any medical therapy, since there is an expectation that medical treatment generally cures. Thus, some amount of improvement from any therapy comes from this learned expectation. It has been estimated that approximately one third of the effect of any medication is related to the placebo effect (Rosenthal & Oparil, 2002). In medical research, a placebo, or inert treatment, is used to estimate the biological effect of new pharmacological treatments. The degree of improvement on placebo treatment is subtracted from that associated with the test medication. The new medication must induce a greater improvement when compared to the placebo to be considered an effective therapy.

Such learned associations can also trigger the body's physiological responses, inducing the release of hormones, neuropeptides, and neurotransmitters, which can in turn affect the immune system (Dantzer, 2003; Sternberg, 2000a). The earliest evidence that the immune system could be conditioned was shown in the 1920s when a Russian investigator paired one conditioned stimulus (heat) with injection of a foreign protein that led to antibody production. Subsequently, the presentation of the conditioned stimulus (heat) alone also elicited antibody production (Ader & Cohen, 1992). In a classic experiment in 1970 in rats with SLE, using a taste-aversion conditioning paradigm, a saccharin solution was used as the conditioned stimulus and was paired with an injection of the immuno-suppressant cyclophosphamine. In these studies, the conditioned stimulus was found to induce immunosuppression even when the cyclophosphamide was withdrawn (Ader & Cohen, 1975). The individual or combined actions of hormones, neuropeptides, and neurotransmitters on the immune system may play a role in the process of immune conditioning. Although further studies are needed, it may be that conditioning is the intermediate process that links positive emotions with beneficial health effects through the different patterns of neuroendocrine and autonomic responses activated during these states (Ader & Cohen, 2001).

SUMMARY

In the last few decades, the bidirectional communication between the neuroendocrine system and the immune system has been elucidated. Hormones, neuropeptides, neurotransmitters, and cytokines all play an important role in the modulation of immune and neuroendocrine functions. This complex network involves numerous biological pathways, through which emotions can influence the balance between health and disease. Physical and psychosocial stress has been described as altering immune responsiveness and sometimes increasing susceptibility to disease. Conversely, epidemiological studies have shown the influence of positive emotions on disease and resilience. Social factors, such as religiousness, spirituality, social support, sociability, and altruistic behavior, have been shown to help patients to cope with illness and also have been related to better health outcomes. In this chapter, we summarized some biological pathways that link social interactions and positive emotions with immune response and improvement of health.

Neural and neuroendocrine pathways associated with social interactions, such as mother-infant interactions, monogamy, affiliation, paternal care, and pair bonding, have been extensively studied. Dopamine, oxytocin, vasopressin, and prolactin have been implicated in the modulation of affiliative behaviors,

although other molecules, such as serotonin, endogenous opioids, norepinephrine, and acetylcholine, have also been described. Several neural and neuroendocrine factors may mediate the effects of positive emotions and affiliative
behaviors on immune responses and health. These include neural and neuroendocrine factors that modulate and attenuate the stress responses' negative effects on immunity (acetylcholine, endogenous opioids, OT, prolactin, GABA)
and endogenous mediators that directly positively affect immune responses (endogenous opioids, dopamine, OT, AVP, prolactin). Finally, the biology of the
placebo, the process of active learning and conditioning of the immune response,
was discussed as a possible process linking positive emotional responses and
health.

REFERENCES

Ader, R. (1985). Conditioned taste aversions and immunopharmacology. *Annals of the New York Academy of Sciences, 443*, 293–307.

Ader, R., & Cohen, N. (1975). Behaviorally conditioned immunosuppression. *Psychosomatic Medicine, 37*(4), 333–340.

Ader, R., & Cohen, N. (1992). Conditioned immunopharmacologic effects on cell-mediated immunity. *International Journal of Immunopharmacology, 14*(3), 323–327.

Ader, R., & Cohen, N. (1993). Psychoneuroimmunology: Conditioning and stress. *Annual Review of Psychology, 44*, 53–85.

Ader, R., & Cohen, N. (2001). *Conditioning and immunity.* San Diego, CA: Academic.

Altemus, M. (1995). Neuropeptides in anxiety disorders: Effects of lactation. *Annals of the New York Academy of Sciences, 771*, 697–707.

Altemus, M., Deuster, P. A, Galliven, E., Carter, C. S., & Gold, P. W. (1995). Suppression of hypothalamic-pituitary-adrenal axis responses to stress in lactating women. *Journal of Clinical Endocrinology and Metabolism, 80*(10), 2954–2959.

Altemus, M., Jacobson, K. R., Debellis, M., Kling, M., Pigott, T., Murphy, D. L., & Gold, P. W. (1999). Normal CSF oxytocin and NPY levels in OCD. *Biological Psychiatry, 45*(7), 931–933.

Altemus, M., Pigott, T., Kalogeras, K. T., Demitrack, M., Dubbert, B., Murphy, D. L., & Gold, P. W. (1992). Abnormalities in the regulation of vasopressin and orticotropin releasing factor secretion in obsessive compulsive disorder. *Archives of General Psychiatry, 49*(1), 9–20.

Amenta, F., Bronzetti, E., Felici, L., Ricci, A., & Tayebati, S. K. (1999). Dopamine D2-like receptors on human peripheral blood lymphocytes: A radioligand binding assay and immunocytochemical study. *Journal of Autonomic Pharmacology, 19*(3), 151–159.

Antoni, F. A. (1993). Vasopressinergic control of pituitary adrenocorticotropin secretion comes of age. *Frontiers in Neuroendocrinology, 14*(2), 76–122.

Antoni, M. H. (2003). Psychoneuroendocrinology and psychoneuroimmunology of cancer: Plausible mechanisms worth pursuing? Brain Behavior, *and Immunity*, *17*(Suppl. 1), S84–91.

Appenrodt, E., Schnabel, R., & Schwarzberg, H. (1998). Vasopressin administration modulates anxiety-related behavior in rats. *Physiology & Behavior, 64*(4), 543–547.

Arolt, V., Weitzsch, C., Wilke, I., Nolte, A., Pinnow, M., Rothermundt, M., & Kirchner, H. (1997). Production of interferon-gamma in families with multiple occurrence of schizophrenia. *Psychiatry Research, 66*(2–3): 145–152.

Aubry, J. M., Turnbull, A. V., Pozzoli, G., Rivier, C., & Vale, W. (1997). Endotoxin decreases corticotropin-releasing factor receptor 1 messenger ribonucleic acid levels in the rat pituitary. *Endocrinology, 138*(4): 1621–1626.

Bachner-Melman, R., Gritsenko, I., Nemanov, L., Zohar, A. H., Dina, C., & Ebstein, R. P. (2005). Dopaminergic polymorphisms associated with self-report measures of human altruism: A fresh phenotype for the dopamine D4 receptor. *Molecular Psychiatry, 10*(4), 333–335.

Baker, C., Richards, L. J., Dayan, C. M., & Jessop, D. S. (2003). Corticotropin-releasing hormone immunoreactivity in human T and B cells and macrophages: Colocalization with arginine vasopressin. *Journal of Neuroendocrinology, 15*(11), 1070–1074.

Banks, W. A., Satin, A. J., & Broadwell, R. D. (1995). Passage of cytokines across the blood-brain barrier. *Neuroimmunomodulation, 2*, 241–248.

Basu, S., &. Dasgupta, P. S. (2000). Dopamine, a neurotransmitter, influences the immune system. *Journal of Neuroimmunology, 102*(2), 113–124.

Bell, J., Adler, M. W., & Greenstein, J. I. (1992). The effect of arginine vasopressin on the autologous mixed lymphocyte reaction. *International Journal of Immunopharmacology, 14*(1), 93–103.

Benz, D., Cadet, P., Mantione, K., Zhu, W., & Stefano, G. (2002). Tonal nitric oxide and health: Anti-bacterial and -viral actions and implications for HIV. *Medical Science Monitor: International Medical Journal of Experimental and Clinical Research, 8*(2), RA27–31.

Bergquist, J., Tarkowski, A., Ewing, A., & Ekman, R. (1998). Catecholaminergic suppression of immunocompetent cells. *Immunology Today, 19*(12), 562–567.

Besedovsky, H., del Rey, A., Sorkin, E., Da Prada, M., Burri, R., & Honegger, C. (1983). The immune response evokes changes in brain noradrenergic neurons. *Science, 221*(4610), 564–566.

Bielsky, I. F., Hu, S. B., Szegda, K. L., Westphal, H., & Young, L. (2004). Profound impairment in social recognition and reduction in anxiety-like behavior in vasopressin V1a receptor knockout mice. *Neuropsychopharmacology, 29*(3), 483–493.

Blalock, J. E. (1989). A molecular basis for bidirectional communication between the immune and neuroendocrine systems. *Physiological Reviews, 69*(1): 1–32.

Blandini, F., Cosentino, M., Mangiagalli, A., Marino, F., Samuele, A., Rasini, E., Fancellu, R., Tassorelli, C., Pacchetti, C., Martignoni, E., Riboldazzi, G., Calandrella, D., Lecchini, S., Frigo, G., & Nappi, G. (2004). Modifications of apoptosis-related protein levels in lymphocytes of patients with Parkinson's disease: The effect of dopaminergic treatment. *Journal of Neural Transmission, 111*(8), 1017–1030.

Bodnar, R. J., &. Klein, G. E. (2004). Endogenous opiates and behavior: 2003. *Peptides, 25*(12), 2205–2256.

Bokor, M., Farago, A., Schnabel R., & Garam, T. (1992). Relationship between the immune system and the diseases of the central nervous system. *Therapia Hungarica, 40*(2), 51–57.

Bole-Feysot, C., Goffin, V., Edery, M., Binart, N., & Kelly P. A. (1998). Prolactin (PRL) and its receptor: Actions, signal transduction pathways and phenotypes observed in PRL receptor knockout mice. *Endocrine Review, 19*(3), 225–268.

Borovikova, L. V., Ivanova, S., Zhang, M., Yang, H., Botchkina, G. I., Watkins, L. R., Wang, H., Abumrad, N., Eaton, J. W., & Tracey, K. J. (2000). Vagus nerve stimulation attenuates the systemic inflammatory response to endotoxin. *Nature, 405*(6785): 458–462.

Brandspiegel, H. Z., Marinchak, R. A., Rials, S. J., & Kowey, P. R. (1998). A broken heart. *Circulation, 98*(13): 1349.

Bridges, R. S., &. Ronsheim, P. M. (1990). Prolactin (PRL) regulation of maternal behavior in rats: Bromocriptine treatment delays and PRL promotes the rapid onset of behavior. *Endocrinology, 126*(2), 837–848.

Broadbent, D. E., Broadbent, M. H., Phillpotts, R. J., & Wallace J. (1984). Some further studies on the prediction of experimental colds in volunteers by psychological factors. *Journal of Psychosomatic Research, 28*(6), 511–523.

Bryant, H. U., & Roudebush, R. E. (1990). Suppressive effects of morphine pellet implants on in vivo parameters of immune function. *Journal of Pharmacology and Experimental Therapeutics, 255*(2), 410–414.

Bugajski, J., Gadek-Michalska, A., & Bugajski, A. J. (2004). Nitric oxide and prostaglandin systems in the stimulation of hypothalamic-pituitary-adrenal axis by neurotransmitters and neurohormones. *Journal of Physiology and Pharmacology, 55*(4), 679–703.

Bussiere, J. L., Adler, M. W., Rogers, T. J., & Eisenstein, T. K. (1992). Differential effects of morphine and naltrexone on the antibody response in various mouse strains. *Immunopharmacology and Immunotoxicology, 14*(3), 657–673.

Caldji, C., Diorio, J., & Meaney, M. J. (2003). Variations in maternal care alter GABA(A) receptor subunit expression in brain regions associated with fear. *Neuropsychopharmacology, 28*(11), 1950–1959.

Carr, D. B., Bullen, B. A., Skrinar, G. S., Arnold, M.A., Rosenblatt, M., Beitins, I. Z., Martin, J. B., & McArthur, J. W. (1981). Physical conditioning facilitates the exercise-induced secretion of beta-endorphin and beta-lipotropin in women. *New England Journal of Medicine, 305*(10), 560–563.

Carr, D. J., DeCosta, B. R., Kim, C. H., Jacobson, A. E., Guarcello, V., Rice, K. C., & Blalock, J. E. (1989). Opioid receptors on cells of the immune system: Evidence for delta- and kappa-classes. *Journal of Endocrinology, 122*(1), 161–168.

Carter, C. S. (1992). Oxytocin and sexual behavior. *Neuroscience and Biobehavioral Review 16*(2): 131–144.

Carter, C. S., & Altemus, M. (1997). Integrative functions of lactational hormones in social behavior and stress management. *Annals of the New York Academy of Sciences, 807*, 164–174.

Carter, D. A., & Lightman, S. L. (1987). Oxytocin responses to stress in lactating and hyperprolactinaemic rats. *Neuroendocrinology, 46*(6), 532–537.

Cesario, T. C., Yousefi, S., Carandang, G., Sadati, N., Le, J., & Vaziri, N. (1994). Enhanced yields of gamma interferon in prolactin treated human peripheral blood mononuclear cells. *Proceedings of the Society for Experimental Biology and Medicine, 205*(1), 89–95.

Chakroborty, D., Sarkar, C., Mitra, R. B., Banerjee, S., Dasgupta, P. S., & Basu, S. (2004). Depleted dopamine in gastric cancer tissues: Dopamine treatment retards growth of gastric cancer by inhibiting angiogenesis. *Clinical Cancer Research, 10*(13), 4349–4356.

Champoux, M., Bennett, A., Shannon, C., Higley, J. D., Lesch, K. P., & Suomi, S. J. (2002). Serotonin transporter gene polymorphism, differential early rearing, and behavior in rhesus monkey neonates. *Molecular Psychiatry, 7*(10), 1058–1063.

Charney, D. S. (2004). Psychobiological mechanisms of resilience and vulnerability: Implications for successful adaptation to extreme stress. *American Journal of Psychiatry, 161*(2), 195–216.

Cho, M. M., DeVries, A. C., Williams, J. R., & Carter, C. S. (1999). The effects of oxytocin and vasopressin on partner preferences in male and female prairie voles (Microtus ochrogaster). *Behavioral Neuroscience, 113*(5), 1071–1079.

Chowdrey, H. S., Lightman, S. L., Harbuz, M. S., Larsen, P. J., & Jessop, D. S. (1994). Contents of corticotropin-releasing hormone and arginine vasopressin immunoreactivity in the spleen and thymus during a chronic inflammatory stress. *Journal of Neuroimmunology, 53*(1), 17–21.

Chrousos, G. P. (1998). Ultradian, circadian, and stress-related hypothalamic-pituitary-adrenal axis activity: A dynamic digital-to-analog modulation. *Endocrinology, 139*(2), 437–440.

Chrousos, G. P. (2000). The stress response and immune function: Clinical implications. The 1999 Novera H. Spector Lecture. *Annals of the New York Academy of Sciences, 917*, 38–67.

Chuang, T. K., Killam, K. F., Jr., Chuang, L. F., Kung, H. F., Sheng, W. S., Chao, C. C., Yu, L., & Chuang, R. Y. (1995). Mu opioid receptor gene expression in immune cells. *Biochemical and Biophysical Research Communications, 216*(3), 922–930.

Cohen, S., Doyle, W. J., Skoner, D. P., Rabin, B. S., & Gwaltney, J. M., Jr. (1997). Social ties and susceptibility to the common cold. *Journal of the American Medical Association, 277*(24), 1940–1944.

Cohen, S., Doyle, W. J., Turner, R., Alper, C. M., Skoner, D. P., et al. (2003). Sociability and susceptibility to the common cold. *Psychological Science, 14*(5), 389–395.

Cohen, S., & Rabin, B. S. (1998). Psychologic stress, immunity, and cancer. *Journal of National Cancer Institute, 90*(1), 3–4.

Colombo, C., Cosentino, M., Marino, F., Rasini, E., Ossola, M., Blandini, F., Mangiagalli, A., Samuele, A., Ferrari, M., Bombelli, R., Lecchini, S., Nappi, G., & Frigo, G. (2003). Dopaminergic modulation of apoptosis in human peripheral blood mononuclear cells: Possible relevance for Parkinson's disease. *Annals of the New York Academy of Sciences, 1010,* 679–682.

Cook-Mills, J. M., Cohen, R. L., Perlman, R. L., & Chambers, D. A. (1995). Inhibition of lymphocyte activation by catecholamines: Evidence for a non-classical mechanism of catecholamine action. *Immunology, 85*(4), 544–549.

Cunningham, E. T., Jr., Wada, E., Carter, D. B., Tracey, D. E., Battey, J. F., & De Souza, E. B. (1992). In situ histochemical localization of type I interleukin-1 receptor messenger RNA in the central nervous system, pituitary, and adrenal gland of the mouse. *Journal of Neuroscience, 12*(3), 1101–1114.

Czura, C. J., & Tracey, K. J. (2005). Autonomic neural regulation of immunity. *Journal of Internal Medicine, 257*(2), 156–166.

Dantzer, R. (2003). Cytokines and sickness behavior. Ann Arbor, MI: Kluwer Academic.

Dantzer, R., Bluthe, R. M., Koob, G. F., & Le Moal, M. (1987). Modulation of social memory in male rats by neurohypophyseal peptides. *Psychopharmacology (Berlin), 91*(3), 363–368.

Dardenne, M., & Savino, W. (1994). Control of thymus physiology by peptidic hormones and neuropeptides. *Immunology Today, 15*(11), 518–523.

Dasgupta, P. S., & Lahiri, T. (1987). Stimulation of tumorcidal activity of peritoneal macrophage by dopamine treatment. *Medical Science Research, 15,* 1301–1302.

Davis, B. J., Flanagan, B. F., Gilfillan, A. M., Metcalfe, D. D., & Coleman, J. W. (2004). Nitric oxide inhibits IgE-dependent cytokine production and Fos and Jun activation in mast cells. *Journal of Immunology, 173*(11), 6914–6920.

Deleplanque, B., Vitiello, S., Le Moal, M., & Neveu, P. J. (1994). Modulation of immune reactivity by unilateral striatal and mesolimbic dopaminergic lesions. *Neuroscience Letters, 166*(2), 216–220.

de Quervain, D. J., Fischbacher, U., Treyer, V., Schellhammer, M., Schnyder, U., Buck, A., & Fehr, E. (2004). The neural basis of altruistic punishment. *Science, 305*(5688), 1254–1258.

Deuschle, M., Schweiger, U., Weber B., Gotthardt, U., Korner, A., Schmider, J., Standhardt, H., Lammers, C. H., & Heuser, I. (1997). Diurnal activity and pulsatility of the hypothalamus-pituitary-adrenal system in male depressed patients and healthy controls. *Journal of Clinical Endocrinology and Metabolism, 82*(1), 234–238.

Devoino, L., Alperina, E., & Idova, G. (1988). Dopaminergic stimulation of the immune reaction: Interaction of serotoninergic and dopaminergic systems in neuroimmunomodulation. *International Journal of Neuroscience, 40*(3–4), 271–288.

Devoino, L., Cheido, M., Alperina, E., & Idova G. (2003). Evidence for a role of dopaminergic mechanisms in the immunostimulating effect of mu-opioid receptor agonist DAGO. *International Journal of Neuroscience, 113*(10), 1381–1394.

Devoino, L., Idova, G., et al. (1994). Brain neuromediator systems in the immune response control: Pharmacological analysis of pre- and postsynaptic mechanisms. *Brain Research, 633*(1–2): 267–274.

Dhabhar, F. S., & McEwen, B. S. (1999). Enhancing versus suppressive effects of stress hormones on skin immune function. *Proceedings of the National Academy of Sciences of the United States of America, 96*, 1059–1064.

Dhabhar, F. S., & McEwen, B. S. (2001). *Bidirectional effects of stress and glucocorticoid hormones on immune function: Possible explanations for paradoxical observations.* San Diego, CA: Academic.

Ebner, K., Bosch, O. J., Kromer, S. A., Singewald, N., & Neumann, I. D. (2005). Release of oxytocin in the rat central amygdala modulates stress-coping behavior and the release of excitatory amino acids. *Neuropsychopharmacology, 30*(2), 223–230.

Ebner, K., Wotjak, C. T., Landgraf, R., Engelmann, M., et al. (2000). A single social defeat experience selectively stimulates the release of oxytocin, but not vasopressin, within the septal brain area of male rats. *Brain Research, 872*(1–2), 87–92.

Ekman, R., Gobom, J., Persson, R., Mecocci, P., Nilsson, C. L., et al. (2001). Arginine vasopressin in the cytoplasm and nuclear fraction of lymphocytes from healthy donors and patients with depression or schizophrenia. *Peptides, 22*(1), 67–72.

Elenkov, I. J., Webster, E. L., Torpy, D. J., & Chrousos, G. P. (1999). Stress, corticotropin-releasing hormone, glucocorticoids, and the immune/inflammatory response: Acute and chronic effects. *Annals of the New York Academy of Sciences, 876*, 1–11; discussion 11–13.

Elenkov, I. J., Wilder, R. L., Chrousos, G. P., & Vizi, E. S. (2000). The sympathetic nerve: An integrative interface between two supersystems: The brain and the immune system. *Pharmacological reviews, 52*(4), 595–638.

Elmquist, J. K., Scammell, T. E., & Saper, C. B. (1997). Mechanisms of CNS response to systemic immune challenge: The febrile response. *Trends in Neuroscience, 20*, 565–570.

Engelmann, M., Ebner, K., Landgraf, R., Holsboer, F., & Wotjak, C. T. (1999). Emotional stress triggers intrahypothalamic but not peripheral release of oxytocin in male rats. *Journal of Neuroendocrinology, 11*(11), 867–872.

Engelmann, M., Landgraf, R., & Wotjak, C. T. (2004). The hypothalamic-neurohypophysial system regulates the hypothalamic-pituitary-adrenal axis under stress: An old concept revisited. *Frontiers in Neuroendocrinology, 25*(3–4), 132–149.

Engelmann, M., Wotjak, C. T., Neumann, I., Ludwig, M., & Landgraf, R. (1996). Behavioral consequences of intracerebral vasopressin and oxytocin: Focus on learning and memory. *Neuroscience and Biobehavioral Reviews, 20*(3), 341–358.

Everitt, B. J., & Wolf, M. E. (2002). Psychomotor stimulant addiction: A neural systems perspective. *Journal of Neuroscience, 22*(9), 3312–3320.

Everts, H. G., & Koolhaas, J. M. (1999). Differential modulation of lateral septal vasopressin receptor blockade in spatial learning, social recognition, and anxiety-related behaviors in rats. *Behavioural Brain Research, 99*(1), 7–16.

Faraone, S. V., Doyle, A. E., Mick, E., & Biederman, J. (2001). Meta-analysis of the association between the 7–repeat allele of the dopamine D(4) receptor gene and attention deficit hyperactivity disorder. *American Journal of Psychiatry, 158*(7), 1052–1057.

Fauci, A. S. (1979). Immunosuppressive and anti-inflammatory effects of gluco-corticoids. *Monographs on Endocrinology, 12*, 449–465.

Fehr, E., & Rockenbach, B. (2004). Human altruism: Economic, neural, and evolutionary perspectives. *Current Opinion in Neurobiology, 14*(6), 784–790.

Forner, M. A., Barriga, C., Rodriguez, A. B., & Ortega, E. (1995). A study of the role of corticosterone as a mediator in exercise-induced stimulation of murine macrophage phagocytosis. *Journal of Physiology, 488*(pt. 3), 789–794.

Francis, D., Diorio, J., Liu, D., & Meaney, M. J. (1999). Nongenomic transmission across generations of maternal behavior and stress responses in the rat. *Science, 286*(5442), 1155–1158.

Fries, E., Moragues, N., Caldji, C., Hellhammer, D. H., & Meaney, M. J. (2004). Preliminary evidence of altered sensitivity to benzodiazepines as a function of maternal care in the rat. *Annals of the New York Academy of Sciences, 1032*, 320–323.

Gainer, H., & Wray, S. (1994). *Cellular and molecular biology of oxytocin and vasopressin.* New York: Raven.

Ganguli, R., Brar, J. S., Chengappa, K. R., DeLeo, M., Yang, Z. W., Shurin, G, & Rabin, B. S. (1995). Mitogen-stimulated interleukin-2 production in never-medicated, first-episode schizophrenic patients: The influence of age at onset and negative symptoms. *Archives of General Psychiatry, 52*(8), 668–672.

Geen, R. G. (1997). *Psychophysiological approaches to personality psychology.* New York: Academic.

Geenen, V., Defresne, M. P., Robert, F., Legros, J. J., Franchimont, P., & Boniver, J. (1988). The neurohormonal thymic microenvironment: Immunocytochemical evidence that thymic nurse cells are neuroendocrine cells. *Neuroendocrinology, 47*(4), 365–368.

Ghosh, M. C., Mondal, A. C., Basu, S., Banerjee, S., Majumder, J., Bhattacharya, D., & Dasgupta, P. S. (2003). Dopamine inhibits cytokine release and expression of tyrosine kinases, Lck and Fyn in activated T cells. *International Immunopharmacology, 3*(7), 1019–1026.

Gibbs, D. M., Vale, W., Rivier, J., & Yen, S. S. (1984). Oxytocin potentiates the ACTH-releasing activity of CRF(41) but not vasopressin. *Life Science, 34*(23), 2245–2249.

Gingrich, B., Liu, Y, Cascio, C., Wang, Z., & Insel, T. R. (2000). Dopamine D2 receptors in the nucleus accumbens are important for social attachment in female prairie voles (Microtus ochrogaster). *Behavioral Neuroscience, 114*(1), 173–183.

Giovenardi, M., Padoin, M. J., Cadore, L. P., & Lucion, A. B. (1997). Hypothalamic paraventricular nucleus, oxytocin, and maternal aggression in rats. *Annals of the New York Academy of Sciences, 807*, 606–609.

Goehler, L. E., Gaykema, R. P., Hansen, M. K., Anderson, K., Maier, S. F., & Watkins, L. R. (2000). Vagal immune-to-brain communication: A visceral chemosensory pathway. *Autonomic Neuroscience: Basic and Clinical, 85*(1–3), 49–59.

Goehler, L. E., Relton, J. K., Dripps, D., Kiechle, R., Tartaglia, N., Maier, S. F., & Watkins, L. R. (1997). Vagal paraganglia bind biotinylated interleukin-1 receptor antagonist: A possible mechanism for immune-to-brain communication. *Brain Research Bulletin, 43*(3), 357–364.

Gold, P. W., Goodwin, F. K., & Chrousos, G. P. (1988). Clinical and biochemical manifestations of depression: Relation to the neurobiology of stress (1). *New England Journal of Medicine, 319*(6), 348–353.

Goldfien, A. (1994). *Adrenal medulla*. Norwalk, CT: Appleton & Lange.

Gomez-Serrano, M., Tonelli, L., Listwak, S., Sternberg, E., & Riley, A. L. (2001). Effects of cross fostering on open-field behavior, acoustic startle, lipopolysaccharide-induced corticosterone release, and body weight in Lewis and Fischer rats. *Behavior Genetics, 31*(5), 427–436.

Graves, F. C., Wallen, K., & Maestripieri, D. (2002). Opioids and attachment in rhesus macaque (Macaca mulatta) abusive mothers. *Behavioral Neuroscience, 116*(3), 489–493.

Handa, R. J., Nunley, K. M., Lorens, S. A., Louie, J. P., McGivern, R. F., & Bollnow, M. R. (1994). Androgen regulation of adrenocorticotropin and corticosterone secretion in the male rat following novelty and foot shock stressors. *Physiology & Behavior, 55*(1), 117–124.

Hansen, S., &. Ferreira, A. (1986). Food intake, aggression, and fear behavior in the mother rat: Control by neural systems concerned with milk ejection and maternal behavior. *Behavioral Neuroscience, 100*(1), 64–70.

Hansenne, I., Rasier, G., Charlet-Renard, C., DeFresne, M. P., Greimers, R., Breton, C., Legros, J. J., Geenen, V., & Martens, H. (2004). Neurohypophysial receptor gene expression by thymic T cell subsets and thymic T cell lymphoma cell lines. *Clinical & Developmental Immunology, 11*(1), 45–51.

Harris, J. C. (2003). Social neuroscience, empathy, brain integration, and neurodevelopmental disorders. *Physiology & Behavior, 79*(3), 525–531.

Harte, J. L., Eifert, G. H., & Smith, R. (1995). The effects of running and meditation on beta-endorphin, corticotropin-releasing hormone and cortisol in plasma, and on mood. *Biological Psychology, 40*(3), 251–265.

Hartmann, D. P., Holaday, J. W., & Bernton, E. W. (1989). Inhibition of lymphocyte proliferation by antibodies to prolactin. *FASEB Journal, 3*(10), 2194–2202.

Herbert, T. B., & Cohen, S. (1993a). Depression and immunity: A meta-analytic review. *Psychological Bulletin, 113*(3), 472–486.

Herbert, T. B., & Cohen, S. (1993b). Stress and immunity in humans: A meta-analytic review. *Psychosomatic Medicine, 55*(4), 364–379.

Hiestand, P. C., Mekler, P., Nordmann, R, Grieder, A., & Permmongkol, C. (1986). Prolactin as a modulator of lymphocyte responsiveness provides a possible mechanism of action for cyclosporine. *Proceedings of the National Academy of Sciences of the United States of America, 83*(8), 2599–2603.

Houghtling, R. A., & Bayer, B. M. (2002). Rapid elevation of plasma interleukin-6 by morphine is dependent on autonomic stimulation of adrenal gland. *Journal of Pharmacology and Experimental Therapeutics, 300*(1), 213–219.

House, J. S., Landis, K. R., & Umberson, D. (1988). Social relationships and health. *Science, 241*(4865), 540–545.

Hsueh, C. M., Chen, S. F., Ghanta, V. K., & Hiramoto, R. N. (1995). Expression of the conditioned NK cell activity is beta-endorphin dependent. *Behavioural Brain Research*, *678*(1–2), 76–82.

Hu, S. B., Zhao, Z. S., Yhap, C., Grinberg, A., Huang, S. P., Westphal, H., & Gold, P. (2003). Vasopressin receptor 1a-mediated negative regulation of B cell receptor signaling. *Journal of Neuroimmunology*, *135*(1–2), 72–81.

Idler, E. L., & Kasl, S. V. (1997). Religion among disabled and nondisabled persons II: Attendance at religious services as a predictor of the course of disability. The journals of gerontology. Series B, *Psychological Sciences and Social Sciences*, *52*(6), S306–316.

Insel, T. R. (2003). Is social attachment an addictive disorder? *Physiology & Behavior*, *79*(3), 351–357.

Insel, T. R., & Winslow, J. T. (1998). Serotonin and neuropeptides in affiliative behaviors. *Biological Psychiatry*, *44*(3), 207–219.

Insel, T. R., Winslow, J. T., Wang, Z. X., Young, L., & Hulihan, T. J. (1995). Oxytocin and the molecular basis of monogamy. *Advances in Experimental Medicine and Biology*, *395*, 227–234.

Insel, T. R., Young, L., & Wang, Z. (1997). Central oxytocin and reproductive behaviours. *Reviews of Reproduction*, *2*(1), 28–37.

Irwin, M. (2002). Psychoneuroimmunology of depression: Clinical implications. *Brain, Behavior, and Immunity*, *6*(1), 1–16.

Janiak, P., Kasson, B. G., & Brody, M. J. (1989). Central vasopressin raises arterial pressure by sympathetic activation and vasopressin release. *Hypertension*, *13*(6 Pt. 2), 935–940.

Johnson, H. M., Smith, E. M., Torres, B. A., & Blalock, J. E. (1982). Regulation of the in vitro antibody response by neuroendocrine hormones. *Proceedings of the National Academy of Sciences of the United States of America*, *79*(13), 4171–4174.

Johnson, H. M., & Torres, B. A. (1985). Regulation of lymphokine production by arginine vasopressin and oxytocin: Modulation of lymphocyte function by neurohypophyseal hormones. *Journal of immunology* *135*(2 Suppl.), 773s–775s.

Kavelaars, A., Ballieux, R. E, & Heijnen, C. J. (1989). The role of IL-1 in the corticotropin-releasing factor and arginine-vasopressin-induced secretion of immunoreactive beta-endorphin by human peripheral blood mononuclear cells. *Journal of Immunology*, *142*(7), 2338–2342.

Kemper, T. L., & Bauman, M. (1998). Neuropathology of infantile autism. *Journal of Neuropathology and Experimental Neurology*, *57*(7), 645–652.

Kendrick, K. M., Da Costa, A. P., Broad, K. D., Ohkura, S., Guevara, R., Levy, F., & Keverne, E. B. (1997). Neural control of maternal behaviour and olfactory recognition of offspring. *Brain Research Bulletin*, *44*(4), 383–395.

Keverne, E. B., & Martensz, N. D. (1989). Beta-endorphin concentrations in cerebrospinal fluid of monkeys are influenced by grooming relationships. *Psychoneuroendocrinology*, *14*(1–2), 155–161.

Kiecolt-Glaser, J. K., Robles, T. F., Heffner, K. L., Loving, T. J., & Glaser, R. (2002). Psycho-oncology and cancer: Psychoneuroimmunology and cancer. *Annals of Oncology: Official Journal of the European Society for Medical Oncology*, *13*(Suppl. 4), 165–169.

Kim, S. J., Young, L. J., Gonen, D., Veenstra-VanderWeele, J., Courchesne, R.,

Courchesne, E., Lord, C., Leventhal, B. L., Cook, E. H., & Insel, T. R. (2002). Transmission disequilibrium testing of arginine vasopressin receptor 1A (AVPR1A) polymorphisms in autism. *Molecular Psychiatry, 7*(5), 503–507.

Klein, D. F. (1994). Pregnancy and panic disorder. *Journal of Clinical Psychiatry, 55*(7), 293–294.

Koenig, H. G., George, L. K., & Peterson, B. L. (1998). Religiosity and remission of depression in medically ill older patients. *American Journal of Psychiatry, 155*(4), 536–542.

Koenig, H. G., George, L. K., Titus, P., & Meador, K. G. (2004a). Religion, spirituality, and acute care hospitalization and long-term care use by older patients. *Archives of Internal Medicine, 164*(14), 1579–1585.

Koenig, H. G., George, L. K., & Titus, P. (2004b). Religion, spirituality, and health in medically ill hospitalized older patients. *Journal of the American Geriatrics Society, 52*(4), 554–562.

Koenig, H. G., Shelp, F., Goli, V., Cohen, H. J., & Blazer, D. G. (1989). Survival and health care utilization in elderly medical inpatients with major depression. *Journal of the American Geriatrics Society, 37*(7), 599–606.

Kohm, A. P., & Sanders, V. M. (2001). Norepinephrine and beta 2-adrenergic receptor stimulation regulate CD4+ T and B lymphocyte function in vitro and in vivo. *Pharmacological Reviews, 53*(4), 487–525.

Kubzansky, L. D., Wright, R. J., Cohen, S., Weiss, S., Rosner, B., & Sparrow, D. (2002). Breathing easy: A prospective study of optimism and pulmonary function in the normative aging study. *Annals of Behavioral Medicine, 24*(4), 345–353.

Kumar, A., Singh, S. M., & Sodhi, A. (1997). Effect of prolactin on nitric oxide and interleukin-1 production of murine peritoneal macrophages: Role of Ca2+ and protein kinase C. *International Journal of Immunopharmacology, 19*(3), 129–133.

Landgraf, R., Gerstberger, R., Montkowski, A., Probst, J. C., Wotjak, C. T., Holsboer, F., & Engelmann, M. (1995). V1 vasopressin receptor antisense oligodeoxynucleotide into septum reduces vasopressin binding, social discrimination abilities, and anxiety-related behavior in rats. *Journal of Neuroscience, 15*(6), 4250–4258.

Lang, R. E., Heil, J. W., Ganten, D., Hermann, K., Unger, T., & Rascher, W. (1983). Oxytocin unlike vasopressin is a stress hormone in the rat. *Neuroendocrinology, 37*(4), 314–316.

Leckman, J. F., Goodman, W. K., North, W. G., Chappell, P. B., Price, L. H., Pauls, D. L., Anderson, G. M., Riddle, M. A., McSwiggan-Hardin, M., & McDougle, C. J. (1994). Elevated cerebrospinal fluid levels of oxytocin in obsessive-compulsive disorder: Comparison with Tourette's syndrome and healthy controls. *Archives of General Psychiatry, 51*(10), 782–792.

Lee, Y., & Voogt, J. L. (1999). Feedback effects of placental lactogens on prolactin levels and Fos-related antigen immunoreactivity of tuberoinfundibular dopaminergic neurons in the arcuate nucleus during pregnancy in the rat. *Endocrinology, 140*(5), 2159–2166.

Le Moal, M., Dantzer, R., Michaud, B., & Koob, G. F. (1987). Centrally injected arginine vasopressin (AVP) facilitates social memory in rats. *Neuroscience Letters, 77*(3), 353–359.

Lesch, K. P., & Mossner, R. (1998). Genetically driven variation in serotonin up-take: Is there a link to affective spectrum, neurodevelopmental, and neuro-degenerative disorders? *Biological Psychiatry, 44*(3), 179–192.

Levine, S. (2001). Primary social relationships influence the development of the hypothalamic-pituitary-adrenal axis in the rat. *Physiology & Behavior, 73*(3), 255–260.

Levo, Y., Harbeck, R. J., & Kirkpatrick, C. H. (1985). Regulatory effect of hydro-cortisone on the in vitro synthesis of IgE by human lymphocytes. *International Archives of Allergy and Applied Immunology, 77*, 413–415.

Lightman, S. L., & Young, W. S. III. (1989). Lactation inhibits stress-mediated se-cretion of corticosterone and oxytocin and hypothalamic accumulation of cor-ticotropin-releasing factor and enkephalin messenger ribonucleic acids. *Endocrinology, 124*(5), 2358–2364.

Liu, D., Diorio, J., Tannenbaum, B., Caldji, C., Francis, D., Freedman, A., Sharma, S., Pearson, D., Plotsky, P. M., & Meaney, M. J. (1997). Maternal care, hip-pocampal glucocorticoid receptors, and hypothalamic-pituitary-adrenal re-sponses to stress. *Science, 277*(5332), 1659–1662.

Lonstein, J. S., Simmons, D. A., Swann, J. M., & Stern, J. M. (1998). Forebrain expression of c-fos due to active maternal behaviour in lactating rats. *Neuro-science, 82*(1), 267–281.

Lorton, D., Bellinger, D., Duclos, M., Felten, S. Y., & Felten, D. L. (1996). Appli-cation of 6–hydroxydopamine into the fatpads surrounding the draining lymph nodes exacerbates adjuvant-induced arthritis. *Journal of Neuroimmunology, 64*(2), 103–113.

Lorton, D., Lubahn, C., Klein, N., Schaller, J., & Bellinger, D. L. (1999). Dual role for noradrenergic innervation of lymphoid tissue and arthritic joints in adju-vant-induced arthritis. *Brain, Behavior, and Immunity, 13*(4), 315–334.

MacLean, P. (1990). *The triune brain in evolution: Role in paleocerebral functions.* New York: Plenum.

Madden, K. S., Sanders, V. M., & Felten, D. L. (1995). Catecholamine influences and sympathetic neural modulation of immune responsiveness. *Annual Review of Pharmacology and Toxicology, 35*, 417–448.

Maes, M., Bosmans, E, Calabrese, J., Smith, R., & Meltzer, H. Y. (1995). Interleukin-2 and interleukin-6 in schizophrenia and mania: Effects of neuroleptics and mood stabilizers. *Journal of Psychiatric Research, 29*(2), 141–152.

Mahalati, K., Okanoya, K., Witt, D. M., & Carter, C. S. (1991). Oxytocin inhibits male sexual behavior in prairie voles. *Pharmacology, Biochemistry, and Behav-ior, 39*(1), 219–222.

Makara, G. B., Mergl, Z., & Zelena, D. (2004). The role of vasopressin in hypothalamo-pituitary-adrenal axis activation during stress: An assessment of the evidence. *Annals of the New York Academy of Sciences, 1018*, 151–161.

Makman, M. H. (1994). Morphine receptors in immunocytes and neurons. *Advances in Neuroimmunology, 4*(2), 69–82.

Marques-Deak, A., Cizza, G., & Sternberg E. (2005). Brain-immune interactions and disease susceptibility. *Molecular Psychiatry, 10*(3), 239–250.

Marttila, R. J., Eskola, J., Paivarinta, M., & Rinne, U. K. (1984). Immune functions in Parkinson's disease. *Advances in Neurology, 40*, 315–323.

Marx, J. (1995). How the glucocorticoids suppress immunity. *Science, 270*(5234), 232–233.

Masten, A. S., & Coatsworth, J. D. (1998). The development of competence in favorable and unfavorable environments: Lessons from research on successful children. *American Psychologist, 53*(2), 205–220.

McCann, S. M., Kimura, M., Karanth, S., Yu, W. H., Mastronardi, C. A., & Rettori, V. (2000). The mechanism of action of cytokines to control the release of hypothalamic and pituitary hormones in infection. *Annals of the New York Academy of Sciences, 917*, 4–18.

McKenna, F., McLaughlin, P. J., Lewis, B. J., Sibbring, G. C., Cummerson, A., Bowen-Jones, D., & Moots, R. J. (2002). Dopamine receptor expression on human T- and B-lymphocytes, monocytes, neutrophils, eosinophils and NK cells: A flow cytometric study. *Journal of Neuroimmunology, 132*(1–2), 34–40.

McMurray, R. W. (2001). Prolactin in murine systemic lupus erythematosus. *Lupus, 10*(10), 742–747.

Meisenberg, G. (1988). Vasopressin-induced grooming and scratching behavior in mice. *Annals of the New York Academy of Sciences, 525*, 257–269.

Miller, B. D., & Wood, B. L. (1994). Psychophysiologic reactivity in asthmatic children: A cholinergically mediated confluence of pathways. *Journal of the American Academy of Child and Adolescent Psychiatry, 33*(9), 1236–1245.

Miller, B. D., & Wood, B. L. (1997). Influence of specific emotional states on autonomic reactivity and pulmonary function in asthmatic children. *Journal of the American Academy of Child and Adolescent Psychiatry, 36*(5), 669–677.

Mitchell, B. F., & Schmid, B. (2001). Oxytocin and its receptor in the process of parturition. *Journal of the Society for Gynecologic Investigation, 8*(3), 122–133.

Molitor, T. W., Morilla, A., Risdahl, J. M., Murtaugh, M. P., Chao, C. C., & Peterson, P. K. (1992). Chronic morphine administration impairs cell-mediated immune responses in swine. *Journal of Pharmacology and Experimental Therapeutics, 260*(2), 581–586.

Moll, U. M., Lane, B. L., Robert, F., Geenen, V., & Legros, J. J. (1988). The neuroendocrine thymus: Abundant occurrence of oxytocin-, vasopressin-, and neurophysin-like peptides in epithelial cells. *Histochemistry, 89*(4), 385–390.

Mong, J. A., &. Pfaff, D. W. (2003). Hormonal and genetic influences underlying arousal as it drives sex and aggression in animal and human brains. *Neurobiology of Aging, 24*(Suppl. 1), S83–88; discussion S91–92.

Mong, J. A., & Pfaff, D. W. (2004). Hormonal symphony: Steroid orchestration of gene modules for sociosexual behaviors. *Molecular Psychiatry, 9*(6), 550–556.

Morikawa, K., Oseko, F., & Morikawa, S. (1994). Immunosuppressive activity of bromocriptine on human T lymphocyte function in vitro. *Clinical and Experimental Immunology, 95*(3), 514–518.

Moskowitz, D. S., Pinard, G., Zuroff, D. C., Annable, L., & Young, S. N. (2001). The effect of tryptophan on social interaction in everyday life: A placebo-controlled study. *Neuropsychopharmacology, 25*(2), 277–289.

Moskowitz, D. S., Pinard, G., Zuroff, D. C., Annable, L., & Young, S. N. (2003). Tryptophan, serotonin and human social behavior. *Advances in Experimental Medicine and Biology, 527,* 215–224.

Nanda, N., & Pal, G. K. (2005). Effect of dopamine injection into caudate nucleus on immune responsiveness in rats: A pilot study. *Immunology Letters, 96*(1), 151–153.

Nelson, E. E., & Panksepp, J. (1998). Brain substrates of infant-mother attachment: Contributions of opioids, oxytocin, and norepinephrine. *Neuroscience and Biobehavioral Reviews, 22*(3), 437–452.

Nestler, E. J. (2001). Molecular neurobiology of addiction. *American Journal on Addictions, 10*(3), 201–217.

Neumann, I. D. (2001). Alterations in behavioral and neuroendocrine stress coping strategies in pregnant, parturient and lactating rats. *Progress in Brain Research, 133,* 143–152.

Neumann, I. D., Kromer, S. A., Toschi, N., & Ebner, K. (2000). Brain oxytocin inhibits the (re)activity of the hypothalamo-pituitary-adrenal axis in male rats: Involvement of hypothalamic and limbic brain regions. *Regulatory Peptides, 96*(1–2), 31–38.

Neveu, P. J. (1993). Brain lateralization and immunomodulation. *International Journal of Neuroscience, 70*(1–2), 135–143.

Newton, M., & Newton, N. (1948). The let-down reflex in human lactation. *Journal of Pediatrics, 33,* 698–704.

Nistico, G., Caroleo, M. C., Arbitrio, M., & Pulvirenti, L. (1994). Dopamine D1 receptors in the amygdala enhance the immune response in the rat. *Annals of the New York Academy of Sciences, 741,* 316–323.

Odendaal, J. S., & Meintjes, R. A.. (2003). Neurophysiological correlates of affiliative behaviour between humans and dogs. *Veterinary Journal, 165*(3), 296–301.

O'Doherty, J. P. (2004). Reward representations and reward-related learning in the human brain: Insights from neuroimaging. *Current Opinion in Neurobiology, 14*(6), 769–776.

Offen, D., Ziv, I., Gorodin, S., Barzilai, A., Malik, Z., & Melamed, E. (1995). Dopamine-induced programmed cell death in mouse thymocytes. *Biochimica et Biophysica Acta, 1268*(2), 171–177.

Ogawa, S., Robbins, A., Kumar, N., Pfaff, D. W., Sundaram, K., & Bardin, C. W. (1996). Effects of testosterone and 7 alpha-methyl-19–nortestosterone (MENT) on sexual and aggressive behaviors in two inbred strains of male mice. *Hormones and Behavior, 30*(1), 74–84.

Osaki, M. Y., Castellan-Baldan, L., Calvo, F., Carvalho, A. D., Felippotti, T. T., de Oliveira, R., Ubiali, W. A., Paschoalin-Maurin, T., Elias-Filho, D. H., Motta, V., da Silva, L. A., & Coimbra, N. C. (2003). Neuroanatomical and neuropharmacological study of opioid pathways in the mesencephalic tectum: Effect of mu(1)- and kappa-opioid receptor blockade on escape behavior induced by electrical stimulation of the inferior colliculus. *Brain Research, 992*(2), 179–192.

Patchev, V. K., Mastorakos, G., Brady, L. S., Redwine, J., Wilder, R. L., & Chrousos, G. P. (1993). Increased arginine vasopressin secretion may participate in the enhanced susceptibility of Lewis rats to inflammatory disease. *Neuroendocrinology, 58*(1), 106–110.

Pavin, D., Le Breton, H., & Daubert, C. (1997). Human stress cardiomyopathy mimicking acute myocardial syndrome. *Heart, 78*(5), 509–511.

Pavlov, V. A., & Tracey, K. J. (2004). Neural regulators of innate immune responses and inflammation. *Cellular and Molecular Life Sciences, 61*(18), 2322–2331.

Peeva, E., Venkatesh, J., Michael, D., & Diamond, B.. (2004). Prolactin as a modulator of B cell function: Implications for SLE. *Biomedical Pharmacotherapy, 58*(5), 310–319.

Pellegrini, I., Lebrun, J. J., Ali, S., & Kelly, P. A. (1992). Expression of prolactin and its receptor in human lymphoid cells. *Molecular Endocrinology, 6*(7), 1023–1031.

Pfaff, D. W. (1999). *Drive: Neural and molecular mechanism for sexual motivation.* Cambridge, MA: MIT Press.

Pitkow, L. J., Sharer, C. A., Ren, X., Insel, T. R., Terwilliger, E. F., & Young, L. J. (2001). Facilitation of affiliation and pair-bond formation by vasopressin receptor gene transfer into the ventral forebrain of a monogamous vole. *Journal of Neuroscience, 21*(18), 7392–7396.

Qureshi, G. A., Hansen, S., & Sodersten, P. (1987). Offspring control of cerebrospinal fluid GABA concentrations in lactating rats. *Neuroscience Letters, 75*(1), 85–88.

Rabin, B. S., Ganguli, R., Cunnick, J. E., & Lysle, D. T. (1988). The central nervous system–immune system relationship. *Clinics in Laboratory Medicine, 8*(2), 253–268.

Reder, A. T. (1992). Regulation of production of adrenocorticotropin-like proteins in human mononuclear cells. *Immunology, 77*(3), 436–442.

Reiche, E. M., Nunes, S. O., & Morimoto, H. K. (2004). Stress, depression, the immune system, and cancer. *The Lancet Oncology, 5*(10), 617–625.

Ricci, A., Veglio, F., & Amenta, F. (1995). Radioligand binding characterization of putative dopamine D3 receptor in human peripheral blood lymphocytes with [3H]7–OH-DPAT. *Journal of Neuroimmunology, 58*(2), 139–144.

Richardson, G. E., & Waite, P. J.. (2002). Mental health promotion through resilience and resiliency education. *International Journal of Emergency Mental Health, 4*(1), 65–75.

Rizzolatti, G., & Arbib, M. A. (1998). Language within our grasp. *Trends in Neurosciences, 21*(5), 188–194.

Rogers, T. J., Steele, A. D., Howard, O. M., & Oppenheim, J. J. (2000). Bidirectional heterologous desensitization of opioid and chemokine receptors. *Annals of the New York Academy of Sciences, 917*, 19–28.

Rosenthal, T., & Oparil, S. (2002). The effect of antihypertensive drugs on the fetus. *Journal of Human Hypertension, 16*(5), 293–298.

Rutter, M., Andersen-Wood, L., Beckett, C., Bredenkamp, D., Castle, J., Groothues, C., Kreppner, J., Keaveney, L., Lord, C., & O'Connor, T. G. (1999). Quasi-autistic patterns following severe early global privation: English and Romanian Adoptees (ERA) study team. *Journal of Child Psychology and Psychiatry, and Allied Disciplines, 40*(4), 537–549.

Sabharwal, P., Glaser, R, Lafuse, W., Varma, S., Liu, Q., Arkins, S., Kooijman, R., Kutz, L., Kelley, K. W., & Malarkey, W.B. (1992). Prolactin synthesized and secreted by human peripheral blood mononuclear cells: An autocrine growth factor for lymphoproliferation. *Proceedings of the National Academy of Sciences of the United States of America, 89*(16), 7713–7716.

Saha, B., Mondal, A. C., Basu, S., & Dasgupta, P. S. (2001). Circulating dopamine level, in lung carcinoma patients, inhibits proliferation and cytotoxicity of CD4+ and CD8+ T cells by D1 dopamine receptors: An in vitro analysis. *International Immunopharmacology, 1*(7), 1363–1374.

Sanders, V. M.,. Baker, R. A., Ramer-Quinn, D. S., Kasprowicz, D. J., Fuchs, B. A., & Street, N. E. (1997). Differential expression of the beta2-adrenergic receptor by Th1 and Th2 clones: Implications for cytokine production and B cell help. *Journal of Immunology, 158*(9), 4200–4210.

Sanders, V. M., Kasprowicz, D. J., Kohm, A. P., Swanson, M. A., et al. (2001). *Neurotransmitter receptors on lymphocytes and other lymphoid cells.* San Diego, CA: Academic.

Sanders, V. M., & Kohm, A. P. (2002). Sympathetic nervous system interaction with the immune system. *International Review of Neurobiology, 52,* 17–41.

Sasaki, S., Watanobe, H., & Takebe, K. (1995). The role of arginine vasopressin in interleukin-1 beta-induced adrenocorticotropin secretion in the rat. *Neuroimmunomodulation, 2*(3), 134–136.

Scantamburlo, G., Ansseau, M., et al. (2001). Implication de la neurohypophyse dans le stress psychique. *Encephale, 27*(3), 245–259.

Schmidt, M., Oitzl, M. S., Levine, S., & de Kloet, E. R. (2002). The HPA system during the postnatal development of CD1 mice and the effects of maternal deprivation. *Developmental Brain Research, 139*(1), 39–49.

Schwartz, C., Meisenhelder, J. B, Ma, Y., & Reed, G. (2003). Altruistic social interest behaviors are associated with better mental health. *Psychosomatic Medicine, 65*(5), 778–785.

Scott, L. V., & Dinan, T. G. (1998). Vasopressin and the regulation of hypothalamic-pituitary-adrenal axis function: Implications for the pathophysiology of depression. *Life Sciences, 62*(22), 1985–1998.

Sephton, S. E., Sapolsky, R. M., Kraemer, H. C., & Spiegel, D. (2000). Diurnal cortisol rhythm as a predictor of breast cancer survival. *Journal of the National Cancer Institute, 92*(12), 994–1000.

Sephton, S., & Spiegel, D. (2003). Circadian disruption in cancer: A neuroendocrine-immune pathway from stress to disease? *Brain Behavior Immunity, 17*(5), 321–328.

Shavit, Y., Depaulis, A., Martin, F. C., Terman, G. W., Pechnick, R. N., Zane, C. J., Gale, R. P., & Liebeskind, J. C. (1986). Involvement of brain opiate receptors in the immune-suppressive effect of morphine. *Proceedings of the National Academy of Sciences of the United States of America, 83*(18), 7114–7117.

Shibasaki, T., Hotta, M., Sugihara, H., & Wakabayashi, I. (1998). Brain vasopressin is involved in stress-induced suppression of immune function in the rat. *Brain Research, 808*(1), 84–92.

Sperner-Unterweger, B., Barnas, C., Fuchs, D., Kemmler, G., Wachter, H., Hinterhuber, H., & Fleischhacker, W. W. (1992). Neopterin production in acute schizophrenic patients: An indicator of alterations of cell-mediated immunity. *Psychiatry Research, 42*(2), 121–128.

Spiegel, D. (2002). Effects of psychotherapy on cancer survival. *Nature Reviews Cancer, 2*(5), 383–389.

Stack, E. C., Balakrishnan, R., Numan, M. J., & Numan, M. (2002). A functional neuroanatomical investigation of the role of the medial preoptic area in neural circuits regulating maternal behavior. *Behavioural Brain Research, 131*(1–2), 17–36.

Stern, J. M., Goldman, L., & Levine, S. (1973). Pituitary-adrenal responsiveness during lactation in rats. *Neuroendocrinology, 12*(3), 179–191.

Sternberg, E. (2000a). *The balance within: The science connecting health and emotions.* New York: Freeman.

Sternberg, E. M. (2000b). Interactions between the immune and neuroendocrine systems. *Progress in Brain Research, 122*, 35–42.

Sternberg, E. M., Chrousos, G. P., Wilder, R. L., & Gold, P. W. (1992). The stress response and the regulation of inflammatory disease. *Annals of Internal Medicine, 117*(10), 854–866.

Sternberg, E. M., Hill, J. M., Chrousos, G. P., Kamilaris, T., Listwak, S. J., Gold, P. W., & Wilder, R. L. (1989). Inflammatory mediator-induced hypothalamic-pituitary-adrenal axis activation is defective in streptococcal cell wall arthritis-susceptible Lewis rats. *Proceedings of the National Academy of Sciences of the United States of America, 86*(7), 2374–2378.

Sternberg, E. M., Wedner, H. J., Leung, M. K., & Parker, C. W. (1987). Effect of serotonin (5–HT) and other monoamines on murine macrophages: Modulation of interferon-gamma induced phagocytosis. *Journal of Immunology, 138*(12), 4360–4365.

Sternberg, E. M., Young, W. S., Bernardini, R., Calogero, A. E., Chrousos, G. P., Gold, P. W., & Wilder, R. L. (1989). A central nervous system defect in biosynthesis of corticotropin-releasing hormone is associated with susceptibility to streptococcal cell wall-induced arthritis in Lewis rats. *Proceedings of the National Academy of Sciences of the United States of America, 86*(12), 4771–4775.

Stevens, J. A., Fonlupt, P., Shiffrar, M., & Decety, J. (2000). New aspects of motion perception: Selective neural encoding of apparent human movements. *Neuroreport, 11*(1), 109–115.

Swedo, S. E., Leonard, H. L., Kruesi, M. J., Rettew, D. C., Listwak, S. J., Berrettini, W., Stipetic, M., Hamburger, S., Gold, P. W., & Potter, W. Z. (1992). Cerebrospinal fluid neurochemistry in children and adolescents with obsessive-compulsive disorder. *Archives of General Psychiatry, 49*(1), 29–36.

Taub, D. D., Eisenstein, T. K., Geller, E. B., Adler, M. W., & Rogers, T. J. (1991). Immunomodulatory activity of mu- and kappa-selective opioid agonists. *Proceedings of the National Academy of Sciences of the United States of America, 88*(2), 360–364.

Torner, L., Toschi, N., Nava, G., Clapp, C., & Neumann, I. D. (2002). Increased hypothalamic expression of prolactin in lactation: Involvement in behavioural and neuroendocrine stress responses. *European Journal of Neuroscience, 15*(8), 1381–1389.

Totman, R., Kiff, J., Reed, S. E., & Craig, J. W. (1980). Predicting experimental colds in volunteers from different measures of recent life stress. *Journal of Psychosomatic Research, 24*(3–4), 155–163.

Tracey, K. J. (2002). The inflammatory reflex. *Nature, 420*(6917), 853–859.

Tracey, K. J., & Warren, H. S. (2004). Human genetics: An inflammatory issue. *Nature, 429*(6987): 35–37.

Tsao, C. W., Lin, Y. S., & Cheng, J. T. (1997). Effect of dopamine on immune cell proliferation in mice. *Life Sciences, 61*(24), PL361–371.

Tubaro, E., Borelli, G., Croce, C., Cavallo, G., & Santiangeli, C. (1983). Effect of morphine on resistance to infection. *Journal of Infectious Diseases, 148*(4), 656–666.

Tyrell, J. B., Aron, D. C., & Forsham, P. H. (1994). *Glucocorticoid & adrenal androgens.* Norwalk, CT: Appleton & Lange.

Tyrell, J. B., Finding, J. W., Aron, D. C., et al. (1994). *Hypothalamus and pituitary.* Norwalk, CT: Appleton & Lange.

Uchino, B. N., Cacioppo, J. T., & Kiecolt-Glaser, J. K. (1996). The relationship between social support and physiological processes: A review with emphasis on underlying mechanisms and implications for health. *Psychological Bulletin, 119*(3), 488–531.

Vallejo, R., de Leon-Casasola, O., & Benyamin, R. (2004). Opioid therapy and immunosuppression: A review. *American Journal of Therapeutics, 11*(5), 354–365.

van der Poll, T., Coyle, S. M., Barbosa, K., Braxton, C. C., & Lowry, S. F. (1996). Epinephrine inhibits tumor necrosis factor-alpha and potentiates interleukin 10 production during human endotoxemia. *Journal of Clinical Investigation, 97*(3), 713–719.

Vera-Lastra, O., Jara, L. J., & Espinoza, L. R. (2002). Prolactin and autoimmunity. *Autoimmunity Reviews, 1*(6) 360–364.

Wandinger, K. P., Hagenah, J. M., Kluter, H., Rothermundt, M., Peters, M., & Vieregge, P. (1999). Effects of amantadine treatment on in vitro production of interleukin-2 in de-novo patients with idiopathic Parkinson's disease. *Journal of Neuroimmunology, 98*(2), 214–220.

Wang, Z., Yu, G., Cascio, C., Liu, Y., Gingrich, B., & Insel, T. R. (1999). Dopamine D2 receptor-mediated regulation of partner preferences in female prairie voles (Microtus ochrogaster): A mechanism for pair bonding? *Behavioral Neuroscience, 113*(3), 602–611.

Wassink, T. H., Piven, J., Vieland, V. J., Pietila, J., Goedken, R. J., Folstein, S. E., & Sheffield, V. C. (2004). Examination of AVPR1a as an autism susceptibility gene. *Molecular Psychiatry, 9*(10), 968–972.

Watkins, L. R., &. Maier, S. F. (2005). Immune regulation of central nervous system functions: From sickness responses to pathological pain. *Journal of Internal Medicine, 257*(2), 139–155.

Weaver, I. C., Cervoni, N., Champagne, F. A., D'Alessio, A. C., Sharma, S., Seckl, J. R., Dymov, S., Szyf, M., & Meaney, M. J. (2004). Epigenetic programming by maternal behavior. *Nature Neuroscience, 7*(8), 847–854.

Webster, J. I., Tonelli, L., & Sternberg, E. M. (2002). Neuroendocrine regulation of immunity. *Annual Review of Immunology, 20,* 125–163.

Weisenfeld, A. R., Malatesta, C. Z., Whitman, P. B., Granrose, C., & Uili, R. (1985). Psychophysiological response of breast and bottle-feeding mothers to their infants' signal. *Psychophysiology, 22,* 79–86.

Whitfield, J. F., MacManus, J. P., & Gillan, D. J. (1970). The possible mediation by cyclic AMP of the stimulation of thymocyte proliferation by vasopressin and the inhibition of this mitogenic action by thyrocalcitonin. *Journal of Cellular Physiology, 76,* 65–76.

Wiegers, G., & Reul, J. (1998). Induction of cytokine receptors by glucocorticoids: Functional and pathological significance. *Trends in Pharmacological Sciences, 19,* 317–321.

Wiegers, G. J., Reul, J. M., Holsboer, F., & de Kloet, E. R. (1994). Enhancement of rat splenic lymphocyte mitogenesis after short term preexposure to corticosteroids in vitro. *Endocrinology 135,* 2351–2357.

Wilckens, T. (1995). Glucocorticoids and immune function: Physiological relevance and pathogenic potential of hormonal dysfunction. *Trends in Pharmacological Sciences, 16*(6), 193–197.

Wilder, R. L. (1995). Neuroendocrine-immune system interactions and autoimmunity. *Annual Review of Immunology, 13,* 307–338.

Williams, J. H., Whiten, A., Suddendorf, T., & Perrett, D. I. (2001). Imitation, mirror neurons and autism. *Neuroscience and Biobehavioral Reviews, 25*(4), 287–295.

Windle, R. J., Kershaw, Y. M., Shanks, N., Wood, S. A., Lightman, S. L., & Ingram, C. D. (2004). Oxytocin attenuates stress-induced c-fos mRNA expression in specific forebrain regions associated with modulation of hypothalamo-pituitary-adrenal activity. *Journal of Neuroscience, 24*(12), 2974–2982.

Windle, R. J., Shanks, N., Lightman, S. L., & Ingram, C. D. (1997). Central oxytocin administration reduces stress-induced corticosterone release and anxiety behavior in rats. *Endocrinology, 138*(7), 2829–2834.

Winslow, J. T., Hastings, N., Carter, C. S., Harbaugh, C. R., & Insel, T. R. (1993). A role for central vasopressin in pair bonding in monogamous prairie voles. *Nature, 365*(6446), 545–548.

Winslow, J. T., Noble, P. L., Lyons, C. K., Sterk, S. M., & Insel, T. R. (2003). Rearing effects on cerebrospinal fluid oxytocin concentration and social buffering in rhesus monkeys. *Neuropsychopharmacology, 28*(5), 910–918.

Witt, D. M., Winslow, J. T., & Insel, T. R. (1992). Enhanced social interactions in rats following chronic, centrally infused oxytocin. *Pharmacology, Biochemistry, and Behavior, 43*(3), 855–861.

Wittstein, I. S., Thiemann, D. R., Lima, J. A., Baughman, K. L., Schulman, S. P., Gerstenblith, G., Wu, K. C., Rade, J. J., Bivalacqua, T. J., & Champion, H. C. (2005). Neurohumoral features of myocardial stunning due to sudden emotional stress. *New England Journal of Medicine, 352*(6), 539–548.

Won, S. J., Chuang, Y. C., Huang, W. T., Liu, H. S., & Lin, M. T. (1995). Suppression of natural killer cell activity in mouse spleen lymphocytes by several dopamine receptor antagonists. *Experientia, 51*(4), 343–348.

Wong, M. L., Bongiorno, P. B., Gold, P. W., & Licinio, J. (1995). Localization of interleukin-1 beta converting enzyme mRNA in rat brain vasculature: Evidence that the genes encoding the interleukin-1 system are constitutively expressed in brain blood vessels: Pathophysiological implications. *Neuroimmunomodulation, 2*(3), 141–148.

Wotjak, C. T., Ganster, J., Kohl, G., Holsboer, F., Landgraf, R., & Engelmann, M. (1998). Dissociated central and peripheral release of vasopressin, but not oxytocin, in response to repeated swim stress: New insights into the secretory capacities of peptidergic neurons. *Neuroscience, 85*(4), 1209–1222.

Young, L. J., Toloczko, D., & Insel, T. R. (1999). Localization of vasopressin (V1a) receptor binding and mRNA in the rhesus monkey brain. *Journal of Neuroendocrinology, 11*(4), 291–297.

Young, L. J., Wang, Z., & Insel, T. R. (1998). Neuroendocrine bases of monogamy. *Trends in Neuroscience, 21*(2), 71–75.

Yu-Lee, L. (2001). Stimulation of interferon regulatory factor-1 by prolactin. *Lupus 10*(10), 691–699.

Zhang, T. Y., Parent, C., Weaver, I., & Meaney, M. J. (2004). Maternal programming of individual differences in defensive responses in the rat. *Annals of the New York Academy of Sciences, 1032*, 85–103.

Zorrilla, E. P., Luborsky, L., McKay, J. R., Rosenthal, R., Houldin, A.,Tax, A., McCorkle, R., Seligman, D. A., & Schmidt, K. (2001). The relationship of depression and stressors to immunological assays: A meta-analytic review. *Brain Behavior and Immunity, 15*(3), 199–226.

10 Integrating Positive Psychology Into Epidemiologic Theory: Reflections on Love, Salutogenesis, and Determinants of Population Health

Jeff Levin

This chapter seeks to integrate the emerging field of positive psychology into epidemiologic theory. It is demonstrated that the putative health effects of positive-psychological constructs, exemplified by altruistic and compassionate love, can be understood in terms of concepts implicit in existing theoretical perspectives on the psychosocial determinants of population health. An ostensibly salutary impact of giving and receiving love on health indicators makes sense precisely because it is consonant with current understanding of how other psychosocial characteristics or phenomena serve to reduce morbidity or to promote health. This, it is believed, is due to providing a sense of coherence, which facilitates a coping response and thus strengthens the host resistance of populations, reducing susceptibility to disease.

The discussion that follows is in four parts. First, it is shown how the effects of constructs taken from the field of positive psychology can be investigated and understood in an epidemiologic context. This discussion emphasizes key concepts in population health, including risk status, the natural history of disease, and pathogenesis. Second, a summary is provided of Antonovsky's views on salutogenesis and coherence. These are key components of any metatheoretical discussion of a potentially salutary role of positive-psychological characteristics. Third, important conceptual distinctions are made among the determinants of morbidity, disease, and health in order to clarify existing confusion regarding the impact of psychosocial variables. This confusion is mostly due to inadequate differentiation of individual versus population-wide levels of analysis, pathogenic versus salutogenic orientations, and determinant versus etiologic factors. Finally, an overview is provided of how the putative health benefits of love might be assessed from several popular theoretical perspectives that specify how psychosocial constructs affect indicators of population health. This discussion summarizes how epidemiologists conceive of the psychosocial determinants of morbidity, disease, and health. It is asserted that an observed health effect of love, and of positive-psychological constructs generally, can be accommodated by traditional epidemiologic thinking and is thus amenable to systematic investigation.

PSYCHOSOCIAL EPIDEMIOLOGY AND THE NATURAL HISTORY OF DISEASE

The past several years have seen a dramatic growth of interest in health-related research on topics related to altruism, such as helping behavior, supportive resources, compassion, and love. The increasing popularity of these topics is part of a wider recognition of the relevance of constructs developed within the positive psychology movement to theory and research on determinants of physical- and mental-health outcomes (Snyder & McCullough, 2000). An excellent set of papers, published in a special issue of the *Journal of Social and Clinical Psychology*, made the case for investigators to pay closer attention to underinvestigated virtues such as hope, self-control, forgiveness, gratitude, humility, wisdom, and love (McCullough & Snyder, 2000). For most of these classical sources of human strength, including love, contributors documented existing theory and, in some cases, measurement approaches that could be utilized to explore protective or otherwise salutary impacts. Empirical investigations of these constructs in relation to health-related outcomes, however, were found to be lacking.

This is not surprising in light of the historically "negative" polarity of research in psychosocial epidemiology. Constructs typically studied by epidemiologists conducting social research and by social scientists conducting health-related research are characterized by a presumptive risk-enhancing status. Social, psychosocial, and behavioral epidemiologists by convention tend to focus on exposures (epidemiologese for "independent variables") whose presence is posited to heighten the risk of morbidity or mortality, or other adverse outcomes. If borne out by data analyses, such constructs are denoted as risk factors, whose eradication or restriction can then be targeted by public-health interventions, such as behavior-change programs. Examples are myriad: stressful life events, the Type A behavioral pattern, bereavement, job stress, daily hassles, external locus of control, dysfunctional social networks, and various unhealthy practices (smoking, drinking, poor diet, lack of exercise, etc.).

The traditional focus, in the context of the natural history of disease, is on factors that hasten pathogenesis, or the process of becoming diseased. That is, what is emphasized in psychosocial-epidemiologic theory and research is the

identification of detrimental characteristics of people or their social environments whose presence, over time, is associated with greater risk or odds of moving
across the clinical threshold from a status of well to a status of ill. This focus on
describing or predicting pathophysiology is the default orientation of epidemiology and is so tacitly accepted that it is rarely acknowledged. In psychosocial
epidemiology, a field dominated by social scientists without explicit training in
epidemiology or biomedicine (Zielhuis & Kiemeney, 2001), it may be that many
researchers are not even aware of the concept of natural history or of its clinical
significance (Freer & McWhinney, 1983).

The pathogenic process is conventionally depicted in diagrams of the natural history of disease (see Figure 10.1) as movement from left to right, in a "forward" direction, from the realm of normal healthy populations to the domain
of disease and, ultimately, death (Leavell & Clark, 1965). Holding back the tide
of pathogenesis, at the population-wide level, is believed to be best achieved by
preventing or mitigating the effects of deleterious experiences or characteristics: reducing job stress, comforting the bereaved, offering smoking cessation
programs, etc. In this way, healthy people who exhibit these characteristics
(populations at risk, in epidemiologese) can be protected against subsequent
morbidity. This is known as primary prevention.

But what about helping people who are already ill? And what about members of healthy populations who wish to attain something more—a state of wellness
or high-level healthiness? Epidemiologists rarely explore this issue, whether they
are psychosocial epidemiologists or otherwise. The emphasis is rather on how
people become ill, or remain healthy, not on how they become well. An unspoken presumption in the consensus understanding of natural history and the pathogenic process is that movement from a diseased to a healthy state is movement
from right to left, in a "backward" direction, so to speak, and involves action taken
in furtherance of the flipside of a respective risk factor. For example, if smoking
cigarettes leads to cancer morbidity and smoking cessation prior to the appearance of signs or markers of disease prevents morbidity, then presumably smoking
cessation also contributes to recovery. If stress and hostility contribute to coro-

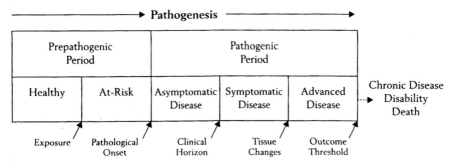

Figure 10.1. The natural history of disease.

nary artery disease, then the removal of stress and reduction of hostility may help to reduce symptoms or, better, to reverse the disease process itself.

Sometimes this makes sense, but in other instances may not. Those factors that cause illness and whose absence may prevent illness may not, when flipped over, or inverted, cure people or help them to attain an even healthier state than their baseline level of health. For certain types of morbidity with known physical or physiological causes, this point is obvious. For example, cigarette smoking is associated with coronary artery disease and early myocardial infarction, and smoking cessation may mitigate heart-related symptoms. But it is unlikely that smoking cessation in a patient with advanced disease could be expected, by itself, to produce a cure, much less a state of wellness beyond that experienced by a person who never smoked. A more obvious example: Exposure to venom from a poisonous spider bite can cause a life-threatening wound; avoiding such spiders will not help an existing wound to heal. That requires an array of therapies: debridement of the wound, antibiotics, and perhaps antivenin. These treatments, moreover, while components of a cure—a "leftward" movement through the natural history of disease—can only take a person so far; they would not constitute a therapy of choice for a patient wishing to improve the appearance or function of already healthy tissue.

For psychosocial factors ostensibly associated with physical or psychiatric morbidity, this point may be less apparent. For example, epidemiologic studies show that bereavement due to widowhood is associated with depression and higher mortality. Further, marriage is associated with less morbidity and greater longevity, especially among young and middle-aged males. But would a widow or widower finding a new spouse be able to substantially reverse both a depressive state and physiological changes that compromise survival? Maybe; maybe not. Perhaps depression would be ameliorated in some people. Perhaps longevity could be re-extended, so to speak, as well. But could most folks become happier and live longer than they would have in the first place, had they not been widowed—in the "better than ever" sense implied by engendering a state of wellness? It does not seem likely, but, regardless, this would depend upon other physiological processes, social status,, and psychological states and traits.

In any event, to use coronary artery disease as an example, epidemiologists have unquestioningly focused far more attention on the purported etiologic or risk-enhancing role of Type A behavior than on any ostensibly protective, moderating, or health-promoting effect of the "opposite" Type B pattern (Kaplan, 1992). Other examples can be found among the pool of psychosocial constructs whose health effects are regularly investigated by epidemiologists and medical social scientists. The "rightward," pathogenic focus implicit in how research questions are framed is a carryover from epidemiology's origins investigating outbreaks of epidemic infectious diseases in order to search for a culpable pathogenic agent. The negative polarity of so many psychosocial constructs is a carryover from (a) sociology's postwar disciplinary identity as an applied science of social problems and (b) psychology's historical focus on abnormal behavior. These conceptual conventions limit the questions that psychosocial epidemiologists typically ask, but they are not the only valid approach for this field.

ANTONOVSKY, COHERENCE, AND SALUTOGENESIS

To better clarify how psychosocial factors may influence health in both directions across the natural history of disease, Antonovsky (1987) developed the concept of salutogenesis. This he defined as "not just the other side of the coin from the pathogenic orientation, but, rather, [something] radically different" (p. 2). The assumptions of a salutogenic orientation are not present in the prevailing understanding of the natural history of disease, informed as it is by a pathogenic orientation. These features were summarized in an earlier analysis by the present author (Levin, 1996) and include:

- Presence of a dynamic "health ease/dis-ease continuum," rather than a continuum of healthy versus diseased
- A call for epidemiologic research to focus not on disease but rather on people's "stories," in order to identify salient health-promoting factors
- Assertion that salutogenic factors are not just the opposite categories of pathogenic factors, as noted above, but may be entirely different factors
- Assertion that stressors may be salutary and not exclusively pathological, as they may make demands that produce adaptations with positive health consequences
- A call for epidemiologic research to focus on identifying those factors that facilitate adaptation, rather than solely on potentially etiologic factors
- Heightened curiosity about "deviant" cases—for example, Type A persons who do not develop heart disease, smokers who do not get cancer—rather than a default judgment that these are outliers and thus should be ignored

The advantage to thinking salutogenically, according to Antonovsky (1987), is that it forces epidemiologists and social scientists to "devote our energies to . . . formulation of a theory of coping" (p. 13). Such a theory is necessary because the salutogenic process, as was suggested, may be physiologically and psychosocially distinct from the pathogenic process, and not just its reverse. For researchers, this is the issue in a nutshell: How we heal or attain wellness may invoke altogether different variables—processes, statuses, and characteristics—than those that arise in studies of becoming ill or preventing illness.

Antonovsky's (1979) own theory centered on his concept of the sense of coherence, which he described as "a global orientation to one's inner and outer environments which is hypothesized to be a significant determinant of location and movement on the health ease/dis-ease continuum" (Antonovsky, 1993,

p. 731). This, he proposed, develops over the life course and comprises three elements: (1) comprehensibility (the extent to which internal psychological and
external environmental stimuli make cognitive sense), (2) manageability (the
extent to which available resources are adequate), and (3) meaningfulness (the
extent to which challenging events are seen as worthy of emotional investment
and engagement) (Antonovsky, 1979). In practical terms, any psychosocial characteristic that could provide a context for interpreting the events of one's life and
enable a person to deal with and to derive meaning from such events could be
said to engender coherence. It is worth noting that this description of coherence
resembles both Geertz's (1966) well-known definition of religion and contemporary descriptions of the features and functions of coping (e.g., Pargament, 1997).

The capability of psychosocial characteristics to provide a sense of coherence and thus facilitate coping, as described by Antonovsky, was presaged decades ago by Cassel, the epidemiologist most known for pioneering the study of
the impact of social and psychological exposures on morbidity. Cassel proposed
not only that features of interpersonal relationships could buffer or cushion individuals from noxious stimuli (Cassel, 1964) but, later, that certain psychosocial characteristics may represent independently protective factors that reduce
susceptibility to disease (Cassel, 1976). This, he suggested, is achieved through
bolstering host resistance, or the ability of persons or populations to withstand
exposure to pathogenic agents or conditions. Antonovsky's (1974) own phrase
for this was "generalized resistance resources." In the context of the natural history of disease, host resistance is potentially necessary, although not sufficient,
for "leftward," or salutogenic, movement. At the very least, in theory, it represents a salient force for slowing or halting "rightward" movement, i.e., for preventing complications, improving prognosis, and hastening recovery.

Antonovsky's perspective on coherence and salutogenesis represents a promising template for psychosocial epidemiology, but these concepts have been
underappreciated and underutilized. Psychosocial epidemiology, like the rest
of epidemiology, is mostly about the study of pathogenic exposures, in this instance social-psychological states or traits. Where positive variables, such as social
support, are investigated, they are typically studied as potential mediating factors or moderators of risk in a pathogenic process whose outcome is morbidity
or mortality. One of the few attempts to propose a salutogenic interpretation
of an empirical question in psychosocial epidemiology has been theoretical work
by the present author that attempts to make sense of the literature on the observed effects of religiousness (Levin, 1996, 2003). Even there, however, the
primary focus has been on determining how the exposure variable functions to
reduce the risk of morbidity—more so than to promote healing or wellness.

The most promising application of Antonovsky's ideas would be to effect a
marriage of positive psychology and psychosocial epidemiology. His understanding of the importance of context and meaning in facilitating coping, coupled with
his depictions of the healing or health-promoting process, dovetail nicely with

epidemiologic efforts to understand how psychosocial exposures enhance host resistance and thus mitigate disease risk. Positive psychology would contribute to psychosocial epidemiology by encouraging a refocus away from pathogenesis and on salutogenesis. Psychosocial epidemiology would contribute to positive psychology by providing a context and methods for evaluating and understanding the salutary aspects of human psychology at a population-wide rather than individual level. The marriage of these fields would contribute to public health and medicine, ideally by encouraging more systematic investigation of linkages between mental and emotional states and plausible biological mechanisms of disease causation, an issue rarely engaged by epidemiologists (Weed & Hursting, 1998).

Among positive-psychological constructs, scholarly discourse on love is the most theory-dense, due to three decades of research and writing by psychologists (Sternberg & Barnes, 1988) and by the provocative and recently rediscovered work of the sociologist Sorokin (1954). Thus, consideration of love can serve as the vanguard of a new, positive-psychosocial epidemiology that investigates factors that promote salutogenesis and not just factors that heighten the risk of pathogenesis. While longitudinal studies of factors that promote healing among ill people, or wellness among healthy people, are not the traditional orientation of epidemiology, existing methodologies are applicable to such research. That is, this new approach would by no means challenge existing procedures related to sampling or research design or data analysis. Methodology, therefore, would not present a barrier.

Theoretically, however, it is an open question whether current models of psychosocial factors in disease risk are applicable for framing research questions and positing hypotheses about potentially salutogenic effects. A pressing need exists for theory development focusing on how positive-psychosocial constructs and variables, exemplified by love, might be expected to contribute to a sense of coherence and thus strengthen host resistance and influence the course of salutogenesis. Just what precisely is meant by the word "contribute" is an important issue that must be explored before an explicit theoretical statement can be formulated. Almost all existing research in psychosocial epidemiology focuses on risk factors for rates of morbidity. This is not the same thing as a focus on the determinants of individual cases of disease or of positive health states. Moreover, conceptual distinctions among risk factors, statistical determinants or predictors, and putative etiologic factors are typically glossed over or ignored.

PSYCHOSOCIAL DETERMINANTS OF MORBIDITY, DISEASE, AND HEALTH

The discussion in this section may seem obscure, counterintuitive, or even confusing to many physicians and medical social scientists. Such confusion is due, in large part, to the lack of clarity with which epidemiologists have articulated the parameters of their discipline to researchers outside of public health.

Modern epidemiology is conventionally defined as the investigation of the distribution and determinants of morbidity and mortality in populations. This is not the same as searching for the determinants of cases of disease; epidemiology is not a branch of medicine nor directly concerned with identifying etiologic factors in individuals (Stallones, 1987). Epidemiologists focus on the determinants of morbidity, i.e., population-wide rates of disease. The objective is to identify patterns and determinants of rates of disease as manifest across population systems, or large social networks—not in any individual person (Koopman & Lynch, 1999). Myriad exposures may determine population-wide morbidity for certain diseases; the well-known "web of causation" metaphor comes to mind (McMahon, Pugh, & Ipsen, 1960). But this multifactorial web pertains only to that set of environmental or host exposure variables that separately or together elevate the risk or odds of morbidity disparities—which can then be targeted for public-health intervention. Such interventions may be population-wide, such as efforts to change environmental health policies, or, like many health promotion programs, may seek to change discrete health-related behaviors of individuals. Epidemiologic studies which identify social, psychosocial, or environmental risk factors for morbidity thus serve a critical function in focusing applied public-health efforts in the policy and practice arenas (Shy, 1997).

But this does not imply that risk factors, as population-wide determinants are known, are necessarily disease-causing entities in any given person. At the individual level, psychosocial risk factors do indeed contribute to disease susceptibility in many people in certain situations (see Schwartz & Diez-Roux, 2001). As Taylor (1990) has noted, "Research that examines whether or not psychological and social factors are involved in health and illness has largely made its point" (p. 46). No serious academic scientist would question this any more. But it is hard to imagine how such factors could directly cause disease—a pathophysiological state—in the absence of (a) a pathogenic biological, chemical, or physical agent; (b) an injury to, an impact of stress upon, or the senescence of a physiological system or organ; or (c) a genetic trait that predisposes one to a particular disease. Not everything that adds to the burden of morbidity in a population is necessarily etiologic in an individual, or, put differently, the causes of incidence are not necessarily the causes of cases (see Rose, 1985).

In one specific sense, negative psychosocial characteristics may perhaps be considered partially etiologic: in the context of mitigating host resistance and thus enabling a fertile ground for potentially harmful exposures to initiate pathogenesis. One is reminded of the debate more than a century ago between Pasteur and Bernard over "the seed or the soil"—that is, whether the germ or the flesh, or, in epidemiologic terms, whether pathogenic exposures or host resistance, are of greater salience in disease causation. In modern epidemiology, both elements are acknowledged as part of the equation. Accordingly, certain deleterious psychosocial states or traits may antecede cases of disease in individuals by inducing psychophysiological reactivity that works to compromise host defenses and inhibit host resistance (Steptoe, 1998), thus exacerbating the impact of other risk factors or elevating susceptibility to opportunistic agents seeking to gain a foothold. This can be true both for acute, communicable diseases and for what are currently considered to be chronic, degenerative diseases of noninfectious origin. The concomitant cascade of physiological effects more or less defines the well-known stress response (Dodge & Martin, 1970), accounts for cases of what is known vernacularly as psychosomatic or psychogenic illness (Lipowski, 1984), and is becoming a well-accepted and scientifically validated framework for contextualizing mental and emotional impacts on health and disease (Sternberg, 2001).

The key take-away point: Whether serving as antecedents to individual cases of disease, through triggering a pathogenic process, or as risk factors for population-wide rates of morbidity, where psychosocial factors are implicated in contributing to the production of disease is through their compromising of host resistance. Such factors are not themselves disease-causing agents but rather may exert a deleterious impact on the overall constitution of individual hosts or host populations and thus increase their susceptibility to pathogenic agents or processes, resulting in asymptomatic, symptomatic, or advanced disease; disability; or death.

Epidemiologists' inattention to spelling out these issues for physicians, biomedical researchers, and social and behavioral scientists has created needless conflict and confusion. Considerable energy, for example, has been expended to carefully dissect and critique the overstated and misinterpreted web-of-causation idea (Krieger, 1994, 2001)—which, to reiterate, remains a heuristically useful public-health concept but is not as meaningful etiologically and may not even make sense in that context (see Stallones, 1980). To wit, it was recently suggested that "social conditions" are "fundamental causes of disease" (Link & Phelan, 1995). Social-structural characteristics of populations indisputably antecede disparities in population-wide indices, such as morbidity and mortality; this has been known at least since Graunt (1662/1939) indexed London's Bills of Mortality in the 17th century. But to be a "fundamental" cause of cases of disease would seem to imply both an identity as a primary source of pathogenesis and an unmediated effect on human physiology, which, in this instance, does not make biological sense. Poverty, poor education, inadequate social resources, and lack of supportive social networks, for example, are indeed key features of the web of determinants of population-wide rates of morbidity and mortality due to many diseases, just as are many psychological constructs. But these characteristics cannot in and of themselves directly produce diseases inside of individual bodies in the absence of exposure to a specific pathogen, an inherited trait, or medical or stress-related sequelae that impair functioning of a physiological system or organ. Moreover, many more chronic, degenerative diseases thought to include a psychogenic or sociogenic etiologic component may be of infectious origin than has been commonly believed (Ewald, 2002), including atherosclerosis and cancer, leading causes of death in the socioeconomically developed world.

At the population-wide level, social conditions can be rightly seen as vital "upstream," or distal, risk factors (Kaplan, 1995), changes in which may be more appropriate, just, and effective targets for public-health intervention than more proximal variables, such as physiological states or biomarkers. The latter may be intransigent to change, or may be cofactors of advanced cases of disease and thus not appropriate foci for primary prevention. The communitarian and social-justice orientation of public health thus calls for intervention at levels beyond the individual when this can prevent the greatest suffering among the greatest number of people (Barry, 1975). But social conditions are themselves not pathogenic agents—they are social-environmental characteristics—and they cannot account for exposure to all pathogens, to their transmission, or to the subsequent course of disease.

Another result of epidemiologists' inattention to delineating the parameters and nuances of population-health concepts has been ceaseless debate about the psychosocial versus biological origin of disease. On one side are social and behavioral scientists, and some physicians, espousing variations of a biopsychosocial model of the determinants of disease (Engel, 1977). Pitted against them, in defense of the traditional medical model of disease, are those physicians and biomedical scientists asserting that any purported empirical evidence implicating psychosocial factors, such as mental states, in the pathogenesis of disease is "folklore" (Angell, 1985). Ironically, each side may be more or less correct, depending upon whether one is speaking of the web of risk factors at the population-wide level or the pathogenic process at the level of individual patients, especially in terms of the most proximal, or "downstream," physiological statuses or cofactors. Yet because each side speaks a different language and because the context is different, neither sees the validity of the other side.

A rare exception to these polarized discussions can be found in the sophisticated theoretical model put forth by Jenkins (1985), who is uniquely credentialed as a psychologist, epidemiologist, and clinical and population-health researcher. His understanding of the patterning of morbidity in individuals and populations accommodates the interaction of biological, psychological, and behavioral characteristics and processes with aspects of cultural, social, biological, and physical environments. These interactions occur in diverse ways that heighten the risk of certain diseases, and the scope and magnitude of such effects vary across the natural history of disease—that is, depending upon whether one is investigating predisposition, precipitation, signs and/or symptoms of early disease, or full clinical disease and whether one's endpoint is recovery, rehabilitation, disability, or death. Moreover, the confluence of the potential determinants of disease or morbidity is dependent upon the disease entity in question and the stage of the life course, among other contextual factors.

If speaking of the social and psychosocial determinants of morbidity in populations is not the same as speaking of the social and psychosocial determinants of disease in individuals, what of the emerging field referred to as the "social determinants of health"? Notwithstanding an excellent base of empirical findings dating back a half century, coupled with a heartening renaissance of interest since the 1990s (e.g., Amick, Levine, Tarlov, & Walsh, 1995; Berkman & Kawachi, 2000; Evans, Barer, & Marmor, 1994; Marmot & Wilkinson, 1999; Tarlov & St. Peter, 2000), some conceptual and theoretical confusion exists within this field. Specifically, evidence of the social determinants of health is typically presented in the form of observed disparities in morbidity and mortality rates—rarely in terms of indices of health or positive well-being. These include population-wide differences in morbidity and mortality attributable to social-structural or sociodemographic variables, such as poor working conditions or inequality in income; to psychosocial constructs, such as stress or social support; and to behaviors, such as cigarette smoking. Positive study results thus point presumably to these social and psychological characteristics being implicated among the web of factors antecedent to population-level morbidity. Such results say nothing about their hypothetical role in causing or leading to health, which the field's name seems to promise. In this field, as in epidemiology in general, the most common measures of "health status" are actually measures of disease or death status (Wolfson, 1994), typically at the population-wide level.

This conceptual confusion about psychosocial exposures and putative health-related outcomes has more than semantic implications. A case in point: The thousand-plus studies showing differences in morbidity and mortality rates by categories of religious affiliation and participation (Koenig, McCullough, & Larson, 2001) have created needless controversy, with competing camps alternately promoting these studies as proving that religion is good for one's health or disparaging them as scientifically unsound or impossible (see Levin, 2001a). Neither side is correct, the underlying problem being that each camp advances straw men and each speaks a different language. For one, epidemiologic studies are based on observation, not experiment, produce findings based on probabilistic associations, and thus cannot "prove" relationships between exposures and outcomes. Second, studies have for the most part identified religious differences in population-wide rates of morbidity and mortality, not health. Third, whether something is "good" or "bad" for a particular person is a value judgment outside the purview of epidemiology, which can only estimate risks that exist on average across a population. Fourth, nearly all comprehensive scholarly reviews have vetted the methodological soundness of most large-scale studies in this field; the labeling of this work as unscientific is purely ideological. Fifth, positive results may seem impossible only if they are misinterpreted as providing evidence of a clinical outcome, such as a healing power over disease, which they do not. This distinction—between the prevention of morbidity (which this research addresses) and the healing of disease (which this research does not address)—is apparently not obvious to the clinicians and scientists who continue to disbelieve and disparage significant findings showing a religious effect on the former on the grounds that a religious effect on the latter seems implausible. In fairness, such confusion may result because this distinction is rarely articulated by the physicians and social and behavioral scientists producing these findings, perhaps due to a similar lack of awareness.

In short, four distinct outcomes can be differentiated for psychosocial epidemiology (see Figure 10.2). One distinction can be made by level of analysis, whether individual or population-wide. A second distinction can be made by the direction that one is moving through the natural history of disease, whether pathogenic ("rightward") or salutogenic ("leftward").

For psychosocial exposures, the following classes of outcomes can be investigated. Biomedical researchers have focused considerable attention on cell a, both clinically and in the laboratory, leading to much of the controversy surrounding the ostensible psychosocial causation of disease. Because the focus is on individual patients or on discrete systems within the human organism, the role of psychosocial, macrolevel, or otherwise socially contexted variables may seem implausible. Social and psychosocial epidemiologists have focused predominantly on cell b: studies of psychosocial risk factors for morbidity and mortality. Examples include research on stress and chronic disease morbidity, the Type A behavioral pattern and morbidity due to coronary artery disease, and social support and overall mortality. Very little work has targeted cell c, although interesting basic-science research has begun to probe possible neurophysiological (D. F. Smith, 2002) and molecular (Lohff, Schaefer, Nierhaus, Peters, Schaefer, & Vos, 1998; Schaefer, Nierhaus, Lohff, Peters, Schaefer, & Vos, 1998) correlates or mechanisms of salutogenesis. For biomedicine, this is an exciting frontier.

What is proposed is something akin to cell d, along with a variation on cell b, namely, investigation of the potentially salutogenic impact of psychosocial exposures at the population-wide level (cell d), as well as the use of psychosocial exposures of positive polarity (e.g., love, gratitude, forgiveness) in lieu of

Direction Through the Natural History of Disease

		Pathogenesis	Salutogenesis
Level of Analysis	Individual	a Disease Status	c Normal Status or Wellness
	Population	b Morbidity and Mortality	d Population Health

Figure 10.2. Typology of health-related outcomes investigated in relation to psychosocial exposures.

the more traditional negatively polarized constructs in conventional epidemiologic investigations of morbidity and mortality (cell b). This is in sharp contrast to conventional psychosocial research in epidemiology and medicine, whereby negatively defined constructs (e.g., stress, Type A behavior) are investigated in relation to rates of morbidity (cell b) or cases of disease (cell a). *The new orientation being proposed here is thus threefold: a combination of positive-psychological exposure variables investigated in relation to population-wide rates of both pathogenic and salutogenic outcomes.*

To summarize: (1) The determinants of morbidity, disease, and health are not all the same thing; (2) the classes of variables used to define these outcomes are quite different; and (3) the effects of positive-psychosocial exposures, such as love, may be investigated at different levels of analysis and in different directions through the natural history of disease. A key corollary of these three summary points is that these distinct types of psychosocial investigation may entail distinctive theoretical approaches.

INTEGRATING LOVE INTO THEORETICAL PERSPECTIVES IN PSYCHOSOCIAL EPIDEMIOLOGY

Psychosocial epidemiology represents a merger of the theories and constructs of social psychology with the approach and methods of epidemiology. It is one of three fields which, historically, fall under the larger rubric of social epidemiology. This metafield—think of it as epidemiology crossed with social science research—also comprises behavioral epidemiology, which focuses on the epidemiologic impact of health-related behaviors, and the study of social-structural and socioeconomic influences on morbidity and mortality, also known, confusingly, as social epidemiology. The salad days of psychosocial epidemiology were from the late 1950s through the 1970s, centered at the University of North Carolina School of Public Health (Brown, 2002). Psychosocial epidemiology became eclipsed by behavioral epidemiology in the 1980s, with the advent of federal funding for health promotion and disease prevention programs, and by a resurgence of interest in the social determinants of health in the 1990s. But the emergence of interest in the epidemiology of positive-psychological constructs, such as faith and love, portends a renaissance of psychosocial-epidemiologic theory and research.

This final section provides (a) an overview of theoretical perspectives that have governed research and writing by psychosocial epidemiologists over the past 40 years and (b) brief summaries of how love can be studied within the framework provided by each respective class of theories. In sociological terms, these are a mix of "grand" and "midrange" theories. The concept of midrange theory derives from Merton (1949/1968), who differentiated between what sociologists call grand theory, or large metatheories of everything, and less-reaching theories specific to particular fields or issues. A grand theory is a paradigmatic statement reflecting a larger world view, usually identified with founding theorists and subsequent expositors. Such statements are competing ways of organizing existing information in order to understand scientifically observable phenomena (see Kuhn, 1970). Examples include the functionalism of Durkheim, Parsons, and Merton; the conflict structuralism identified with Marx and his followers; and the symbolic interactionism that evolved from work by Weber, Mead, and Blumer. Within psychology, the term grand theory is not used, but such perspectives can be identified, e.g., the behaviorism of Watson and Skinner, the psychodynamic schools that followed Freud, and the humanism and transpersonalism of the late 20th century.

A grand theory may spawn various midrange theories, or they may arise independently. Theories of the middle range are less ambitious, posited simply to order hypotheses regarding particular sociological or social-psychological phenomena of concern to certain fields of study, e.g., the theory of relative deprivation, the theory of cognitive dissonance, the disengagement theory of aging. Midrange theories may, in turn, generate theoretical models governing analyses of data bearing on a set of conceptual relationships. Examples include the myriad path models positing relationships among variables, which are found in every area of research in the social sciences. Theory making has never been a priority within epidemiology (Weed, 2001), due to its historical roots in microbiology and emphasis on control of infectious diseases of presumed monofactorial etiology, but theory-driven research has always been normative within social, psychosocial, and behavioral epidemiology.

What follows is not an exhaustive list of theories put forth in psychosocial epidemiology—far from it—but rather the most influential classes of perspectives on how psychosocial exposures are believed to affect health-related outcomes. Some appear to be grand theories, or paradigmatic statements; others seem more like midrange theories. Each has been around for decades, has its associated proponents, and has succeeded in informing the conduct of research studies and the interpretation of empirical findings. Judgment is withheld as to which perspectives are "right" or "wrong"; the objective is simply to demonstrate that constructs associated with love can be accommodated by them. Further, these do not represent discrete theories, but rather classes of overlapping perspectives or, better, approaches to contextualizing a potential relationship between psychosocial variables and health or illness. These perspectives seek to describe and explain how human health and well-being are affected by characteristics of the inner life in relation to the external environment of people and institutions—more or less a working definition of psychosocial epidemiology.

The perspectives summarized here include (a) the biopsychosocial model and systems theory, (b) the stress paradigm and coping, (c) psychosomatic and mind-body medicine, (d) behavioral medicine and health psychology, and (e) social environment and person-environment fit. According to each perspective, a salutary effect of love can be accommodated by the existing theories of how psychosocial characteristics of people and populations affect the prevention of disease and morbidity and the promotion of health and well-being.

The Biopsychosocial Model and Systems Theory

Beginning in the 1970s, critiques appeared which detailed the conceptual limitations of the dominant biomedical model of disease causation. As articulated by Engel (1977), biomedicine was judged to be dogmatically reductionistic by dint of an overreliance on molecular biology as a source of explanations for the origins of diseases. Contemporary developments in social psychiatry, especially, convinced him and others that much more was involved in the production of disease than was captured in the traditional basic sciences. In remedy, Engel proposed a "biopsychosocial model" founded on a more "holistic" perspective on what defines a human being and on what explains health-impacting life processes. This model, in turn, was grounded in the biological school known as systems theory, as first described by von Bertalanffy (1968) and others decades earlier. While subsequent history shows that biomedicine is more resilient than its critics suggested (see Glenn, 1988), and indeed has seen its hegemony grow with recent developments in molecular biology, genomics, and life sciences, variations on a biopsychosocial approach have nonetheless greatly influenced research and writing at the interface of epidemiology, medicine, and the social sciences.

In an explication of his model, Engel (1980) described the biopsychosocial approach as "a scientific model constructed to take into account the missing dimensions of the biomedical model" (p. 535). This he depicted as a metasystem of interpenetrating and integrated component systems, arranged hierarchically and constituting a human life. A human being, he asserted, was embedded in—indeed, defined by—organized systems ranging from those constituting a physical human (subatomic particles, atoms, molecules, organelles, cells, tissues, organs and organ systems, the nervous system) to those extending beyond the body (dyads, families, communities, cultures and subcultures, societies and nations, the biosphere). Intermediating these two classes of system, as he defined things, were the person's behavior and experience. This perspective has proven to be useful and influential, especially for primary care physicians seeking more effective ways to identify disease risks (Engel, 1980) and to manage patients (C. K. Smith & Kleinman, 1983) and for efforts to rationalize health care, planning, and policy (Brody & Sobel, 1979). Its influence can be seen in subsequent theoretical writing within psychosocial epidemiology which takes a multifactorial approach to the determinants of morbidity, including the stress, psychosomatic, and social-environment perspectives described below.

The experience of love can be accommodated at various levels along the systems hierarchy, as defined by this theory. Individual people, of course, can give and receive love—or, in the language of this perspective, experience love and behave lovingly. These experiences and behaviors can occur in interaction with other people and within families. Wider social structures (communities, cultures, nations) can act lovingly toward individual people and family units, expressed through social and health policies and through social-structurally defined statuses and sanctioned mores governing human interaction. People, in turn, can act altruistically and compassionately toward these social structures in a variety of ways, such as through the expression of particular attitudes (e.g., patriotism, advocating progressive reform) and self-sacrificing behaviors (e.g., military service, activism and change agency). These loving interactions are experienced by being cognitively engaged and felt, which may trigger or manifest in psychophysiological and neuroendocrinological changes, which ultimately result in somatic responses, whether the reduction of signs and symptoms or salutogenic reactions.

The Stress Paradigm and Coping

The conception of certain disease risks as stressors engendering by individuals an adaptive response that mediates and ostensibly moderates the impact on pathology is by now a tacit perspective among health scientists. The stress perspective is such an ingrained part of the orientation of sociomedical scientists that it can be termed paradigmatic, as it represents the principal lens through which researchers view the impact of the wider social-psychological world on the health of individuals and groups. The term stress long ago became a buzz word for social scientists, taking on divergent meanings as a stimulus, response, or outcome, depending upon the author. As articulated by Selye (1936), an early proponent of this theory, stress defines a kind of inborn response system that kicks in when demands on the human organism require a protective response. This he encapsulated in his "general adaptation syndrome," a three-step model encompassing an alarm phase followed by an adaptive response phase and, ultimately, by exhaustion or failure of bodily defenses (Selye, 1973).

Subsequent research and writing have expanded these concepts for application to human health, as exemplified by the work of Levi (1971–1987), at the Karolinska Institute, and those who have utilized measurement indices that follow in the "life events" tradition of the Social Readjustment Rating Scale (Holmes & Rahe, 1967). Psychosocial epidemiologists have taken special interest in the adaptation phase, which, through the years, has evolved into the field of research built around coping and social support. Consistent with the appreciation of host resistance as a determinant of morbidity, Cassel (1974b) criticized those who treated the relationship between stressor and disease as equivalent to that between a microorganism and disease; for him, the impact of stressors was clearly "conditional" (p. 473). Clinical manifestations were not solely due to the actions of a given pathogenic stressor, but also to "constitutional factors" (p. 473). In a *Festschrift* to Cassel, his colleagues summarized his working hypothesis that "rapid social change . . . placed stressors on the adaptive capacity of persons at the same time that it tended to disrupt their traditional systems of social and psychological support from others" (Ibrahim, Kaplan, Patrick, Slome, Tyroler, & Wilson, 1980, p. 2). Echoing this theme in a call for renewed focus on stress among social epidemiologists, Graham (1974) suggested, "Loss or gain of statuses in the milieu may be another source of fruitful inquiry" (p. 1048). Those factors—cognitive, affective, behavioral, social-structural—that might mitigate the deleterious impact of stressful circumstances or events and thus foster an effective coping response have been subjected to voluminous research since the influential Institute of Medicine (IOM) report in 1982, which first gave sanction to large-scale studies of this topic (Hamburg, Elliott, & Parron, 1982). A search of the National Library of Medicine's database of peer-reviewed journals uncovered more than 10,000 scholarly articles and reviews linked to both of the keywords "stress" and "coping" since the IOM report.

This mediating or moderating role as a coping resource is not the only possible place for psychosocial factors within the stress paradigm. It has been proposed that positive-psychological states affect health status both indirectly, through facilitating attempts to cope with stress, as described above, and directly, through the effects of what is termed "eustress," or the converse of distress. In an outstanding review, Edwards and Cooper (1988) proposed a theoretical model for the integration of positive psychology into the study of the determinants of physical health, within a eustress-coping context. Drawing upon clinical, epidemiologic, and laboratory evidence, they asserted that positive-psychological states may engender "the direct appraisal of factors in the environment as meeting or exceeding desires" (p. 1448), resulting in eustress that, in turn, "may evoke physiological responses which, in the long run, improve physical health" (p. 1448) through accepted hormonal and biochemical pathways. Examples of such positive states, backed by empirical research, include humor, laughter, and amusement; happiness and euphoria; positive life events; job and life satisfaction; and self-efficacy, optimism, and hope. It is not much of a stretch to envision other positive-psychological constructs, such as gratitude, forgiveness, and love, as engendering the same type of response. This excellent theoretical model has been largely ignored—fewer than 20 scholarly citations in the nearly two decades since its publication—but deserves close scrutiny by every researcher interested in how positive psychology might be relevant to the study of health and illness.

Psychosomatic and Mind-Body Medicine

Speculation about the nature and health impact of interactions between psyche and soma, or mind and body, dates back at least to Hippocrates and was a prominent theme of medical and psychiatric writing throughout the 19th century (Schwab, 1985). Systematic investigation of mind-body connections for the purposes of understanding cases of organic disease began with Alexander (1950) in the 1930s and relied upon psychodynamic methods. Psychosomatic medicine, as a defined field of study focusing on linkages among the brain, behavior, and biological processes (Jenkins, 1985), flowered in subsequent decades and today is represented by a variety of professional societies and scientific journals. The psychosomatic "movement" was especially influential for psychosocial epidemiology in the 1960s and 1970s, with social-psychological and personality perspectives existing alongside of and eventually overtaking the more traditional psychoanalytic perspective as a source of psychological variables for use in large-scale epidemiologic studies (Bahnson, 1974).

As a theoretical basis for psychosocial-epidemiologic research, psychosomatic medicine sits on a foundation of two principles (Lipowski, 1984). These have been termed the "holistic conception," namely, that "the notions of mind and body refer to inseparable and mutually dependent aspects of man" (p. 159), and the "psychogenic conception," which asserts that "certain attributes or functions of the organism, those that be called 'psychologic' or 'mental,' constitute a class of causative agents in morbidity" (p. 162). The psychosomatic approach, then, implies "the inseparability and interdependence of psychosocial and biologic (physiologic, somatic) aspects of humankind" (p. 167). Since the 1980s, these interdependencies have been spelled out in detail, with scientists mapping behaviorally determined patterns of neuroendocrine response (Henry, 1982), neuroendocrine-immune interactions (Reichlin, 1993), and psychological modulation of immunity (Maier, Watkins, & Fleshner, 1994), culminating in the rapidly growing basic science of psychoneuroimmunology (Ader, Felten, & Cohen, 1991).

The phrase psychosomatic medicine is used less today, having been supplanted by "mind-body medicine," meaning essentially the same thing. Its usage was hastened in large part by efforts of the Fetzer Institute, which funded several popular books in the 1990s, including *Healing and the Mind* (Moyers, 1993), based on a PBS television series, and *Mind Body Medicine* (Goleman & Gurin, 1993), published by Consumer Reports. Whichever phrase is used, the intent is the same for epidemiologic research: to investigate the impact of mental and emotional states, including the psychobiological mechanisms by which such effects operate, on the incidence and course of disease. Various multifactorial and step-sequential models have been proposed to account for these connections, ranging from extremely detailed maps of physiological, cellular, and genetic processes drawn up by basic scientists to path models of hypothesized directional effects among groups of psychosocial constructs, more typical of sociomedical or behavioral researchers. The former is exemplified by a proposal integrating the mind modulation of cellular activity via the autonomic nervous system, of mind-gene communication via the endocrine system, of innate immunity, and of neuropeptides (Rossi, 1993); the latter by a model linking affective disturbances and physical disorders through a variety of biological, behavioral, cognitive, and social mediators (Cohen & Rodriguez, 1995).

Taking these models as a cue, positive-psychological constructs with emotional correlates or components, such as compassionate or divine love, have a clear place in theories of mediating links between psyche and soma. Experiencing loving emotions or witnessing loving acts may produce affects resulting in hormonal, neurochemical, or metabolic changes within the body. Experiencing acts of loving kindness—either as giver or receiver—or a sense of God's love may help to reframe cognitive distortions that translate pain, disability, or physical symptoms into mood or anxiety disorders, and vice versa, by mitigating threats to self-esteem, self-efficacy, and sense of control. The interpersonal context of loving interactions may provide similar mediation by helping to preserve role functions and to prevent the deterioration of social networks that regulate life-affirming self-images, positive emotions, and healthy practices. Evidence from experimental and population-based studies provides preliminary support for these connections. One famous study of viewers of a documentary film about Mother Teresa found increased levels of S-IgA (salivary immunoglobulin A) for 1 hour afterward among subjects asked to recall times when they were loved— a finding not present among subjects who viewed a film about Nazis or who did not dwell on love (McClelland, 1986). Two more recent studies by the present author suggest that affirmation of a loving relationship with God is associated with greater perceived health even in the face of chronic disease and disability (Levin, 2001b) and with less depressed affect even in the face of poor health (Levin, 2002).

Behavioral Medicine and Health Psychology

In contemporary psychosocial epidemiology, two divergent perspectives have come to the fore, each influenced by elements of the biopsychosocial model, stress theory, and the basic science of mind-body interactions. One of these perspectives is mostly associated with work by behavioral and clinical psychologists and some psychiatrists; the other is more the province of sociologists. The former, behavioral medicine, emerged as a separate field in the 1970s, bringing together scientists and clinicians who had achieved success in the 1960s in applying behavioral therapy to mental-health problems, developing biofeedback, and identifying behavioral risk factors for the most incident and lethal chronic, degenerative diseases, such as coronary artery disease and cancer (Blanchard,

1982). The emphasis of behavioral medicine, especially in an epidemiologic context, is on ostensibly modifiable behaviors, rather than on cognitive and affective influences on morbidity that may be less salient in their effects and more intractable in terms of public-health intervention. This perspective is influential both clinically and in public health, as interventions targeting changes in the lifestyle behaviors of individuals have been a controversial but principal focus of health promotion programs since the early 1980s (Roberts, 1987; Runyan, DeVellis, DeVellis, & Hochbaum, 1982).

Around the time that behavioral medicine rose to prominence, health psychology emerged as a subspecialty within academic psychology. These two fields overlap quite a bit—in the scope of their research emphases, in key figures, and in "classic" publications. Often, these terms are used interchangeably, developments in one field ascribed to the other, or behavioral medicine is referenced as a perspective within health psychology. Still, clear distinctions exist. To generalize, whereas behavioral medicine focuses expressly on modifiable behaviors, the mission of health psychology is broader, "involving all branches of psychology in virtually every aspect of the health enterprise" (Taylor, 1990, p. 40). In an epidemiologic context, this includes health-related behaviors, personality styles and traits, emotional states, cognitions and attributions, and myriad values, conations, and experiences. The perspective and focus of behavioral medicine have been most influential for behavioral epidemiology; health psychology encompasses more of a social-psychological orientation and has been a rich source of theories and constructs for psychosocial epidemiology.

The greatest evidence of this cross-fertilization of health psychology and epidemiology is seen in the thousands of published studies that implicate a broad swath of psychological constructs as risk or protective factors with respect to morbidity rates or health indicators. As summarized in many popular and scholarly works, such as *Who Gets Sick* (Justice, 1987), these include, but are not limited to, health locus of control, the Type A behavioral pattern, bereavement, hassles and uplifts, hardiness, John Henryism, self-esteem and mastery, and features of health beliefs and personality styles, from optimism to hostility. Some constructs once believed to be etiologically significant, such as the cancer-prone personality, are now in question. Other constructs have been found to be health impacting, but only at specific stages of the natural history of disease. A well-known example: the primary preventive impact of religious participation, in contrast to the persistent and incorrect presumption that studies have identified a consistent effect of religiousness on the curing of disease.

Since the 1990s, health psychologists have shifted attention to how psychological characteristics or states affect immune response and disease susceptibility (Cohen & Herbert, 1996). Mind-body medical scientists have explored bidirectional effects between psychological factors and physiological, biomolecular, and cellular processes (Myers & Benson, 1992). This work brings together theory and research on stress, emotions, personality, and social relationships with developments in psychoneuroimmunology and the basic sciences, blurring distinctions among the theoretical perspectives discussed in this section and creating alliances with neuroepidemiology. These perspectives are becoming synthesized into a thriving and multidisciplinary, if far from unified, field of mind-body research, which is slowly moving toward the investigation of topics in population health. One example is the recent proposal for epidemiologic research on the transcendent experience (Levin & Steele, 2005). Such topics are an exciting frontier for psychosocial epidemiology, as they promise a cross-fertilization of areas as diverse as behavioral neuroscience, social psychology, and consciousness research.

The call for an epidemiology of the transcendent experience exemplifies how a spiritually contexted positive-psychological state with validated psychophysiological correlates might be engaged in population-health research (Levin & Steele, 2005). The authors defined two classes of transcendent experience: one fleeting yet characterized by spiritual ecstasy, bliss, and joy; the other more permanent and characterized by heightened awareness and a transformational shift in consciousness. Both are associated with alterations in perception, with intense and pleasurable affects, and with a unitive sense of connection to God or the loving source of being. Diverse theoretical models have been proposed for the neurophysiological processes underlying these experiences, drawing on concepts associated with neuropsychological, psychoanalytic, Jungian, humanistic, transpersonal, perceptual-cognitive, and contextual perspectives and schools. These concepts represent a cross-section of the cutting edge of mind-body research in biomedicine: neurobiofeedback, neurotransmitters, conditioning, neurocognition, consciousness, and psychophenomenology. These varied approaches to the connections among mind, brain, and body represent a rich source of hypotheses for epidemiologists and a stepping-off point for the formulation of research programs.

Social Environment and Person-Environment Fit

Among psychosocial epidemiologists with a disciplinary background in sociology or a medical specialty in social, community, or family medicine, the dominant theoretical perspective differs in important ways from the orientation of social, behavioral, and health psychologists. Identified with the work of Kark and Cassel, fathers of the larger field of social epidemiology, epidemiologists of the "North Carolina school" have been most interested in how the characteristics and disruptions of the human social environment serve to elevate morbidity and to promote pathophysiological responses. Constructs of interest include social disorganization, social hierarchy, social mobility, urbanization, acculturation, social support networks, and other social and interpersonal resources that buffer socioecologic stress (Cassel, 1974a). This approach is psychosocial-epidemiologic and not strictly social-epidemiologic in the sense that the latter term is used today—for studies of social-structural and sociodemographic variables, such as social class status and socioeconomic indicators. What sets the North Carolina school apart is attention to the population-health impact of transactions between the inner life of people and the larger social context in which they live, rather than a focus on one or the other.

While this social-environmental perspective has guided the work of sociologists in the field of psychosocial epidemiology, parallels can be observed in social psychology, notably in theories of person-environment fit (or P-E fit). Derived from the work of Lewin (1936), which he termed field theory, the P-E fit perspective holds that any psychological event, such as a behavior, is an outcome of interactions between the characteristics of the person and his or her environment. It has generated a variety of theories and measures and has been influential in occupational psychology, child development, and several other fields. Health-related research based explicitly on P-E fit has been less common, although it has been an influential perspective in population-based studies of occupational stress (Edwards & Cooper, 1990).

Guided by these perspectives, contemporary psychosocial epidemiologists have elaborated on the work of Cassel and colleagues in the tradition of the North Carolina school. A representative example is Vernon and Buffler's (1988) excellent synthesis of sociological and epidemiologic research on status inconsistency, or incongruities in social status between an individual and his or her social and cultural environment. The authors' sophisticated model combines social, psychological, and biological variables leading from incongruities and discrepancies in status to chronic disease morbidity. This process is mediated, sequentially, by a pathway from conflicting expectations to uncertainty to perceived stress to coping responses to psychophysiological symptoms and changes in autonomic nervous system and endocrine activity to chronic arousal to increased disease susceptibility. But this is not the only way that the P-E relationship bears on morbidity. Characteristics of the social environment may themselves "*moderate* or *mediate* the physiological effects of other ecological characteristics of an environment" (Kiritz & Moos, 1974, p. 110), such as population density (Wardwell, 1974).

In mapping out precisely how social environment can affect the epidemiology of disease, two roles, then, can be identified. First, disrupted social relationships may compromise host resistance, which mediates the impact of exposure risks on disease status and morbidity (Syme, 1986). Second, social statuses and relationships may lead to physical morbidity through the mediating effects of behavioral or psychological processes (e.g., health practices, coping styles) or through effecting physiological changes (e.g., cardiovascular indicators, such as increased blood pressure or heart rate; Berkman, 1981). These roles provide a template for hypothesizing how positive-psychological exposures might protect against morbidity.

A creative take on this issue was provided by Kaplan (1992), a colleague of Cassel at North Carolina and a pioneering figure in psychosocial epidemiology. In an essay on the salutogenic properties of the Type B behavioral pattern, Kaplan identified "protective processes" associated with Type B that might mitigate the incidence and course of coronary artery disease. He zeroed in on a set of constructs familiar to students of positive psychology, each of which, in an ecological context, are directly relevant to psychosocial epidemiology and to research on the determinants of well-being. These constructs are (a) uniqueness, autonomy, and self-esteem, which Kaplan believed to be associated with the capability to give and receive appreciation and to seek honest assessment of personal skills and limitations; (b) wisdom, which he viewed as a coping resource due to its positive influence on realistic cognitions that might influence salutary behavioral outcomes; (c) forgiveness, which he saw as a correlate of generosity and humility that fosters the avoidance of unhealthy demands and helps to forgo hostility and resentment; and (d) sociability, which for him is rooted in love and manifests in friendships and healthy attachments that relieve isolation, bolster morale, and are therapeutic. Accordingly, love is integral for adaptive fitness and thus for the prevention of morbidity and maintenance of well-being. Yet in the literature on social support, Kaplan laments, agreeing with Leighton (1959), "the most neglected dimension is the capacity to love and be loved" (Kaplan, 1992, p. 11).

SUMMARY AND INTEGRATION

It is challenging but not impossible to offer a single, integrative statement summarizing the role of positive-psychological factors, such as love, across these five classes of theoretical perspectives. These perspectives vary in how they contextualize health and disease, to be sure, and thus in the constructs and variables considered to be potential determinants. Still, each theorizes, at minimum, that characteristics of the human psyche—cognitive, affective, behavioral—alone or in interaction with features of the social environment influence the probability and subsequent course of health-related events. Concomitantly, it has been shown that each perspective can accommodate a role for positive-psychological states in the prevention of morbidity or disease and the promotion of health in individuals or populations. A preliminary effort is made to capture the proposed salutogenic sequelae of positive psychology in the model depicted in Figure 10.3.

In this figure, several key psychosocial and biological constructs featured as elements in the reviewed perspectives are arrayed sequentially. They are posited to mediate a hypothetical salutary effect of positive psychology, exemplified by love. Experiencing love—that is, exchanging love with other people or beings, or with God—is hypothesized to foster a sense of coherence, as described by Antonovsky. By being a loving person, and receiving love in return, one may derive meaning from human interactions and thus experience the stresses and

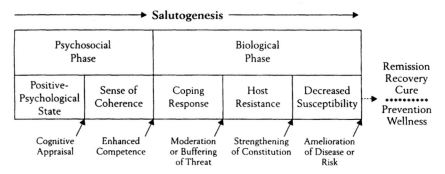

Figure 10.3. The natural history of health (for psychosocial exposures).

vicissitudes of life as comprehensible and manageable. Continued success may validate this appraisal and enhance a sense of competence that is characteristic of successful coping, thus buffering or moderating the impact of potential disease risks. This protective influence may, in turn, bolster the resistance of individuals, through established physiological mechanisms, and of populations and thus decrease susceptibility to disease. The culmination, in theory, is the successful primary prevention of disease in individuals or of elevated morbidity in populations; the hastening of movement toward remission, recovery, or cure among already diseased people or populations; or the attainment of wellness among the already healthy. This model thus posits a hypothetical sequence by which love and other positive-psychological factors engender the maintenance or improvement of health among individuals or populations regardless of disease status. The pathways depicted in this model represent a preliminary take on a proposed "natural history of health" (Levin, 2003) for psychosocial exposures. It should be noted that this salutogenic model or map is not merely the reverse of the more familiar pathogenic model—that is, not simply a "leftward" trek across the same terrain by which disease is produced. This feature of the salutogenic model was by explicit design and recapitulates the main points that have been put forth in this chapter.

To summarize, the integration of positive psychology into psychosocial epidemiology is not just desirable, but feasible. Positive-psychological constructs, such as aspects, domains, or expressions of love, can be accommodated by existing theoretical perspectives and incorporated into epidemiologic studies. For this marriage to succeed, the nuances of the fundamental principles of population health, detailed earlier, must be acknowledged and dealt with exactingly. If this is done, then no intrinsic theoretical or methodological barriers prevent the ascendancy of a positive psychosocial epidemiology. Such a development would herald not just the birth of a new field of study, but would constitute an important step toward the integration of mind-body medicine and public health, lay-ing a foundation for our understanding of the processes by which psychosocial exposures contribute to the health of populations.

The author would like to thank Lea Steele, Ph.D., for her helpful comments on earlier drafts of this manuscript.

REFERENCES

Ader, R., Felten, D. L., & Cohen, N. (Eds.). (1991). *Psychoneuroimmunology* (2nd ed.). San Diego, CA: Academic.

Alexander, F. (1950). *Psychosomatic medicine.* New York: Norton.

Amick, B. C., III, Levine, S., Tarlov, A. R., & Walsh, D. C. (Eds.). (1995). *Society and health.* New York: Oxford University Press.

Angell, M. (1985). Disease as a reflection of the psyche. *New England Journal of Medicine, 312,* 1570–1572.

Antonovsky, A. (1974). Conceptual and methodological problems in the study of resistance resources and stressful life events. In B. Dohrenwend & B. Dohrenwend (Eds.), *Stressful life events: Their nature and effects* (pp. 245–258). New York: Wiley.

Antonovsky, A. (1979). *Health, stress, and coping: New perspectives on mental and physical well-being.* San Francisco: Jossey-Bass.

Antonovsky, A. (1987). *Unraveling the mystery of health: How people manage stress and stay well.* San Francisco: Jossey-Bass.

Antonovsky, A. (1993). The structure and properties of the Sense of Coherence Scale. *Social Science and Medicine, 36,* 725–733.

Bahnson, C. B. (1974). Epistemological perspectives of physical disease from the psychodynamic point of view. *American Journal of Public Health, 64,* 1035–1040.

Barry, P. Z. (1975). Individual versus community orientation in the prevention of injuries. *Preventive Medicine, 4,* 47–56.

Berkman, L. F. (1981). Physical health and the social environment: A social epidemiological perspective. In L. Eisenberg & A. Kleinman (Eds.), *The relevance of social science to medicine* (pp. 51–75). Dordrecht, Holland: Reidel.

Berkman, L. F., & Kawachi, I. (Eds.). (2000). *Social epidemiology.* New York: Oxford University Press.

Blanchard, E. B. (1982). Behavioral medicine: Past, present, and future. *Journal of Consulting and Clinical Psychology, 50,* 795–796.

Brody, H., & Sobel, D. S. (1979). A systems view of health and disease. In D. S. Sobel (Ed.), *Ways of health: Holistic approaches to ancient and contemporary medicine* (pp. 87–104). New York: Harcourt Brace Jovanovich.

Brown, T. M. (2002). Sidney Kark and John Cassel: Social medicine pioneers and South African émigrés. *American Journal of Public Health, 92,* 1744–1745.

Cassel, J. (1964). Social science theory as a source of hypotheses in epidemiological research. *American Journal of Public Health, 54,* 1482–1488.

Cassel, J. (1974a). An epidemiological perspective of psychosocial factors in disease etiology. *American Journal of Public Health, 64,* 1040–1043.

Cassel, J. (1974b). Psychosocial processes and "stress": Theoretical formulation. *International Journal of Health Services, 4,* 471–482.

Cassel, J. (1976). The contribution of the social environment to host resistance. *American Journal of Epidemiology, 104,* 107–123.

Cohen, S., & Herbert, T. B. (1996). Health psychology: Psychological factors and physical disease from the perspective of psychoneuroimmunology. *Annual Review of Psychology, 47,* 113–142.

Cohen, S., & Rodriguez, M. S. (1995). Pathways linking affective disturbances and physical disorders. *Health Psychology, 14,* 374–380.

Dodge, D. L., & Martin, W. T. (1970). Beyond the germ theory: Psychosomatic and sociosomatic conceptions. In D. L. Dodge & W. T. Martin, *Social stress and chronic illness: Mortality patterns in industrial society* (pp. 26–51). South Bend, IN: Notre Dame University Press.

Edwards, J. R., & Cooper, C. L. (1988). The impacts of positive psychological states on physical health: Review and theoretical framework. *Social Science and Medicine, 27,* 1447–1459.

Edwards, J. R., & Cooper, C. L. (1990). The person-environment fit approach to stress: Recurring problems and some suggested solutions. *Journal of Organizational Behavior, 11,* 293–307.

Engel, G. L. (1977). The need for a new medical model: A challenge for biomedicine. *Science, 196,* 129–136.

Engel, G. L. (1980). The clinical application of the biopsychosocial model. *American Journal of Psychiatry, 137,* 535–544.

Evans, R. G., Barer, M. L., & Marmor, T. R. (Eds.). (1994). *Why are some people healthy and others not? The determinants of health of populations.* New York: de Gruyter.

Ewald, P. W. (2002). *Plague time: The new germ theory of disease.* New York: Anchor.

Fine, P. E. M. (1993). Herd immunity: History, theory, practice. *Epidemiologic Reviews, 15,* 265–302.

Frank, J. D. (1975). Mind-body relationships in illness and healing. *Journal of the International Academy of Preventive Medicine, 2*(3), 46–59.

Freer, C. B., & McWhinney, I. R. (1983). Natural history of disease. In R. B. Taylor (Ed.), *Family medicine: Principles and practice* (2nd ed., pp. 97–104). New York: Springer-Verlag.

Geertz, C. (1966). Religion as a cultural system. In M. Banton (Ed.), *Anthropological approaches to the study of religion* (pp. 1–46). London: Tavistock.

Glenn, M. L. (1988). The resurgence of the biomedical model. *Family Medicine, 20,* 324–325.

Goleman, D., & Gurin, J. (1993). *Mind body medicine: How to use your mind for better health.* Yonkers, NY: Consumer Reports Books.

Graham, S. (1974). The sociological approach to epidemiology. *American Journal of Public Health, 64,* 1046–1049.

Graunt, J. (1939). *Natural and political observations made upon the Bills of Mortal-*

ity: London, 1662. Baltimore: Johns Hopkins University Press. (Original work published 1662)

Hamburg, D. A., Elliott, G. R., & Parron, D. L. (Eds.). (1982). Stress, coping, and health. In *Health and behavior: Frontiers of research in the biobehavioral sciences* (pp. 63–87). Washington, DC: National Academy Press.

Henry, J. P. (1982). The relation of social to biological processes in disease. *Social Science and Medicine, 16,* 369–380.

Holmes, T. H., & Rahe, R. H. (1967). The Social Readjustment Rating Scale. *Journal of Psychosomatic Research, 11,* 213–218.

Ibrahim, M. A., Kaplan, B. H., Patrick, R. C., Slome, C., Tyroler, H. A., & Wilson, R. N. (1980). The legacy of John C. Cassel. *American Journal of Epidemiology, 112,* 1–7.

Jenkins, C. D. (1985). New horizons for psychosomatic medicine. *Psychosomatic Medicine, 47,* 3–25.

Justice, B. (1987). *Who gets sick: How beliefs, moods, and thoughts affect your health.* Los Angeles: Tarcher.

Kaplan, B. H. (1992). Social health and the forgiving heart: The Type B story. *Journal of Behavioral Medicine, 15,* 3–14.

Kaplan, G. A. (1995). Where do shared pathways lead? Some reflections on a research agenda. *Psychosomatic Medicine, 57,* 208–212.

Kiritz, S., & Moos, R. H. (1974). Physiological effects of social environments. *Psychosomatic Medicine, 36,* 96–114.

Koenig, H. G., McCullough, M. E., & Larson, D. B. (2001). *Handbook of religion and health.* New York: Oxford University Press.

Koopman, J. S., & Lynch, J. W. (1999). Individual causal models and population system models in epidemiology. *American Journal of Public Health, 89,* 1170–1174.

Krieger, N. (1994). Epidemiology and the web of causation: Has anyone seen the spider? *Social Science and Medicine, 39,* 887–903.

Krieger, N. (2001). Theories for social epidemiology in the 21st century: An ecosocial perspective. *International Journal of Epidemiology, 30,* 668–677.

Kuhn, T. S. (1970). *The structure of scientific revolutions* (2nd ed.). Chicago: University of Chicago Press.

Leavell, H. R., & Clark, E. G. (1965). Levels of application of preventive medicine. In *Preventive medicine for the doctor in his community* (3rd ed., pp. 14–38). New York: McGraw-Hill.

Leighton, A. H. (1959). *My name is Legion: Foundations for a theory of man in relation to culture.* New York: Basic.

Levi, L. (Ed.). (1971–1987). *Society, stress, and disease* (Vols. 1–5). New York: Oxford University Press.

Levin, J. S. (1996). How religion influences morbidity and health: Reflections on natural history, salutogenesis and host resistance. *Social Science and Medicine, 43,* 849–864.

Levin, J. (2001a). Etiology recapitulates ontology: Reflections on restoring the spiritual dimension to models of the determinants of health. *Subtle Energies and Energy Medicine, 12,* 17–37.

Levin, J. (2001b). God, love, and health: Findings from a clinical study. *Review of Religious Research, 42,* 277–293.

Levin, J. (2002). Is depressed affect a function of one's relationship with God?: Findings from a study of primary care patients. *International Journal of Psychiatry in Medicine, 32,* 379–393.

Levin, J. (2003). Spiritual determinants of health and healing: An epidemiologic perspective on salutogenic mechanisms. *Alternative Therapies in Health and Medicine, 9*(6), 48–57.

Levin, J., & Steele, L. (2005). The transcendent experience: Conceptual, theoretical, and epidemiologic perspectives. *EXPLORE: The Journal of Science and Healing, 1*(2), 89–101.

Lewin, K. (1936). *Principles of topological psychology.* New York: McGraw-Hill.

Link, B. G., & Phelan, J. (1995). Social conditions as fundamental causes of disease. *Journal of Health and Social Behavior,* Extra Issue, 80–94.

Lipowski, Z. J. (1984). What does the word "psychosomatic" really mean? A historical and semantic inquiry. *Psychosomatic Medicine, 46,* 153–171.

Lohff, B., Schaefer, J., Nierhaus, K. H., Peters, T., Schaefer, T., & Vos, R. (1998). Natural defenses and autoprotection: Naturopathy, an old concept of healing in a new perspective. *Medical Hypotheses, 51,* 147–151.

Maier, S. F., Watkins, L. R., & Fleshner, M. (1994). Psychoneuroimmunology: The interface between behavior, brain, and immunity. *American Psychologist, 49,* 1004–1017.

Marmot, M., & Wilkinson, R. G. (Eds.). (1999). *Social determinants of health.* Oxford: Oxford University Press.

McClelland, D. C. (1986). Some reflections on the two psychologies of love. *Journal of Personality, 54,* 334–353.

McCullough, M. E., & Snyder, C. R. (2000). Classical sources of human strength: Revisiting an old home and building a new one. *Journal of Social and Clinical Psychology, 19,* 1–10.

McMahon, B., Pugh, T. F., & Ipsen, J. (1960). *Epidemiologic methods.* Boston: Little Brown.

Merton, R. K. (1968). Sociological theories of the middle range. In R. K. Merton, *Social theory and social structure* (pp. 39–72). New York: Free Press. (Original work published 1949)

Moyers, B. (1993). *Healing and the mind.* Garden City, NY: Doubleday.

Myers, S. S., & Benson, H. (1992). Psychological factors in healing: A new perspective on an old debate. *Behavioral Medicine, 18,* 5–11.

Pargament, K. I. (1997). *The psychology of religion and coping: Theory, research, practice.* New York: Guilford.

Reichlin, S. (1993). Neuroendocrine-immune interactions. *New England Journal of Medicine, 329,* 1246–1253.

Roberts, M. C. (1987). Public health and health psychology: Two cats of Kilkenny? *Professional Psychology: Research and Practice, 18,* 145–149.

Rose, G. (1985). Sick individuals and sick populations. *International Journal of Epidemiology, 14,* 32–38.

Rossi, E. L. (1993). *The psychobiology of mind-body healing: New concepts of therapeutic hypnosis* (Rev. ed.). New York: Norton.

Runyan, C. W., DeVellis, R. F., DeVellis, B. M., & Hochbaum, G. M. (1982). Health psychology and the public health perspective: In search of the pump handle. *Health Psychology, 1,* 169–180.

Schaefer, J., Nierhaus, K. H., Lohff, B., Peters, T., Schaefer, T., & Vos, R. (1998). Mechanisms of autoprotection and the role of stress-proteins in natural defenses, autoprotection, and salutogenesis. *Medical Hypotheses, 51,* 153–163.

Schwab, J. J. (1985). Psychosomatic medicine: Its past and present. *Psychosomatics, 26,* 583–593.

Schwartz, S., & Diez-Roux, R. (2001). Commentary: Causes of incidence and causes of cases: A Durkheimian perspective on Rose. *International Journal of Epidemiology, 30,* 435–439.

Selye, H. (1936). A syndrome produced by diverse nocuous agents. *Nature, 138,* 32.

Selye, H. (1973). The evolution of the stress concept. *American Scientist, 61,* 692–699.

Shy, C. M. (1997). The failure of academic epidemiology: Witness for the prosecution. *American Journal of Epidemiology, 145,* 479–484.

Smith, C. K., & Kleinman, A. (1983). Beyond the biomedical model: Integration of psychosocial and cultural orientations. In R. B. Taylor (Ed.), *Family medicine: Principles and practice* (2nd ed., pp. 88–97). New York: Springer-Verlag.

Smith, D. F. (2002). Functional salutogenic mechanisms of the brain. *Perspectives in Biology and Medicine, 45,* 319–328.

Snyder, C. R., & McCullough, M. E. (2000). A positive psychology: "If you build it, they will come . . . " *Journal of Social and Clinical Psychology, 19,* 151–160.

Sorokin, P. A. (1954). *The ways and power of love: Types, factors, and techniques of moral transformation.* Boston: Beacon.

Stallones, R. A. (1980). To advance epidemiology. *Annual Review of Public Health, 1,* 69–82.

Stallones, R. A. (1987). The concept of cause in disease [Letter]. *Journal of Chronic Disease, 40,* 279.

Steptoe, A. (1998). Psychophysiological bases of disease. In D. W. Johnston & M. Johnston (Eds.), *Comprehensive clinical psychology* (pp. 39–78). New York: Elsevier.

Sternberg, E. M. (2001). *The balance within: The science connecting health and emotions.* New York: Freeman.

Sternberg, R. J., & Barnes, M. L. (Eds.). (1988). *The psychology of love.* New Haven, CT: Yale University Press.

Syme, S. L. (1996). The social environment and disease prevention. *Advances in Health Education and Promotion, 1*(A), 237–265.

Tarlov, A. R., & St. Peter, R. F. (Eds.). (2000). *The society and population health reader: Vol. 2. A state and community perspective.* New York: New Press.

Taylor, S. E. (1990). Health psychology: The science and the field. *American Psychologist, 45,* 40–50.

Vernon, S. W., & Buffler, P. A. (1988). The status of status inconsistency. *Epidemiologic Reviews, 10,* 65–86.

von Bertalanffy, L. (1968). *General system theory: Foundations, development, applications.* New York: Braziller.

Wardwell, W. I. (1974). Population density and mobility. *American Journal of Public Health, 64,* 1052–1055.

Weed, D. L. (2001). Theory and practice in epidemiology. In M. Weinstein, A. I. Hermalin, & M. A. Sato (Eds.), *Population health and aging: Strengthening the dialogue between epidemiology and demography* (pp. 52–62). New York: New York Academy of Sciences.

Weed, D. L., & Hursting, S. D. (1998). Biologic plausibility in causal inference: Current method and practice. *American Journal of Epidemiology, 147,* 415–425.

Wolfson, M. C. (1994). Social proprioception: Measurement, data, and information from a population health perspective. In R. G. Evans, M. L. Barer, & T. R. Marmor (Eds.), *Why are some people healthy and others not? The determinants of health of populations* (pp. 287–316). New York: de Gruyter.

Zielhuis, G. A., & Kiemeney, L. A. L. M. (2001). Social epidemiology? No way. *International Journal of Epidemiology, 30,* 43–44.

11 Generativity: A Form of Unconditional Love

George E. Vaillant

This chapter will address two questions. First, should we distinguish the unself-ish love associated with Erikson's concept of generativity from the capacity for warm relationships? Put differently, is there a meaningful difference between altruistic leadership and loving attachment per se? Second, sentimentally, we believe that unselfish love should lead to good physical health in late life. But is this belief true?

The evidence for my answers will come from a 60-year prospective study of men's lives: the Study of Adult Development at Harvard Medical School. The study consisted of a cohort of Harvard sophomores, the college cohort, and a cohort of socioeconomically deprived youth, the inner-city cohort. Because of its association with maturity and leadership, generativity is more than the capacity for warm relationships. But before I begin, I will need to define what I mean—and perhaps what Erikson really meant—by the concept of *generativity* and by *capacity for warm relationships*.

As I am defining it, the Eriksonian task of generativity means assuming sustained responsibility for the growth and well-being of others. Generativity involves the demonstration of a clear capacity to care for and guide the next generation without expectation of reciprocity. One of the most difficult facets of generativity is to be in a caring relationship in which one gives up much of the control that parents retain over young children. Mastery of this develop-mental task approximates the Greek and Christian ideal of *agape*, but generativity also involves community building and leadership. Loving mentors and good leaders both learn to "hold loosely" and to share responsibility. Depending on the opportunities that the society makes available, generativity can mean serving as a consultant, guide, mentor, or coach to young adults in the larger society. And it is this association with maturity and with leadership—often highly paid—that makes generativity somewhat different than loving attachment per se.

In contrast, the capacity for warm relationships, whether reflected by the "secure attachment" of a loving toddler or the sometimes possessive attachment of a doting grandmother, has everything to do with love, attachment, and often "emotional intelligence." But loving attachment does not require the maturity, the unselfishness, or the community building associated with generativity.

A member of the college cohort, the product of a caring family, wrote of the first half of his adult life, "From twenty to thirty I learned how to get along with my wife. From thirty to forty I learned how to be a success in my job, and at forty to fifty I worried less about myself and more about the children." He went on to spend the rest of his life as the dean of a small college. He not only looked after students but, as he matured, he also looked after the young faculty. At 82, his adaptation to aging is brilliant. For him, there seems to be little distinction between his generativity and his success at loving relationships. And his physical health is excellent.

But, of course, one swallow does not make a summer.

In old age, there are inevitable losses, and these may overwhelm us if we have not continued to grow beyond our immediate families—and if we have not cast our bread unselfishly upon the waters. Thus, in theory, the mastery of generativity should be strongly correlated with successful adaptation to old age, for to keep it, you have to give it away. *There is no question that generativity leads to and results from good mental health, but the question addressed here is: Does generativity lead to physical health?*

TWO CLARIFYING ANECDOTES

Before turning to statistical evidence, let me offer two case examples to illustrate that generativity is not an artifact of social privilege and that it does not always lead to good physical health in old age.

As a child, inner-city cohort member Bill Dimaggio had to share a bed with his brother in a tenement apartment without central heating. When Bill was 16, his mother died; and his father, a laborer, became disabled and unemployable. With a Wechsler Bellevue IQ of 82 and a Stanford reading IQ of 71, Bill completed 10 grades of school—with difficulty.

Nevertheless, at an interview more than 30 years later, Bill Dimaggio was a charming, responsible, and committed man. If he was short and noticeably overweight, he still retained much of his youthful vigor. Bill's face was expressive; there was a twinkle to his eyes; he conveyed a good sense of humor and a healthy appetite for good conversation.

By continuing without remuneration of any kind to participate for 35 years in the Study of Adult Development, Dimaggio felt that he was contributing something to other people. Until age 40, Dimaggio had worked as a laborer for the Massachusetts Department of Public Works. Then, a position had opened for a carpenter. Although he had no formal qualifications, Dimaggio was able to get the position by seniority. He learned the necessary skills on the job; and of his work, he said, "I like working with my hands." Indeed, he had always enjoyed working with wood, and he pointed out to the interviewer how he had remodeled the inside of his own house. He took pride in his role in maintaining some of Boston's historic municipal buildings. My point is that occupational self-esteem and generativity are not just the prerogatives of CEOs and rocket scientists. But generativity usually can only occur after one has achieved Eriksonian intimacy and one's job has become a source of compensation, commitment, contentment, and competence—what I have called elsewhere the hallmarks of "career consolidation" (Vaillant, 1993). Fewer of us can be generative at 25 than at age 50.

Over the last year, Dimaggio explained that his bosses had been trying to get along better with him. Because he had become one of the few really experienced men on the job, he noted, "They depend on me more." He had become a union steward and so, if he felt that certain jobs were dangerous, he would not allow his men to work on the job. Under union rules, management would listen to him. Management also depended on his experience to help teach other men. In short, with maturity, he had learned to speak with authority. Put differently, after the age of 40, IQ does not count for much. It is what you have learned along the way and your willingness to share it generously with others that society values.

But generativity does not just exist in the workplace. As Dimaggio explained, "It's only a job. I'm more concerned about my wife and kids. Once I leave work I forget about it." He described taking his sons fishing and taking them to all sorts of places as they were growing up. "We spent a lot of time together. I have had more time for my children than my father had for me."

He knew that his children smoked marijuana (the year was 1976), and he said that he could accept that. But if adolescents had to be allowed to learn from mistakes, his children could not smoke pot in the family house. He was accepting of the fact that his youngest son had moved in with a girlfriend. He chalked this up to "him being very immature," and he felt that his son would get more mature as time went on. A vital ingredient of generativity is hope in the species, but such hope is only possible if one's mind can encompass human development. Unselfish love means granting autonomy to those for whom we care as well as protecting them from self-destructive behavior.

When Dimaggio was asked to describe his wife, this inarticulate man then proceeded to offer the interviewer a string of simple words: "sweetheart—very understanding—everything you want in a woman—she loves to talk and argue and I like this." For Dimaggio, loving attachment was not a problem. Dimaggio said that probably what pleased him the most about his wife is her "sense of humor—without it we couldn't have survived." When Dimaggio's wife came back into the room to join in the interview, he was asked to discuss the question of "which child was most like him." Bill suggested that the oldest son had "some of my qualities," but his wife disagreed. She nominated the youngest boy because he has "your sense of humor."

On family disagreements, Dimaggio acknowledged, "We don't settle them readily, but we don't let them overcome us." He explained that when he and his wife had arguments, they did not last very long. "We don't hold grudges." Forgiveness is a vital element of unselfish love. Again, Dimaggio mentioned using a sense of humor to help take the bite out of arguments and disagreements. He said that he and his wife have had to realize that each has his or her own opinions; and so they tried to respect the other's opinions and not force their own opinions on the other. Asked whether he turns to anybody in times of trouble, Bill Dimaggio said, "We turn to each other." His wife then chimed in, "Bill is my best friend." Generativity and attachment often go together. But respect for a mentee's autonomy is a complex balancing act that develops in its own time. Sometimes, the possessiveness of love, as in eros or secure attachment, can get in the way of generativity.

Bill Dimaggio belonged to the Sons of Italy. He had been quite active in that organization, and he regularly helped out with bingo night. He and another member, a close friend, regularly cooked for the club on Saturdays, when the club hosted a lunch for members. Dimaggio said he liked to do the cooking; he liked the feeling of people being happy with his food. In addition, he and his wife also signed up to work for one of the candidates for mayor who was challenging the old-guard city boss; and he expected to donate his time to campaign for the candidate in the coming election. Finally, Dimaggio was quite active in the Council of Organizations, which is sort of an umbrella organization for all of the charitable clubs in Boston's North End. Generativity means giving yourself, not money, to others.

There was no difficulty for the independent raters to agree that Bill Dimaggio was generative. I wanted him to live forever. But Bill Dimaggio—overweight, hypertensive, and a former heavy smoker—died in his 50s from a heart attack.

Butch Bishop was another inner-city man who illustrated Eriksonian generativity. On a study home visit in 1940, Butch Bishop's home was "drab, noisy, and disorderly." His mother was described as a "stout, flabby woman with disheveled hair, and her dirty apron and sloppy slippers did not enhance her uncouth appearance." Her husband, an abusive, alcoholic father, had abandoned the family long before the interview. On the one hand, a son and a daughter were Salvation Army officers; on the other hand, another son was a serious delinquent.

Our study member, Butch Bishop, was her youngest child. He had repeated 1st and 5th grades and then left school in the 11th grade. His tested intelligence revealed a Stanford reading IQ of 78 and a math IQ of 63. In regular school, he got a B for conduct and a D for effort. His dominant traits were "slovenly," "tardy," and "lazy." In contrast, in Salvation Army Sunday school, he was more conscientious. He earned a perfect 12-year attendance record. When Butch Bishop wasn't in school or baby-sitting for his younger siblings, he spent most of his time working for the Salvation Army. His ambition was to grow up to be a minister in the Salvation Army. But adolescent wishes are cheap. A capacity for effective generativity takes time.

After dropping out of high school, Bishop spent 9 months in the Salvation Army College, and then took several 4–week summer courses at Boston University to become a "supply minister" for the Methodist church. (Supply ministers work in parishes too small to pay a "real" minister.)

With the help of his minister brother-in-law, Butch Bishop got a small parish and then as he matured spent the next four decades in charge of larger and larger parishes. What he enjoyed about his work was "helping and teaching people," but as he grew older he found that he preferred to work with the elderly rather than with young people. Consistent with my suggestion that generativity may be different from attachment per se, Bishop worried that he neglected his own small children for his church work. In spite of this and their father's IQ, his children all completed high school and obtained 1–2 years of college.

Currently, Bishop is also active with the Kiwanis Club and his church youth group, and he enjoys looking after his five grandchildren. Each year, he gives the blessing at the high school graduation—a ceremony in which he as a student had been too intellectually challenged to take part. He belongs to a men's group of ministers from which he gets a good deal of emotional support and which he used to comfort himself when his daughter died of a brain tumor. At 70, Butch Bishop described his marriage as excellent, and he still enjoyed counseling others. (Used as an adaptive defense, altruism is giving to others good things not given to you.) At 70, Bishop still could not spell, but he was an elder in the Methodist church and on the board of directors of the Salvation Army. His wife, also a former Salvation Army minister, has had to run the business side of his progressively larger parishes, for maturation and generativity do not improve your skill at math—only at living. Sadly, Butch Bishop died, relatively young, at 72 while this chapter was being written.

THE STUDY OF ADULT DEVELOPMENT
AND ITS METHODOLOGY

Elsewhere, I have noted (Vaillant, 2002) that generativity in both men and women was strongly predictive of successful aging 25 years later. But does this mean that mental health is an inevitable result of unselfish love? Or is it the other way around, and do mental health and maturity lead to unselfish love?

And whichever the causal direction between generativity and mental health, does unselfish love cause physical health? Case histories will not answer the question. I must turn to statistics.

Of the many studies cited in this volume, perhaps the study by Oman and colleagues (Oman et al., 1999) that altruism enhances longevity is the most convincing. Using a 3- to 6-year follow-up, they managed to exclude most of the confounders that might explain the almost threefold difference in mortality that they observed between the elderly who volunteered and those who did not. I shall begin by using the Study of Adult Development to examine Oman's conclusions. The college cohort of 268 Harvard sophomores, selected for relative mental and physical health, has been studied since 1940 (Heath, 1945; Vaillant, 1977). The inner-city cohort consisted of 456 economically and educationally disadvantaged Boston youth who were chosen as a nondelinquent control group for a longitudinal study of delinquency. They were first studied between 1940 and 1945 at an average age of 14 plus or minus 2 years (Glueck & Glueck, 1968). The Gluecks obtained assessments of ethnicity, multiple measures of IQ, school achievement, social class, and family history of learning difficulties. Equally important, the study provided prospectively gathered information on the men's ability to love and to work until age 75. Finally, the sample was homogeneous for potential confounders of tested IQ, such as school system (inner city), race (Caucasian), gender (male), and parental educational disadvantage. The men have been reinterviewed at approximately ages 25, 30, and 47. Since age 45, the men have been followed by biennial questionnaires. Assessment of volunteer activities, generativity, and mature coping styles has been central to both follow-up studies. For both samples, physical exams have been obtained every 5 years for active members, and death certificates have been obtained even for the "drops."

Based on Erikson's (1950) model, generativity was defined as taking responsibility for the development of the next generation (e.g., as coach, parent of adolescents, organization leader, or manager). In addition, such individuals had to have achieved intimacy with a significant other for 10 years and achieved a stable career identity (Vaillant & Milofsky, 1980). For the college men, the rating was by a senior clinician; for the inner-city men, the rating was the consensus judgment of two clinicians. For both cohorts, when the judgment of two raters was obtained, they disagreed in about 25% of the cases. Table 11.1 demonstrates the face validity of our necessarily arbitrary classification of generativity (aka unselfish love).

Assessment of warm relationships was based on a 25-point scale summing each individual's relative success in accomplishing eight different tasks of adult object relations, excluding marriage. One task each reflected enjoyment of children, family of origin, and workmates; three tasks reflected friendship network; and two tasks reflected participation in group activities (Vaillant & Vaillant, 1981).

Table 11.1. Face Validity of Generativity as Assessed for the Inner-City Men

	Generative (N = 109)	Intermediate (N = 95)	Not Generative (N = 110)
Volunteer activities at age 47	54%	17%	12%
Altruism	54%	22%	6%
Good marriage at ages 50–65	70%	59%	35%
Gave kids 2+ years of college	56%	36%	18%
Responsible for care of children	96%	90%	51%
Managerial responsibility at work	40%	17%	4%
Warm objective relations at age 47	50%	15%	6%

Note: The differences between the generative and not-generative groups are all significant at $p = .000$, x^2

The mature defenses of altruism, suppression, anticipation, sublimation, and humor (ages 45–50) were assessed as follows. Based on review of the subjects' adult lives from ages 20 to 47 by a 2-hour interview at age 47, these five adaptive coping styles were each assessed on a 4-point scale by two independent raters. Methods, rationale, and reliability are described elsewhere (Vaillant, 1992, 2000).

Parental social class, parental education, IQ, and multiproblem family membership exerted no effect on whether the participants achieved generativity. Rather, men needed positive familial relationships, sanguine temperament, and the capacity to "take others inside," as it were, to become generative. Such men not only enjoyed warm relationships, they were likely to have enjoyed school and to have found role models.

In general, our efforts replicated the findings reported by Oman et al. (1999) that volunteering (correlated with generativity) leads to extended longevity. Of 72 college men with no voluntary activities at 65, 31 (43%) were dead over the next 20 years; of the 57 men with volunteer activities, only 13 (23%) men were dead ($x^2 = 5.8$, $df .1$, $p < .02$). However, if the single additional confounder, alcohol abuse (ignored by Oman's group), was controlled, the significant association of volunteer activities with reduced mortality disappeared. For example, of the 7 alcohol-dependent men who survived until 65, 6 engaged in no volunteer activities, and 5 were dead by age 75. Twelve other alcohol-dependent men had died before their 65th birthdays; they, too, had been relatively inactive in volunteer activities. In other words, alcoholism both is a lethal disease and interferes with unselfish community activities, and its influence must be controlled before one surmises a causal relationship between volunteering and mortality.

Nevertheless, I was surprised that for both the inner-city and the college cohorts, there was little association between generativity per se and mortality. For the college cohort, the correlation between mortality from 65 to 80 was .00 with generativity at 47, .02 with charitable giving at 65, and .01 with altruism at 47. Confirming my theoretical position that generativity involves giving of the self and not of money, generativity and charitable giving were not significantly associated. Nor was there an association between childhood social class and generativity. By age 50, however, social class was highly associated with generativity ($r = .44$, $p < .001$).

Not surprisingly, generativity was strongly associated with a capacity for warm relationships and with mental health. These latter variables *were* significantly associated with physical health at every age. Like generativity, the mature coping styles of suppression, humor, sublimation, and especially altruism were important to mental health and maturity (Vaillant, 1977), but were unassociated with physical health at ages 75 and 80.

Table 11.2 breaks down the difference between the correlates of warm relationships (i.e., love per se) and the correlates of generativity (i.e., unselfish love). As noted by numerous others, the capacity to love and to be loved is associated with positive physical health. But when a capacity for warm relationships was statistically controlled, then even the weak relationship between generativity and physical health at 70 disappeared, but the strong relationships among generativity, altruism, income, and occupational status (aka leadership) remained.

Generativity ($r = .28$; $p < .001$), religious satisfaction ($r = .22$, $p < .01$), and altruism ($r = .21$, $p < .01$) were all associated with subjective good physical health if not with objective health. In other words, our subjective health (how we, not

Table 11.2. Differences Between the Correlates of Generativity and Warm Relationship When Each Variable Is Separately Controlled for the Inner-City Cohort

	Correlation With Generativity, Controlling for Warm Relationships	Correlation With Warm Relationships, Controlling for Generativity
Generativity More Important Than Warm Relationships		
Likes school	.20**	.04
Years of education	.18	.03
Role model	.18*	.01
Altruism	.30***	.20**
Income age 50	.24***	.10
Occupational status age 50	.34***	.08
Social class age 50	.30***	.09
Warm Relationships More Important Than Generativity		
Warm marriage ages 50–65	.01	.23***
Not clinically depressed	.04	.25***
Objective health age 60	.00	.15*
Objective health age 70	.02	.15*
Active physically age 70	.05	.20***
Alive/Dead	.03	.14*

Note: *$p < .05$; **$p < .01$; ***$p < .001$.

our internist, report our health) has as much to do with our emotional and spiritual health as with our physical health.

DISCUSSION

Perhaps the dilemma of why generativity should be good for "aging well" but not for reducing mortality can be resolved in this fashion. Good habits are very important to objective physical health: loving, not smoking, not abusing alcohol, and pursuing education. For such variables, maturation is not essential. In contrast, maturity, whether measured as the opposite of narcissism or of being "over 30" has little to do with physical health and everything to do with unselfish love. In addition, the habit of putting the welfare of others ahead of one's own does not always lead to good self-care. The fact that subjective physical health was as highly associated with mature defenses as it was with objective physical health helps to explain the illusion that unselfish love is linked to physical health. To use a metaphor, the saints often die young. But in the decade before death, they feel so much better about themselves than do the self-absorbed and the stingy.

Another surprising finding was that unselfish love led so strongly to upward social mobility and was so well rewarded by society. Although we may view deans, matriarchs, bishops, generals, and business magnates as the sometimes lonely products of crass striving and infantile narcissism, in doing so we ignore the ego skills necessary to allow one individual to assume sensitive responsibility for other adults. Leadership looks like nothing more than self-aggrandizement and blind ambition until we try to do it ourselves. Then we discover how much prestigious responsibility reflects the capacity to "wipe other people's noses" and to care for those younger and weaker than ourselves.

Compared to mental health per se, generativity was more highly associated with promotions, marked upward social mobility, and earned income. It was as if bread cast upon the waters literally does return tenfold. But there was often a price. Unlike the majority of people with good mental health and with the capacity for secure attachment, generative individuals and leaders had not always been given to themselves. In contrast to mental health per se, generativity was not always associated with warm childhoods or, when such men were adults, with freedom from depression and psychiatric care. Perhaps we should not be surprised that altruism, another facet of giving without expectation of return, was strongly associated with generativity but not with either mental or physical health.

A provocative paradox was that if unselfish love did not reduce mortality, or necessarily create warm relationships, it was associated with high salaries. To their peers, Field Marshall Bernard Law Montgomery and the Lady of the Lamp (aka Florence Nightingale) were insufferable, selfish egotists. The childhood and adult lives of both individuals were bereft of close attachments. Indeed, even as adults, both individuals overtly hated their mothers. Nevertheless, those younger than Montgomery and Nightingale felt profoundly cared for, and they worshipped Montgomery's and Nightingale's selfless concern for their welfare. At the heart of the developmental task of generativity is the capacity to blend unconditional love and leadership. Indeed, blind ambition rarely makes an effective leader.

Another point that deserves discussion is the association of generativity with maturation. The association of mental health with maturity is mediated not only by progressive brain myelinization into the sixth decade (Benes, 1998) but also by the evolution of emotional and social intelligence through experience. Both processes play a role in the increasing deployment of mature coping mechanisms over time (Vaillant, 1977). The capacity of altruism, humor, and sublimation to transform negative into positive emotions is a cornerstone of maturity as well as of emotional health. All three mechanisms facilitate unselfish love, and the link between mature defenses prior to age 50 and good mental health at 80 (Vaillant, 2000) also underscores the validity of Barbara Fredrickson's (2001) "broaden and build" theory of positive psychology.

Perhaps generativity is more important to the survival of the species than to the survival of the individual. The inexorable march of spiritual development and the unselfish care of the weak has evolved steadily in *Homo sapiens*. The creation of the first Islamic and monastic hospitals occurred more than a millennium ago, and such development is more useful to survival than a clever brain per se. The Benedictine Order whose often obese, hard-drinking, and short-lived members follow a rule that insists that "the care of the sick is to be placed above and before every other duty" has endured for 1,500 years. In contrast, the modern devotees of the "South Beach diet" who spend their free time working out, staying sober, and reading magazines like *SELF* may outlive Benedictine monks by decades, but their health clubs are often of short duration. Thus the race survives through unselfish love even when the individual does not.

REFERENCES

American Psychiatric Association. (1980). *Diagnostic and statistical manual of mental disorders* (3rd ed.). Washington, DC: Author.

Benes, F. M. (1998). Human brain growth spans decades. *American Journal of Psychiatry*, 155:1489.

Brown S., Nesse, R. M., Vonokur, A. D., & Smith, D. N. (2003). Providing social supports may be more beneficial than receiving it. *Psychological Science*, 14:320–327.

Erikson, E. (1950). *Childhood and society*. New York: Norton.

Fredrickson, B. L. (2001). The role of positive emotions in positive psychology. *American Psychologist*, 56:218–226.

Glueck, S., & Glueck, E. (1950). *Unraveling juvenile delinquency*. New York: Commonwealth Fund.

Glueck, S., & Glueck, E. (1968). *Delinquents and nondelinquents in perspective.* Cambridge, MA: Harvard University Press.

Heath, C. (1945). *What people are.* Cambridge, MA: Harvard University Press.

Hollingshead, A. B., & Redlich, F. C. (1958). *Social class and mental illness.* New York: Wiley.

Kotre, J. (1984). *Outliving the self.* Baltimore: Johns Hopkins University Press.

Loevinger, J. (1976). *Ego development.* San Francisco: Jossey-Bass.

Oman, D., Thoresen, C. E., & McMahon, K. (1999). Volunteerism and mortality among the community-dwelling elderly. *Journal of Health Psychology,* 4:301–316.

Schwartz, C., Meisenhelder, J. B., Ma, Y., & Reed, G. (2003). Altruistic social interest behaviors are associated with better mental health. *Psychosomatic Medicine,* 65:778–785.

Vaillant, G. E. (1974). Natural history of male psychological health: II. Some antecedents of healthy adult adjustment. *Archives of General Psychiatry,* 31:15–22.

Vaillant, G. E. (1977). *Adaptation to life.* Boston: Little Brown.

Vaillant, G. E. (1979). Natural history of male psychological health: Effects of mental health on physical health. *New England Journal of Medicine,* 301:1249–1254.

Vaillant, G. E. (1991). The association of ancestral longevity with successful aging. *Journal of Gerontology,* 46:292–298.

Vaillant, G. E. (1992). *Ego mechanisms of defense: A guide for clinicians and researchers.* Washington, DC: American Psychiatric Press.

Vaillant, G. E. (1993). *The wisdom of the ego.* Cambridge, MA: Harvard University Press.

Vaillant, G. E. (1995). *Natural history of alcoholism revisited.* Cambridge, MA: Harvard University Press.

Vaillant, G. E. (2000). Adaptive mental mechanisms: Their role in a positive psychology. *American Psychologist,* 5:89–98.

Vaillant, G. E. (2002). *Aging well.* Boston: Little Brown.

Vaillant, G. E., & Davis, J. T. (2000). Social/emotional intelligence and midlife resilience in schoolboys with low tested intelligence. *American Journal of Orthopsychiatry,* 70:215–222.

Vaillant, G. E., Meyer, S. E., Mukamal, K., & Soldz, S. (1998). Are social supports in late midlife a cause or a result of successful physical aging? *Psychological Medicine,* 28:1159–1168.

Vaillant, G. E., & Milofsky, E. S. (1980). Natural history of male psychological health: IX. Empirical evidence for Erikson's model of the life cycle. *American Journal of Psychiatry,* 137:1348–1359.

Vaillant, G. E., & Vaillant, C. O. (1981). Natural history of male psychological health: X. Work as a predictor of positive mental health. *American Journal of Psychiatry,* 38:1433–1440.

Vaillant, G. E., & Vaillant, C. O. (1990). Natural history of male psychological health: XII. A 45–year study of successful aging at age 65. *American Journal of Psychiatry,* 147:31–37.

Wechsler, D. (1939). *The measurement of adult intelligence.* Baltimore: Williams and Wilkins.

12   The Roles of Love, Attachment, and Altruism in the Adjustment to Military Trauma

Bita Ghafoori
Robert Hierholzer

Posttraumatic stress disorder (PTSD) is a debilitating disorder that affects the lives of a large number of veterans of wartime conflict. In order to prevent the development of PTSD and to treat effectively those who suffer from its symptoms, it is important to determine what factors protect veterans who experienced significant traumas during their military service from being vulnerable to the development of PTSD. Among the factors that have been cited as possibly being protective of PTSD are a secure adult attachment style (Dieperink, Leskela, Thuras, & Engdahl, 2001) and altruistic intent (Kahana, Kahana, & Harel, 1988; Kishon-Barash, Midlarsky, & Johnson, 1999; Midlarsky, 1991).

The primary goals of this chapter are to summarize research on the associations among love in the form of a secure adult attachment, posttraumatic stress disorder, and altruism. The chapter is organized into five sections. The first section briefly reviews PTSD and its symptom clusters. The second section provides an overview of attachment theory and explores evidence that early childhood attachment patterns endure as adult attachment styles. The third reviews efforts to link attachment theory to the concept of adult love. The fourth section explores the relationship between attachment styles and the development of PTSD in those exposed to trauma, suggesting that love and secure attachment may protect against PTSD or ameliorate its course. The final section introduces altruistic intent into the adult attachment equation and examines the relationships among altruism, loving attachments, and PTSD. Implications for treatment, conceptualization, and future research will be discussed.

POSTTRAUMATIC STRESS DISORDER

Exposure to a traumatic event is common. Up to 90% of the general population in the United States has been exposed to a traumatic stressor such as interpersonal violence, automobile accidents, manmade or natural disasters, or wartime combat at some time in their lives (Breslau, Kessler, Chilcoat, Schultz, Davis, & Andreski, 1998). Approximately 10–20% of individuals exposed to a severe trauma will develop PTSD as a result (Kessler, Sonnega, Bromet, Hughes, & Nelson, 1995). PTSD represents the development of characteristic symptoms that result from a traumatic event that is outside the range of normal human experience (Pearce, Schauer, Garfield, Ohlde, & Patterson, 1985). The DSM-IV TR (American Psychiatric Association, 2000) criteria for PTSD specify that the trauma must be such that there was actual or threatened death or serious injury to self or others and that the exposed person's response at the time involved intense fear, helplessness, or horror. Other required features for this diagnosis include persistent reexperiencing of the traumatic event such as nightmares or intrusive thoughts of the event(s) (criterion B of DSM-IV TR); persistent avoidance of stimuli associated with the trauma and numbing of general responsiveness (criterion C of DSM-IV TR); and persistent symptoms of increased arousal not present before the trauma (criterion D of DSM-IV TR).

It is important to note that disturbances in interpersonal relationships are intrinsic to the diagnosis of PTSD. Empirical research bears out that interpersonal disturbances are common with PTSD (Benotsch et al., 2000; Carroll, Rueger, Foy, & Donahoe, 1985; MacDonald, Chamberlain, Long, & Flett, 1999; Nezu & Carnevale, 1987; Roberts et al., 1982). Among the potential manifestations of PTSD as delineated in criterion C of the DSM-IV TR are a "restricted range of affect (unable to have loving feelings)"; a "feeling of detachment or estrangement from others"; and a "sense of a foreshortened future (e.g., does not expect to have a career, marriage, children, or a normal life span)." Impairment in the ability to love and be loved is manifested by stressful interpersonal experiences. Such problems effect relationship dysfunction on a global level (MacDonald, Chamberlain, Long, & Flett, 1999). Interpersonal dysfunction among those with PTSD includes the diminished ability to be emotionally close to others and to express or feel emotions within themselves (Penk et al., 1981). Individuals with PTSD also report more problems relating to social, family, sexual, and work functioning (Solomon & Mikulincer, 1987). Avoidance, emotional numbing, and arousal negatively affect virtually all areas of interpersonal connections. The interactive nature of PTSD symptoms results in various interpersonal problems, each affecting and perpetuating the others in a cyclical pattern, contributing to the longevity of PTSD. PTSD can be seen in an interpersonal context, in which symptoms and love difficulties influence each other in a dismally recurring pattern. When treating such a multifaceted disorder, recognizing the role of love within the conceptualization of PTSD may serve to encompass the interactive complexity of several symptoms.

ATTACHMENT THEORY

Attachment, as described by Bowlby (1977, 1982), refers to the universal, biologically based, emotional bond between the infant and the caregiver, which involves the desire to be close to the attachment figure during times of stress. Early attachments are thought to lay the foundation for future adult relationships. A child is thought to develop a secure attachment to a primary caregiver when clear communication to the caregiver elicits a favorable response (Main, 1990). On the other hand, insecure attachment styles are thought to develop when the child finds that interacting with the caregiver leads to rejection or conflict (Izard & Kobak, 1991). As a result of these early communication responses from the primary caregiver, the child develops an "internal working model" of him- or herself as deserving or undeserving and of others as trustworthy and responsive or as untrustworthy, unresponsive, and rejecting (Bowlby, 1973).

The concept of attachment, whether secure or insecure, has emotional, cognitive, and behavioral elements. Emotionally, a secure attachment has been linked with the ability to tolerate negative emotions (Siegel, 1999). Cognitively, a secure attachment will facilitate a cognitive template of relationships with the expectation that others will be available and responsive during times of need (Siegel, 1999). Behaviorally, a securely attached individual will be able to experience comfort with intimacy, depending on someone and being depended on, and exploring the world without fear of abandonment (Crittendon, 1988).

Longitudinal research has demonstrated the stability of attachment bonds over the lifespan (Main, Kaplan, & Cassidy, 1985). This may be partially due to the fact that internal working models tend to stay outside of conscious awareness and are fairly resistant to change (Bretherton, 1985). In other words, adult attachment may be a manifestation of earlier, primary attachments experienced in infancy and childhood. While attachment patterns are thought to be developed by the original parent-child relationship and to remain fairly stable, the internal working models have been found to change as a consequence of different life circumstances such as severe trauma or war (Bretherton, 1985). Consequently, as one grows, the internal working model may begin to incorporate other attachment relationships. Attachment in adulthood includes a broader range of attachment figures, not only the individual's parents (Csikszentmihalyi & Larson, 1984). Several studies have indicated that attachment patterns influence not only adult romantic relationships, but also friendships and spiritual relationships (Hazen & Shaver, 1987; Kirkpatrick & Shaver, 1992).

LINKING ATTACHMENT AND LOVE:
EVIDENCE FROM EMPIRICAL STUDIES

The idea that attachment and love have something in common has a long history in psychology. Bowlby (1982) contended that attachment patterns continue throughout an individual's life, that if the attachment figure is nearby, accessible, and attentive, an individual will perceive her- or himself as feeling loved and secure. Several researchers have applied the concepts of attachment theory to adult romantic love relationships. Drawing from the ideas of Bowlby, studies examining adult love have found support for a model that conceptualizes love as a parallel to attachment (Bartholomew & Horowitz, 1991; Brennan, Clark, & Shaver, 1998; Hazen & Shaver, 1987; Kirkpatrick & Shaver, 1992).

Hazen and Shaver (1987) studied romantic love as an attachment system in adults. Hazen and Shaver's work in the area of adult attachment has proven to be an important step in the exploration of love experiences. Results from their exploratory analysis indicated that differences in adult attachment styles were related to individuals' experiences and beliefs about romantic love and retrospective reports of subjects' childhood relationships with their parents. Hazen and Shaver built an understanding of adult love by adapting three "love styles" modeled after Ainsworth's (Ainsworth, Blehar, Waters, & Wall, 1978) primary patterns of attachment: secure, avoidant, and anxious/ambivalent. Secure lovers are similar to those who are securely attached, and these individuals are characterized as being comfortable with intimacy and closeness and able to trust and depend on others. Avoidant lovers are similar to those who have an avoidant attachment style, and these individuals are found to be uncomfortable with closeness and intimacy and have difficulty depending on others. Anxious/ambivalent lovers have similarities to those with an anxious/ambivalent attachment style in that they often worry that they will be abandoned or that the other person in their life will not love them.

Bartholomew and Horowitz (1991) also used attachment theory (Ainsworth, Blehar, Waters, & Wall, 1978; Bowlby, 1982) as a springboard for understanding relationships, which they characterized by a four-category model consisting of secure, preoccupied, fearful, and dismissing attachment styles (Bartholomew & Horowitz, 1991). Those with secure attachment display a sense of self-worth along with the belief that people are usually trustworthy and reliable, comparable to Ainsworth's securely attached group. Preoccupied attachment indicates a sense of worthlessness. Preoccupied individuals use the acceptance of others to gain self-acceptance, which corresponds with the anxious/ambivalent group. Those displaying fearful attachment demonstrate feelings of unworthiness along with a negative view of others. This group avoids contact with others to avoid hurt and rejection. Finally, dismissing attachment indicates a positive view of the self along with a negative view of others, leading to a certain level of avoidance. These individuals attempt to maintain their independence while in a relationship. Fearful and dismissing styles each correspond partially with Ainsworth's avoidant group.

Taking the attachment-love connection still further, Kirkpatrick and Shaver (1992) empirically tested the idea that love of God, like romantic love, can be conceptualized in terms of attachment theory. Using Hazen and Shaver's three love styles, they found that individuals characterized as secure lovers of God reported more positive images of God and more religious commitment. Avoidant lovers of God were more likely to characterize themselves as agnostics, and the authors suggested that agnosticism is the opposite of religiousness, just as indifference is characterized as the opposite of love. Individuals whose relationship with God were characterized as anxious/ambivalent were more likely to describe themselves as antireligious and to have had a glossolalia experience. The authors suggest that if glossolalia is viewed as an extreme attempt to "get close to God," then the religiousness of this group is characterized by the extremes one would expect from the ambivalent: antireligious at times and overtly religious, if not clingy, at others. The authors also found that security of attachment to God was positively associated with secure attachment, but only among individuals who reported insecure childhood attachments. The apparent change from childhood attachment style supports the idea that other relationships or life events can alter or influence an otherwise enduring childhood attachment style. The development of a personal relationship with God may influence or change the internal working model initially created by childhood attachments.

We empirically tested the assumption that secure adult attachment is a form of love in veterans. We investigated the relationships between measures of attachment style and measures of love for friends and God. The correlation between Levin's (2001) measure, "the feeling of loving and being loved by God" scale, and the divine relationships measure (Pollner, 1989) was r (99) = .79, p < .001. In addition, the correlation between Rubin's Like Scale (1970), a measure of love between friends, and the relationship rating form, a measure of attachment to friends, was found to range from .368 to .431, p < .01, depending on the specific type of attachment. These results indicate a strong relationship between attachment and love in regard to spiritual relationships and a moderate relationship in regard to friendships. As these results are only preliminary, they should be interpreted cautiously until they are replicated using larger sample sizes.

LOVE, IN THE FORM OF ATTACHMENTS, AND POSTTRAUMATIC STRESS DISORDER

A wealth of research has been conducted on risk factors for the development of PTSD (Foy, Sipprelle, Rueger, & Carroll, 1984). This research has emphasized the importance of trauma exposure and severity of the trauma as well as childhood traumatic experiences as related to subsequent PTSD. Although it has been established that level of combat exposure is predictive of the development of PTSD for veterans of war (Boulanger, 1986), studies that have investigated premilitary vulnerability for PTSD have produced mixed results (e.g., Breslau & Davis, 1992).

Studies also have highlighted the importance and impact of attachments, both secure and insecure, on several different variables. Nonsecure attachments to parents in childhood (e.g., anxious/ambivalent and avoidant attachments as described by Bowlby, 1982) have been linked to stress response syndromes (e.g., Boman, 1986). Insecure attachments also have been linked to a greater propensity for anxiety and depression in adulthood (Amini et al., 1996; Goldberg, 2003). A few researchers have suggested that insecure attachments may also contribute to the development of PTSD (Dieperink, Leskela, Thuras, & Engdahl, 2001; van der Kolk, 1988). Furthermore, two studies (Alexander et al., 1998; Muller, Sicoli, & Lemieux, 2000) have found a relationship between insecure attachment and PTSD symptomatology in adults who were abused as children.

In contrast to insecure attachment findings, it has been found that an inner sense of security derived from having secure adult attachments enhances health and subjective well-being (Shaver, 2002). Boman (1986) found that secure childhood attachment to mothers is associated with less susceptibility to PTSD among in-patient veterans. Other research has found that positive relationships with service mates and spouses weakened painful war memories and stress symptoms in later life for World War II and Korean conflict veterans (Elder & Clipp, 1988). More recent research has demonstrated that a secure relationship with God has beneficial effects on health among family practice out-patients (Levin, 2001). Dieperink and colleagues (2001) conducted a study investigating adult attachment and PTSD and found that former prisoners of war with secure attachment styles reported lower levels of PTSD than those with insecure attachment styles. The study also found that attachment style was a stronger predictor of PTSD symptom intensity than was trauma severity, suggesting that secure attachment style could be protective, in that a positive view of oneself and others may allow for better use of coping skills and support systems.

In addition to these suggestive empirical studies, clinical observations also suggest the importance of attachment in the development of PTSD. Vietnam veterans cite their rejection and vilification by society at large upon their return to this country as playing a role in their distress. We have been impressed by the seeming benefits derived by Vietnam veterans when they become caregivers for their grandchildren (Hierholzer, 2004) and have commented on the importance of investigating the significance of such attachments. Given the paucity of research on the health-promoting effects of veterans' attachments to multiple figures, we studied whether love received from various attachment figures afforded a varied population of out-patient veterans a secure base that was protective of PTSD.

In order to examine the relationship between adult attachment and post-traumatic stress disorder, we studied 99 male veterans with military combat trauma. These study participants were rigorously assessed for PTSD through a clinical interview, which included the clinician-administered Posttraumatic Stress Disorder Scale, version 2 (Weathers, Ruscio, & Keane, 1999). In addition to the clinical interview, participants completed self-report instruments. The measures included the Parental Bonding Index (Parker, Tupling, & Brown, 1979), the Relationship Scales Questionnaire (Griffin & Bartholomew, 1994), the attachment to God measure (Kirkpatrick & Shaver, 1992), and the Experiences in Close Relationships Questionnaire (Brennan, Clark, & Shaver, 1998). Despite all participants having experienced trauma, not all participants had PTSD. Overall, 48.5% met the criteria for current PTSD, meaning that symptoms were present in the last month. In addition, 70% of all participating veterans reported secure attachment to a mother figure as measured by the PBI, and 48% reported a secure attachment to a father figure. One third of the veterans reported a secure attachment to a significant other/spouse as measured by the ECR, and 19% reported an overall secure adult attachment on the RSQ. Forty-six percent of the veterans reported a secure attachment to God as measured by the AGM. Analysis of variance (ANOVA) revealed significant differences in level of PTSD on ECR categories measuring significant other/spousal attachment (F (3,86) = 3.51, p = .019). Tukey's post hoc analyses revealed that veterans who have a dismissing attachment style have higher levels of PTSD (M = 68.62, SD = 21.75) than those with a secure attachment style (M = 46.73, SD = 29.73). ANOVA also revealed differences in level of PTSD on RSQ categories measuring overall adult attachment (F (3,90) = 9.92, p < .001). Tukey's post hoc analyses revealed that veterans with a fearful attachment style had higher levels of PTSD (M = 71, SD = 24.55) than those with a dismissive attachment style (M = 62.74, SD = 19.47) and those with a secure attachment style (M = 33.83, SD = 28.27). The associations between a PTSD diagnosis and attachment to God, friends, and parents yielded nonsignificant results (see Table 12.1).

A stepwise logistic regression was conducted to compare the relative contributions of each attachment style to prediction of PTSD symptoms. Possible confounding variables were measured and controlled for, including history of childhood abuse and level of combat exposure. The model controlled for combat exposure and childhood abuse in the first step. In the second step, adult attachment style was entered with four levels: secure attachment, fearful attachment, dismissive attachment, and preoccupied attachment.

Results are shown in Table 12.2 and indicate that, although degree of combat exposure is significant (p = .04, odds ratio [OR] = 1.04, 95% confidence interval [CI] = 1.00 to 1.08), only fearful attachment (p < .001, OR = 2.96, CI = 1.59 to 5.50) and preoccupied adult attachment (p = .04, OR = .56, CI = .33 to .97) styles were significant predictors of a PTSD diagnosis when adult attachment styles were added to the analysis. Veterans with a fearful attachment

Table 12.1. Adult Attachment Styles in Cases and Controls

Attachment Figure	N	%*	% Cases*	% Control*	F	d	p
God							
AGM	95	46	40	52	1.03	3,91	.384
Parent							
PBI-m	95	70	67	73	.527	3,91	.665
PBI-f	95	48	53	42	.712	4,90	.586
Significant Other							
ECR	90	33	27	42	3.51	3,86	.019
Overall Adult							
RSQ	94	19	7	27	9.92	3,90	.000

Note: * = secure attachment.

style were 2.95 times more likely to have PTSD than veterans with a secure adult attachment style. Veterans with a preoccupied adult attachment style were approximately 56% less likely to have PTSD than veterans with a secure adult attachment style.

The study findings demonstrate that significant other/spousal love is important for individuals with PTSD. The association between PTSD and attachment to God, friends, and parents yielded nonsignificant results. Veterans whose significant other/spousal love relationships were characterized as insecure, in attachment terminology, had higher levels of PTSD than veterans who reported love relationships characterized as secure. Moreover, veterans specifically with

Table 12.2. Logistic Regression (Stepwise) Analysis of Current Chronic PTSD as a Function of Combat Exposure, Childhood Abuse, and Adult Attachment Style

Variable	B	SE	Wald	Significance	Odds Ratio	95° Cl
Added in Step 1						
Combat exposure	.04	.02	4.23	.04	1.04	1.00–1.08
Childhood abuse	−.24	.42	.32	.57	.789	.35–1.80
Added in Step 2						
ATTACHMENT						
Fearful	1.09	.32	11.80	.001	2.96	1.59–5.50
Preoccupied	−.58	.28	4.34	.04	.56	.33–.97
Constant	−2.86	1.26	5.12	.02	.06	

insecure-dismissive love relationships had higher levels of PTSD than those with secure love relationships. Dismissing individuals are thought to be in chronic denial of their attachment needs, yet maintain a positive self-image. Such individuals avoid close relationships and may assert that relationships are relatively unimportant. They may be viewed as quite independent, distant, cool (even cold or arrogant), unemotional, aloof, matter of fact, and rational (Bartholomew, 1990). Previous literature has suggested that individuals with a dismissive style often believe that love does not last and that others will not be available and supportive (Hazen & Shaver, 1987).

According to Bowlby, individuals with insecure attachments during childhood would be expected to develop mental models of attachment relationships that reflect their history of experiences with attachment figures. However, no relationship between perceived parental attachment and PTSD was found. In addition, the majority of individuals in this study reported secure attachments to their parents and an insecure overall attachment style. Main and Goldwyn (1984) stated that individuals may transition from secure to insecure attachment styles during adulthood due to "loss of attachment figures under traumatic circumstances," such as wars. All of the participants in our study participated in wars and experienced combat trauma; therefore, it is plausible that their traumatic experiences may have caused a transformation in their mental models of attachment. In contrast, Main and Goldwyn (1984) also discuss that those who have developed a secure attachment to a significant other/spouse may have undergone a modification of their mental model that has helped them to reduce posttraumatic stress.

While trauma severity independently predicted PTSD, a fearful-avoidant adult attachment style seemed to be the strongest predictor of PTSD. This finding is consistent with other research that found that insecure attachment significantly predicted PTSD (Dieperink et al., 2001). Interestingly, endorsing a preoccupied attachment style was predictive of less PTSD symptomatology. Research has indicated that both fearfully avoidant and preoccupied individuals may be more likely to choose relationships that confirm a negative view of themselves (Carnelley, Pietromonaco, & Jaffe, 1994); however, fearfully avoidant individuals may exhibit an interpersonal avoidance that prevents them from being able to alter their attachment as a function of involvement with a significant other/spouse (Alexander et al., 1998). Alternatively, preoccupied individuals have been described as low in avoidance, anxious, needy, demanding of advice and support, and highly dependent on relationships. These individuals may enter relationships, which ultimately may positively influence their mental health.

Previous work suggests that secure attachments prior to exposure to trauma should help to prevent the development of PTSD. Our work did not confirm this suggestion, but instead highlighted the importance of current attachments. Our work confirms a close association between secure attachment and PTSD. However, our present research cannot establish whether the strong associations between certain attachments and PTSD actually protect against the subsequent development of PTSD, or whether it is post-morbid attachments that ameliorate the course and manifestations of PTSD. The strong association found between PTSD and significant other/spousal attachment but not parental attachment suggests the importance of post-morbid interventions.

As robust as our findings are in this regard, however, our work cannot prove a causal association between secure attachments and a lessened vulnerability to the deleterious effects of trauma. It is possible that the relationship we found between significant other/spousal attachment is simply a fallout of our subjects having PTSD, i.e., severe PTSD perpetuates severe or negative significant other/ spousal relationships, and conversely, no or mild PTSD symptoms may result in less negative impact on intimate relationships. We do not think that this is the case because we found a significant inverse relationship between some individuals with insecure adult attachment style and PTSD. This leads us to believe that the causes of the variations in important adult relationships may be due to possible reorganization of the mental models of attachment.

The effects of combat trauma may reorganize and shift mental models of attachment from secure to insecure. These speculations are consistent with the conditions mentioned by Main and Goldwyn (1984), where the trauma of war is a potential cause for a transformation of mental models. In addition, Main and Goldwyn (1984) state that "gaining a stable attachment figure following a period of vulnerability and chaos," notably a spouse/partner, may help to foster a secure mental model of attachment from a previously insecure mental model of attachment. Our findings are consistent with this scenario. The causes of changes in mental models in the veterans of this study are not known. A prospective study would further clarify the role of mental models of attachment before and after traumatic events and the role of loving relationships as a protective or ameliorating factor for PTSD.

ATTACHMENT, PTSD, AND ALTRUISM

Some research has indicated that Vietnam War veterans who were higher in altruistic intent had lower levels of PTSD as compared to those lower in altruistic intent (Kishon-Barash, Midlarsky, & Johnson, 1999). It has been proposed that secure attachments are an important determinant of altruism (Shaver, 2002) and enable one to be altruistic (e.g., open, kind, and loving toward others). We are currently studying the relationships between attachments and altruism in the context of PTSD.

We have examined the relationships among adult attachments, altruism, and posttraumatic stress disorder symptomatology. More specifically, our study investigated whether altruistic intent was influenced by a relationship with a particular attachment figure (mother, father, friends, significant other/spouse, or God). In addition, this study served as an exploratory analysis of the relationship between altruistic intent and PTSD.

The participants for this study were the same 99 veterans described above. In addition to completing diagnostic interviews and the measures noted above, the subjects also completed the divine relationships measure (Pollner, 1989) and the Self-Report Altruism Scale (Rushton, Chrisjohn, & Fekken, 1981). A series of hierarchical regression analyses were performed to investigate the relationship of attachment to God, attachment to friends, attachment to parents in childhood, and attachment to significant other/spouse variables to altruism (see Table 12.3). None of the attachment to parents in childhood variables in this study was significantly related to altruism. Of the attachment to God variables, "feeling attached to a divine being" was significantly related to altruism (R^2 = .04, $F(1,97)$ = 4.28, p = .04). However, a "sense of religious well-being" did not significantly add to the amount of variance explained. Of the attachment to friends variables, "feeling an intimate attachment to a friend" was significantly related to altruism (R^2 = .09, $F(1,96)$ = 9.91, $p < .002$). Of the attachment to significant other/spouse variables, lower levels of avoidant attachment were significantly related to altruism (R^2 = .05, $F(1,95)$ = 5.45, p = .02).

Bivariate analyses suggested that altruism is significantly correlated with a history of PTSD ($r(99)$ = –.23, $p < .05$), with higher levels of altruism associated with lower levels of lifetime PTSD. Altruism was also correlated with persistent avoidance of stimuli associated with the trauma and numbing of general responsiveness (criterion C of DSM-IV TR) ($r(99)$ = –.26, $p < .05$), with higher levels of altruism associated with lower levels of avoidance and numbing. No relationship was found between altruism and current PTSD (active symptoms

Table 12.3. Regression Analyses of Altruism as a Function of Attachment

Measure	Mean	SD	R^2	df	F	p
ECR anxiety	3.57	1.43				
ECR avoidance	3.76	1.32	.054	1,95	5.45	.02
PBI mother-caring	25.33	8.52				
PBI mother-overprotection	13.96	6.77				
PBI father-caring	18.56	10.41				
PBI father-overprotection	12.55	7.63				
RRF viability	5.11	1.09				
RRF intimacy	4.72	1.04	.094	1,96	9.91	.002
RRF passion	3.09	1.27				
RRF care	4.99	1.37				
RRF global satisfaction	5.07	1.32				
RRF conflict ambivalence	2.46	1.33				
Devine relationships	7.25	3.80	.042	1,97	4.28	.041
Spiritual well-being	43.15	15.57				

within the last month) (r (99) = –.18, p = .079); however, a relationship was found between altruism and current avoidance and numbing (r (99) = –.21, $p <$ .05). Bivariate analyses also indicated that higher levels of altruism were significantly correlated with spiritual well-being (r (99) = .23, $p < .05$) and emotional well-being (r (99) = .35, $p < .05$). A t test did not indicate differences among PTSD and no-PTSD groups in relation to altruism.

Our work underscores prior findings that PTSD does not preclude altruism and that altruism among combat veterans is mostly related to secure adult attachments, among them a secure attachment to a personal God. Our findings suggest that feeling securely attached or loved by a significant other, friend, or God positively predicted veterans' altruistic intent to help. This suggests that rather than being solely the product of early secure attachments, altruistic intent may be related to important adult relationships. In addition, the inverse relationship obtained in this study between altruistic intent and a history of PTSD and, more specifically, the avoidance symptoms of PTSD calls for additional research in this area.

Our findings are limited by the low sample size ($N = 99$) and cross-sectional design of our study. Consequently, we are unable to determine if altruistic intent leads to relief from PTSD or whether PTSD may impede altruism. The benefits of helping others in individuals diagnosed with PTSD are relatively unexplored. Future intervention research could further shed light on this issue by investigating the potential benefits of helping others through the implementation of group therapy that incorporates volunteerism for veterans with PTSD.

CONCLUSION

PTSD related to combat trauma is a lingering disorder that adversely affects many, if not all, aspects of a veteran's life. Not the least of these domains is interpersonal relationships. Current findings suggest many more questions than answers. In turn, these questions suggest avenues for future research. Clearly, prospective studies examining attachment to a variety of figures and the subsequent development of PTSD are needed. As indicated above, our present research cannot establish whether the strong associations between certain attachments and PTSD actually protect against the subsequent manifestations of PTSD. Such studies should be conducted among populations at high risk for trauma exposure: troops prior to deployment, law enforcement officers, emergency workers, and firefighters. While our findings require replication, they argue that psychotherapeutic interventions aimed at couples and families, designed to strengthen less secure relationships, may well be fruitful in the treatment of PTSD.

In addition, the widespread evidence for the beneficial health effects of altruistic acts (reviewed elsewhere in this book), along with clinical observations about the salutary effects of assuming the caregiving role by veterans, suggest the potential for psychotherapeutic interventions which encourage engagement in caring for others or other acts of altruism. Given that so many of the risk factors for the development of PTSD are not readily modifiable, such as extent of combat exposure or severity of trauma, it seems wise to explore the factors that might be modifiable and might lead to clinical improvements. Integrating the concepts of altruistic intent and love attachments into the therapeutic treatment of PTSD may allow positive alteration of the mental models of self and others. Incorporating and highlighting the love of others into treatment may address directly the core symptoms of PTSD that seem to affect interpersonal relationships: continued avoidance and numbing of emotions. Just as PTSD symptoms are cyclical in nature, producing a downward spiral of relationship difficulties, altruistic behavior may produce a positive cycle, serving to improve, strengthen, and create new relationships with self and others.

The authors gratefully acknowledge the dedication and assistance of Ms. Angela Boardman.

REFERENCES

Ainsworth, M. D. S., Blehar, M. C., Waters, E., & Wall, S. (1978). *Patterns of attachment: A psychological study of the strange situation.* Hillsdale, NJ: Erlbaum.

Alexander, P. C., Anderson, C. L., Brand, B., Schaeffer, C. M., Grelling, B. Z., & Kretz, L. (1998). Adult attachment and longterm effects in survivors of incest. *Child Abuse & Neglect, 22,* 45–61.

American Psychiatric Association. (2000). *Diagnostic and statistical manual of mental disorders* (4th ed., rev.). Washington, DC: Author.

Amini, F., Lewis, T., Lannon, R., Louie, A., Baumbacher, G., McGuinness, T., & Schiff, E. Z. (1996). Affect, attachment, memory: Contributions toward psychobiologic integration. *Psychiatry, 59,* 213–239.

Bartholomew, K. (1990). Avoidance of intimacy: An attachment perspective. *Journal of Social and Personal Relationships, 7,* 147–178.

Bartholomew, K., & Horowitz, L. M. (1991). Attachment styles among young adults: A test of a four-category model. *Journal of Personality and Social Psychology, 61,* 226–244.

Benotsch, E. G., Brailey, K. B., Vasterling, J. J., Uddo, M., Constans, J. I., & Sutker, P. B. (2000). War zone stress, personal and environmental resources, and PTSD symptoms in Gulf war veterans: A longitudinal perspective. *Journal of Abnormal Psychology, 109,* 205–213.

Boman, B. (1986). Early experiential environment, maternal bonding and the susceptibility to post-traumatic stress disorder. *Military Medicine, 151,* 528–531.

Boulanger, G. (1986). Predisposition to post-traumatic stress disorder. In G. Boulanger & C. Kadushin (Eds.), *The Vietnam veteran redefined* (pp. 37–50). Hillsdale, NJ: Erlbaum.

Bowlby, J. (1973). *Attachment and loss: Vol. 2. Separation: Anxiety & Anger*. London: Hogarth.

Bowlby, J. (1977) The making and breaking of affectional bonds. *British Journal of Psychiatry*, 130, 201–210 and 421–431.

Bowlby, J. (1982). *Attachment* (2nd ed.) New York: Basic.

Brennan, K. A., Clark, C. L., & Shaver, P. R. (1998). Self-report measurement of adult romantic attachment: An integrative overview. In J. A. Simpson & W. S. Rholes (Eds.), *Attachment theory and close relationships* (pp. 46–76). New York: Guilford.

Breslau, N., & Davis, G. C. (1992). Posttraumatic stress disorder in an urban population of young adults: Risk factors for chronicity. *American Journal of Psychiatry*, 149, 671–675.

Breslau, N., Kessler, R. C., Chilcoat, H. D., Schultz, L. R., Davis, G. C., & Andreski, P. (1998). Trauma and posttraumatic stress disorder in the community: The 1996 Detroit Area Survey of Trauma. *Archives of General Psychiatry*, 55, 626–632.

Bretherton, I. (1985). Attachment theory, retrospect, and prospect. In I. Bretherton & E. Waters (Eds.), *Growing points of attachment theory and research* (pp. 3–38). Chicago: University of Chicago Press.

Carnelley, K. B., Pietromonaco, P. R., & Jaffe, K. (1994). Depression, working models of others, and relationship functioning. *Journal of Personality and Social Psychology*, 66, 127–40.

Carroll, E. M., Rueger, D. B., Foy, D. W., & Donahoe, C. P. (1985). Vietnam combat veterans with posttraumatic stress disorder: Analysis of marital and cohabitating adjustment. *Journal of Abnormal Psychology*, 94, 329–337.

Crittendon, P. M. (1988). Relationships at risk. In J. Belsky & T. Nezworski (Eds.), *Clinical implications of attachment* (pp. 136–174). Hillsdale, NJ: Erlbaum.

Csikszentmihalyi, M., & Larson, R. (1984). *Being adolescent: Conflict and growth in the teenage years*. New York: Basic.

Dieperink, M., Leskela, J., Thuras, P., & Engdahl, B. (2001). Attachment style classification and posttraumatic stress disorder in former prisoners of war. *American Journal of Orthopsychiatry*, 71, 374–378.

Elder, G. H., & Clipp, E. C. (1988). Wartime losses and social bonding: Influences across 40 years in men's lives. *Psychiatry*, 51, 177–198.

Foy, D. W., Sipprelle, R. C., Rueger, D. B., & Carroll, E. M. (1984). Etiology of posttraumatic stress disorder in Vietnam veterans: Analysis of premilitary, military, and combat exposure influences. *Journal of Consulting and Clinical Psychology*, 52, 79–87.

Goldberg, D. (2003). Vulnerability, destabilization and restitution in anxious depression. *Acta Psychiatrica Scandinavica, Supplementum*, 108(Suppl. 418), 81–82.

Griffin, D., & Bartholomew, K. (1994). Models of the self and other: Fundamental dimensions underlying measures of adult attachment. *Journal of Personality and Social Psychology*, 67, 430–445.

Hazen C., & Shaver P. (1987). Romantic love conceptualized as an attachment process. *Journal of Personality and Social Psychology*, 52, 511–524.

Hierholzer, R. W. (2004). Improvement in PTSD patients who care for their grand-children. *American Journal of Psychiatry, 161,* 176.

Izard, C., & Kobak, R. (1991). Emotion system functioning and emotion regula-tion. In J. Garber & K. Dodge (Eds.), *The development of affect regulation* (pp. 303–322). Cambridge: Cambridge University Press.

Kahana, B., Kahana, E., & Harel, Z. (1988). Predictors of psychological well-being among survivors of the Holocaust. In J. P. Wilson, Z. Harel, & B. Kahana (Eds.), *Human adaptation to extreme stress: From the Holocaust to Vietnam* (pp. 171–192). New York: Plenum.

Kessler, R. C., Sonnega, A., Bromet, E., Hughes, M., & Nelson, C. B. (1995). Post-traumatic stress disorder in the National Comorbidity Survey. *Archives of General Psychiatry, 52,* 1048–60.

Kirkpatrick, L. A., & Shaver, P. R. (1992). An attachment-theoretical approach to romantic love and religious belief. *Personality and Social Psychology Bulletin, 18,* 266–275.

Kishon-Barash, R., Midlarsky, E., & Johnson, D. R. (1999). Altruism and the Viet-nam war veteran: The relationship of helping to symptomatology. *Journal of Traumatic Stress, 12,* 655–662.

Levin, J. (2001). God, love, and health: Findings from a clinical study. *Review of Religious Research, 42,* 277–293.

MacDonald C., Chamberlain, K., Long, N., & Flett, R. (1999). Posttraumatic stress disorder and interpersonal functioning in Vietnam war veterans: A mediational model. *Journal of Traumatic Stress, 12,* 701–707.

Main, M. (1990). Cross-cultural studies of attachment organization: Recent stud-ies, changing methodologies, and the concept of conditional strategies. *Human Development, 33,* 48–61.

Main, M., & Goldwyn, R. (1984). Predicting rejection of her infant from mother's representation of her own experience: Implications for the abused-abusing intergenerational cycle. *Child Abuse & Neglect, 8,* 203–217.

Main, M., Kaplan, N., & Cassidy, J. (1985). Security in infancy, childhood, and adulthood: A move to the level of representation. In I. Bretherton & E. Waters (Eds.), *Growing points of attachment theory and research* (pp. 66–106). Chicago: University of Chicago Press.

Midlarsky, E. (1991). Helping as coping. In M. S. Clark (Ed.), *Prosocial behavior: Vol. 12. Review of personality and social psychology* (pp. 238–264). Newbury Park, CA: Sage.

Muller, R. T., Sicoli, L. A., & Lemieux, K. E. (2000). Relationship between at-tachment style and posttraumatic stress symptomatology among adults who report the experience of childhood abuse. *Journal of Traumatic Stress, 13,* 321–322.

Nezu, A. M., & Carnevale, G. J. (1987). Interpersonal problem solving and coping reactions of Vietnam veterans with posttraumatic stress disorder. *Journal of Abnormal Psychology, 96,* 155–157.

Parker, G., Tupling, H., & Brown, L. B. (1979). A parental bonding instrument. *British Journal of Medical Psychology, 52,* 1–10.

Pearce, K. A., Schauer, A. H., Garfield, N. J., Ohlde, C. O., & Patterson, T. W.

(1985). A study of post traumatic stress disorder in Vietnam veterans. *Journal of Clinical Psychology, 41*, 9–14.

Penk, W. E., Robinowitz, R., Roberts, W. R., Patterson, E. T., Dolan, M. P., & Atkins, H. G. (1981). Adjustment differences among male substance abusers varying in degree of combat experience in Vietnam. *Journal of Consulting and Clinical Psychology, 49*, 426–437.

Pollner, M. (1989). Divine relations, social relations, and well-being. *Journal of Health and Social Behavior, 30*, 92–104.

Roberts, W. R., Penk, W. E., Gearing, M. L., Robinowitz, R., Dolan, M. P., & Patterson, E. T. (1982). Interpersonal problems of Vietnam combat veterans with symptoms of posttraumatic stress disorder. *Journal of Abnormal Psychology, 91*, 444–450.

Rubin, Z. (1970). Measurement of romantic love. *Journal of Personality and Social Psychology, 16*, 265–273.

Rushton, J. P., Chrisjohn, R. D., & Fekken, G. C. (1981). The altruistic personality and the Self-Report Altruism Scale. *Personality & Individual Differences, 50*, 1192–1198.

Siegel, D. J. (1999). *The developing mind: Toward a neurobiology of interpersonal experience*. New York: Guilford.

Shaver, P. (2002). *Attachment, compassion, and altruism*. Internet site: University of California, Davis, Department of Psychology, Adult Attachment Lab, Publications, Current Projects and Papers. Accessed September 26, 2006.

Solomon, Z., & Mikulincer, M. (1987). Combat stress reactions, posttraumatic stress disorder, and social adjustment. *Journal of Nervous and Mental Disorders, 175*, 277–285.

van der Kolk, B. A. (1988). The trauma spectrum: The interaction of biological and social events in the genesis of the trauma response. *Journal of Traumatic Stress, 1*, 273–290.

Weathers, F. W., Ruscio, A. M., & Keane, T. M. (1999). Psychometric properties of nine scoring rules for the clinician-administered Posttraumatic Stress Disorder Scale. *Psychological Assessment, 11*, 124–133.

13 Helping Behavior and Longevity: An Emotion Model

Deborah D. Danner
Wallace V. Friesen
Adah N. Carter

A model of emotional behavior is described that builds on research from the Nun Study, which found that written positive emotional expectations in early adulthood predicted longevity more than six decades later. The healing effects of positive emotional responses are proposed as the underlying factor that reinforces helping behavior and reflects an innate, universal mechanism that potentially enhances health and extends life. Evidence for a central nervous system mechanism that innervates a patterned response to emotional arousal continues to mount, as do data supporting the proposition that positive emotion resets and has a healing effect on critical physical systems. Although systematic research focusing on positive emotions is relatively young, the early evidence supports the widely held beliefs that happiness enhances social, psychological, and physical well-being. We propose that research on the health benefits of helping behavior must systematically examine positive emotions as the essential intervening variable between acts of generosity and enhanced health.

The founders of our nation foresaw the personal, social, political, and perhaps health benefits of happiness by guaranteeing the pursuit of happiness in our country's Bill of Rights. Whether our forefathers intuitively understood the relationship between happiness and health is unknown, but this right allows the freedom to strive for the good of all people as part of our pursuit of happiness.

Striving for the good of others without the expectation of personal gain is one definition of altruism. Scientific investigations have examined altruism and the related helping behaviors of volunteerism to uncover possible health benefits associated with such activities. Some studies have found relations between volunteerism and increased longevity (Musick, Herzog, & House, 1999; Oman, Tooresen, & McMahon, 1999), providing strong evidence that such helping behavior may have positive health outcomes. However, these studies await theory and supporting evidence for an underlying neurophysiologic mechanism that might account for the relationship. While research finding that a non-sedentary lifestyle or a balanced diet are related to better health appear to require no theoretical link or additional evidence, the reasons that volunteerism might improve health are less obvious.

With a rapidly increasing elderly population, it is not surprising that an emerging body of research has focused on factors associated with improved health for a generation that for decades has been sold diet, exercise, and chemical and social remedies to ensure better health, feelings of well-being, and even longer lives. For example, recent work found a relationship between recreational gambling and better health in the elderly (Desai et al., 2004). When commenting on the study, Desai and her coauthors emphasized, "Although the underlying reasons remain hypothetical, proposed reasons included the increased activity, socialization, and cognitive stimulation that are related to engaging in gambling" (p. 1678). In the near future, we should expect a proliferation of studies, many with obvious commercial motives, to appear in the literature and in the media without explanation of causal factors. Unlike gambling, diet, or exercise, helping and prosocial behaviors potentially have both personal and societal benefits.

In this chapter, we will focus on a possible mechanism to account for why helping behaviors might have positive health outcomes. We will argue that positive emotional responses, particularly future-oriented positive emotions, form the basis of attitudes that lead to repetitive choices in one's use of time and energy. Such choices related to the arousal of positive emotions secure accompanying cardiovascular and immune physiologic responses capable of improving health and extending life. We will focus primarily on the elderly population, where declining health may be a factor, and where accumulated knowledge and decreased daily demands make providing help to others personally appropriate and socially useful. However, we will suggest that there is no single activity that can provide the panacea of good health for the elderly. In our view, the most likely underlying mechanism linking helping behavior and health is positive emotions, and no single activity or even class of activities will arouse positive emotions in all individuals, especially when responses must be time extended or repetitive.

BRIEF SUMMARY OF NUN STUDY FINDINGS

The generosity and foresight of the School Sisters of Notre Dame and the careful collection of systematic longitudinal data by the Nun Study facilitated an examination of the relationship between autobiographical writings completed at a young age and longevity (Danner, Snowdon, & Friesen, 2001). In this study, sisters who used the greatest number of positive emotion words lived 6 to 10 years longer than those using the fewest positive emotion words. Based on the emotion research of Fredrickson and Levenson (1998), a lifelong pattern of resolving life events with a positive, optimistic attitude was proposed to reduce stresses on the cardiovascular system, resulting in an extended life. The nuns were an ideal population to study this hypothesis because they all had similar diets, housing, and professional responsibilities. Thus, we concluded that the underlying determinant of longevity was attitudinal or emotional. When interpreting the results of this study, we did not consider that differences in altruism might have contributed to better health and longevity. Sisters in this study all spent their working years in helping professions, primarily the education of children, and thus lifelong differences in opportunities or need for generosity would not be expected.

Unfortunately, research using archival data is limited to the records that remain at the time of the study. Details of events during the 60–plus years between the writing of the autobiographies and the deaths of the authors were largely unknown. In particular, evidence of differences between the groups in attitudes or behavior patterns was not available. Although we proposed that the underlying mechanism responsible for the findings in the Nun Study was a pattern of self-activated arousal of positive emotions to reset the potentially harmful effects of negative emotional events in life (Fredrickson & Levenson, 1998), no information was available to confirm such attitudinal differences between the groups. Thus, it is equally probable that the sisters in the high-positive group were more generous or helping as well as more optimistic. What is known is that sisters in the high-positive group reported in their autobiographical writings experiencing more love and admiration in their past and present lives and more enthusiasm and joy when writing of their anticipated future in their chosen profession.

Researchers such as Isen and colleagues (1987) have found positive emotions to enhance creative problem solving. Implicit in such findings is the idea that positive emotions can accelerate problem solving and the reappraisal of circumstances that have aroused negative emotional responses. It is this readiness and capacity to reappraise that underlies retaining a positive attitude throughout adversity. In this chapter, we propose that finding a relationship between helping behavior and good health depends upon the degree to which helpers experience positive emotions.

SUMMARY OF BASIC EMOTION RESEARCH

Charitable organizations offer us the warm feeling of satisfaction of saving a child from disease or starvation and freedom from feelings of guilt for mere pennies a day. So little sacrifice for so much emotional gain! While the goals of most of

these organizations are noble and many of their organizers make personal sacri-
fices to achieve them, their appeals illustrate the power of the emotions and
their importance in motivating helping or prosocial behavior. While the commercial, political, and religious world has, at a very practical level, assumed the
existence of an innate emotion system, scientific psychology denied and neglected
its importance for decades. Clearly, the study of emotions has been elusive and
has required long and tedious effort. Nevertheless, the research of recent decades has provided sufficient evidence to document the existence of a powerful
neurologically based system that motivates our behavior and influences our
thoughts, and the study of emotions has taken its place as a legitimate science.
In this section, we will briefly review some of the findings of emotion research
and emphasize the importance of including the assessment of emotional responses in the study of altruistic behavior.

Darwin (1872) proposed that facial expressions of emotion evolved as a
means of conveying our inner states to others. Such a proposition not only describes overt behaviors but assumes an innate, universal, and neurologically based
system that organizes and drives these behaviors. The anecdotal data that Darwin
provided to support his theory were intriguing but did not meet the standards
of scientific methods. Unfortunately for the early students of facial expressions,
innateness was considered synonymous with reflexive behaviors or fixed action
patterns. When investigators found variability in the interpretations of facial
behaviors assumed to express emotions, an attempt was made to identify a pattern in the variability of interpretation that could be linked to the emotional states
and to some degree the facial patterns for each emotion studied (Woodworth &
Schlosberg, 1954). When variability was found in the expressive behavior of persons during controlled conditions assumed to elicit specific emotions, the search
for universal facial expressions of emotion was disrupted. With the increased
emphasis on learning theory, conditioned responses, and cultural relativism of
the time, efforts to study emotions and their specific expressions came to a halt.
The conclusion was drawn that facial expressions of emotion are culture-specific
habits.

In the mid-20th century, Silvan Tomkins (1962, 1963) made two major
contributions to the study of emotions. First, he began efforts to clarify the interaction between the cognitive and emotional systems. Next, he described in
detail the changes on the face that would occur when happiness, sadness, fear,
anger, shame, disgust, and contempt were aroused. Using depictions of these
emotions that concurred with Tomkins's descriptions, two independent labo-
ratories (those of Paul Ekman and Carroll Izard) developed facial measurement
coding systems and conducted worldwide studies on the interpretation and
expression of the emotions. These studies and numerous replications found
robust evidence for universal expressions of happiness, sadness, anger, fear, surprise, disgust, and, to a limited degree, shame and contempt (e.g., Ekman et al.,
1987). Parallel to these studies, evidence for systematic facial expressions in

nonhuman primates further substantiated Darwin's evolutionary hypothesis (Chevalier-Skolnikoff, 1973).

Following the description of the characteristics of universal facial expressions of emotions, it became evident that "pure" expressions occurred rarely in everyday life. Consequently, emotion theorists developed constructs, such as display rules, to account for the modulation, substitution, and repression of emotional expressions. Most disruptions of the universal expressive and instrumental actions of emotional arousal were found to be associated with learning when and how emotions should be expressed in particular social situations. In other words, not every time that we experience fear do we pull our lips back, lift our brows and pull them together, raise the upper eyelid, and tighten the lower eyelid. Likewise, we may feel a need to run, but we do not always flee when threatened.

Despite the findings of universal elicitors for each of the basic emotions, elicitors of emotions remain dependent upon the individual's appraisal of specific conditions (Boucher & Brandt, 1981; Scherer, Summerfield, & Walbott, 1983). For example, most, but not all, persons are saddened by the death of a parent, but all would be saddened by the loss of a loved object or person. That is, what is appraised as loved and whether it is appraised as lost depends to some degree on the individual's history, emotional propensities, personality, and momentary circumstances. Although promising theoretical and methodological progress has been made in understanding the individual appraisal process, there is no consensus on how to classify appraisals.

The evidence for universal facial expressions of emotions and the description of universal elicitors suggested that patterned nervous system activity would be a prerequisite to action. Subsequently, Robert Levenson and colleagues (e.g., Levenson, Ekman, & Friesen, 1990) identified differentiated, patterned autonomic nervous system activity associated with the emotions of anger, fear, disgust, and sadness in both young and elderly adults from diverse cultures. Further, work by Davidson and collaborators (1990) identified central nervous system activity that distinguishes some emotional states, and other studies found preliminary evidence for the neurological structures responsible for the activation, control, and modulation of emotions.

The development of tools for systematically and objectively measuring the activity of facial muscles facilitated the identification of patterned facial responses in very young infants, which related to the facial expressions of emotion observed in adults. This work provided another important link for establishing an innate basis for human behavior that relies on neurological activation and is not completely dependent upon deliberate action. Finally, the finding by Izard and colleagues (1993) that early tendencies for expressing and presumably experiencing one or a set of emotions more than others provided a strong basis for understanding the development of adult personality.

The quest for evidence of the universality of emotions and for a neurological basis for the commonalities observed in expressive and instrumental behaviors associated with the emotions was long and tedious. The study of a single psychological phenomenon is not accomplished in a vacuum. At times, advances are made only as technology, methodology, and cultural acceptance of ideas evolve. For example, if ideas such as creationism, the dualistic separation of mind and body, or strict behavioral learning theory had pervaded our thinking, advances such as those made in the study of emotions would not have occurred. The study of helping behavior would appear to be even more complex than studying emotions and to a large degree dependent upon further advances in the study of emotions. Because of this interrelatedness, the complementary examination of helping behavior and emotions will likely strengthen the knowledge in both areas of inquiry.

With strong evidence supporting the existence of an innate emotion system and the high probability that emotions are involved in motivating and sustaining helping behavior, it seems reasonable to conclude that an assessment of emotional responses to helping is an essential component for studies of prosocial behavior and its possible relation to health. Unfortunately, the study of emotions is far from complete, and a gold standard for measurement across all contexts is not available. Further, the study of emotions has focused almost exclusively on transient states that are essential for survival and on negative states that affect health adversely. Positive emotions, such as amusement, momentary pride in achievement or success, and contentment, and differences in smiling behavior have received limited attention in the literature. The longer-lasting positive emotional responses to challenges—hope, desire, determination, and enduring satisfaction—have been largely neglected. When considering helping behavior in an older population, these and other positive emotions should be considered. It is these emotions that can open the mind to the reappraisal of negative circumstances and that can relieve the stresses of adverse situations.

Carstensen's socioemotional selection theory (1992) suggests that older persons increasingly choose to participate in activities where they expect to experience positive emotions. Although global assessments of positive and negative affect related to helping provide limited information, we suggest that separate measurements should be made of the emotions experienced in anticipation of the helping situation, during the process of helping, and after the process is completed. Also, care should be taken to avoid socially acceptable responses when gathering data on emotional reactions. Ancillary measures of behavior, such as willingness to continue volunteering, tardiness, absenteeism, and reasons for terminating participation, should be used to support and cross-validate self-reports of emotional responses.

The greatest challenge for the study of emotions will be the development of an understanding of how elicitors and context are appraised for each basic emotion. Such efforts promise to account for and make measurable those instances when two or more emotions are aroused simultaneously and the varied intensities of these emotions, even when eliciting conditions are held constant. To the degree that emotions are involved in motivating helping behavior, understanding the appraisal process in the arousal of emotions is important for the study of helping behavior. More information also is needed about early emotional tendencies and how these tendencies may influence the development of personality. Early tendencies to reappraise adverse circumstances and to see "the bright side" are likely to influence the development of personality. We suspect that psychopathologies beyond those studied to date develop from ineffective appraisals or reappraisals, resulting in patterns of negative emotional experiences that disrupt effective adjustment.

WHAT ARE POSITIVE EMOTIONS?

Most studies of emotions during recent decades have focused on negative or transitory emotions. Emotion-like states of long duration often have been conceptualized as moods in an effort to distinguish the more transitory emotional arousal from sustained emotional states. This conceptualization has had the unfortunate effect of leading some to believe that emotions involve only transitory states. Such a classification is misleading and would not account for the adverse effects of negative emotions on health that have been found by students of psychosomatic medicine. Additionally, less attention has been given to positive emotions, with all positive reactions often combined under the rubric of happiness. Differentiation of the positive emotions has largely been confined to amusement, contentment, satisfaction/achievement, and joy. Even these labels remain largely undefined, and little has been done to identify behavioral responses that might distinguish these emotions.

When examining how positive emotional reactions might improve health, one must assume that these positive reactions involve states that are either repeatedly experienced or that extend beyond a few moments in time. We are proposing that the positive emotions that might be associated with helping behavior and good health are those emotions associated with motivation. We assume that emotions, positive and negative, are the driving force behind motivation and that little or nothing would be learned or accomplished without them. Moreover, we argue that the positive emotions of desire and hope to succeed are forces as powerful as fear or dread of failure.

Assumptions that helping behavior is innate are premature. While the desire to help another when need is clear may be inborn, in most instances, helping involves cognitive problem solving and deliberate decisions. We suggest that fixed helping action patterns would be dysfunctional and even disastrous for the helper and recipient in many situations. If helping is not triggered at this automatic level, then conceptualization is needed for the reasoned and emotional components of a decision to help another. Likewise, a determination of whether the help that is offered or given is appropriate to the recipient's needs is necessary. If situations exist where rational decisions would not be expected to be a part of giving aid, these circumstances require clarification. Further, a description of what constitutes help and what constitutes a need for help must be included in a model of helping. Without information at this level, it will not be possible to identify what, if any, emotions are aroused by the helping behavior in either the helper or the recipient. Separate conceptual models may be needed for different types of helping contexts.

The problem of measuring appraisals is one confronting the study of the influence of helping behaviors on health. Investigation of the appraisal of need, the recipient's readiness to accept aid, the helper's capacity to help, the effectiveness of the helping process, and the success or failure of helping efforts should be included in future work.

Another area important in the study of helping behaviors and health is the degree to which early and perhaps genetic tendencies to experience and to express particular emotions may affect whether negative situations are reappraised, fostering the protective benefits of positive emotions on health.

WHAT HELPING BEHAVIOR IS LIKELY TO ELICIT POSITIVE RESPONSES CAPABLE OF INFLUENCING HEALTH AND EXTENDING LIFE?

To evaluate studies examining expected benefits of helping behavior in the elderly, it is necessary to define what types of helping or altruistic behaviors have been investigated. Penner's (2004) discussion of prosocial behavior provides clarification of the distinction between volunteerism and "bystander interventions," such as helping a stranger in an emergency. Penner describes volunteerism as possessing the following four characteristics: (1) a conscious decision to provide assistance, (2) a long-term commitment, (3) a lack of personal obligation to the individual receiving help at the time the decision is made, and (4) an organizational context. In contrast to volunteerism, the decision to help a stranger is time limited and may involve the feeling of an obligation to provide assistance on the part of the helper. We recommend that when studying volunteerism in the elderly, less formal activities, not necessarily offered through organizations, be included. Additionally, helping behaviors where there is a preexisting relationship with the individual, such as a friend, neighbor, or family member, although not considered to be volunteerism, would be considered helping behavior and, therefore, warrant investigation and description.

WHAT IS UNIQUE FOR STUDIES
OF OLDER PERSONS?

While a 65th birthday or the day of retirement may be major landmarks of life, these events should not be expected to have a significant influence on attitudes, personality, or emotional response patterns. The majority of patterned responses to life's pleasures and difficulties, problem solving, and basic personality characteristics do not change dramatically from earlier years, even though the particular circumstances for older persons may be unique.

Aging may be accompanied by declining physical and/or cognitive capacity. Similarly, retirement from a lifelong profession often reduces or eliminates sources of challenge, success, and satisfaction, which come from using acquired knowledge and skills, and may limit daily contacts. Also, as people age, relationships are lost when spouses and friends die. We propose that the way these changes are managed is usually consistent with earlier life decisions (Antonovsky, 1987). At age 80, there is no longer a 50–year life plan. With increased awareness of mortality comes increased concern about how time is used and greater awareness that some long-term goals cannot be met and perhaps should not be pursued.

The older person is more likely to limit engagement to activities that arouse positive emotions and to avoid situations that are negative or neutral. Although this is not unique to the elderly, Carstensen (1992) has proposed that such selection best accounts for reduced social contact and other activities observed in old age. In old age, as at no earlier period in life, individuals have personal experience and extensive knowledge regarding what arouses positive or negative emotions for them. The selectivity proposed by Carstensen involves well-informed choices about which social activities and relationships to continue and whether to substitute or replace roles. This selectivity may help to explain findings of enhanced physical and psychological well-being observed in studies of helping behavior in the elderly.

How Do the Unique Life Circumstances
of Older Persons Apply to Volunteerism?

Following retirement, there may be less demand to make a living, leaving more time available for selected activities. Volunteerism also may provide opportunities to continue to use knowledge and skills developed during the working years. Volunteering may provide feelings of challenge, accomplishment, and self-worth no longer available from a wage-earning occupation. Most volunteer situations have the potential for social contact and for making new friends and acquaintances. If an organization or charity is candid about the opportunities, expectations, and demands of volunteering, the older person should be able to evaluate whether the volunteer situation offers personally needed opportunities, the degree of need for his/her services, the receptiveness of those needing help, the probability of success or failure, the physical and psychological hazards involved, and whether social support will be available in the event of perceived or real failures. With this information, the older person should be able to select volunteer activities that are most likely to provide positive emotional reactions.

What Is Known About Helping Behaviors Such as Volunteerism in the Elderly?

In this discussion, we will not attempt to provide a comprehensive review of all studies of helping and volunteerism in the elderly. Other chapters in this book will provide this information. Instead, we will examine those studies that deal with variables related to the model of emotions we have described. Our position is that volunteers or helpers who experience positive emotions as a result of helping will have greater health benefits than those who do not. Moreover, we propose that the arousal of positive emotions depends upon appraisals that result in accuracy of the evaluation of need, choosing effective methods of providing help, and feelings of satisfaction with the results of helping. Finally, for there to be health benefits, positive emotions must be of extended duration.

Multiple studies have examined physical, psychological, or well-being measures associated with helping behavior and have investigated differential health outcomes for helpers and recipients. This work suggests that helping behaviors may have more beneficial health effects for the helper than for the recipient. For example, a 5-year study by Brown and others (2003) investigated instrumental and emotional support provided to family and friends and found that those who did not provide support were more than twice as likely to die during the 5 years. A relationship was not found between receiving help and reduced risk of death.

In studies of motives for helping, across all ages, individuals who volunteer for self-oriented rather than other-oriented reasons were more likely to volunteer for longer time periods and were more likely to be satisfied with the experience (e.g., Omoto & Snyder, 1995). Such findings support the proposed emotion model for likely health benefits. Activities would be time extended with volunteers deriving personal satisfaction from the experience. Yet, research with the elderly found that more volunteering, a higher number of different organizations, and more hours spent volunteering were not necessarily better for the helper in relation to health (e.g., Musick, Herzog, & House, 1999). These findings highlight the need for older persons to balance helping activities with other needs so as not to deplete their personal resources. An interesting mathematical modeling game study by Panchanathan and Boyd (2004) attempted to explain why people in a community contribute to the public good, and they offer further support of the above findings. In their work, three different types of game players were identified based on their contribution to the public good—defectors, shunners, and cooperators. Cooperators were those who always helped for the common good and always provided help to others when asked. What these researchers found was that "[t]he cooperators were too nice; they died out. In order to survive, they had to be discriminate about the help they gave" (p. 500).

Several studies suggest that particular types of individuals may be more likely to experience volunteering as positive. Penner (2004) described the prosocial personality and identified two dimensions—helpfulness and other-oriented empathy—that were related to the decision to volunteer, the likelihood of continuing to volunteer, and satisfaction with the experience of volunteering. Similarly, other studies have found that those who volunteer, versus those who do not, were less anxious and more extraverted (Herzog & Morgan, 1993). We suggest that individuals with the characteristics identified in these studies are most likely to receive the health and longevity benefits associated with their helping activities.

Finally, research has found that volunteers, more than nonvolunteers, hold stronger religious beliefs and are more likely to be church members. Becker and Dhingra (2001) found that church attendance and strong religious beliefs both predicted volunteerism. In-depth interviews that were part of the work by Becker and Dhingra provided an explanation of the possible motivations of these participants. "If I am to become more Christ-like, I must serve" seemed to reflect the motivations behind volunteerism in these religious persons. Such findings may mean that positive outcomes associated with helping for religious individuals are somewhat different and may be related to striving to be better in their interactions with others.

CONCLUSIONS

Studies of helping and volunteerism have focused primarily on those who do or do not help others and health and well-being outcomes with some attention given to the characteristics of those who help and to motivations for helping. Little attention has been directed at the emotions involved in the decision to help, the motivation to help, the process of helping, or the outcomes of helping. The role of emotions has not been examined in this research, even though there is evidence that emotions, particularly positive emotions, may be related to health outcomes. The absence of an examination of emotions is conspicuous because many studies have focused on the elderly, an age group likely to select activities that maximize positive emotional responses (see work by Carstensen). Perhaps this lack of research emphasis is due to a conceptualization that has focused primarily on motives and helping contexts, while the conceptualization of the decision and helping process has been neglected. If future research integrates the study of emotions, motivation, cognition, personality, helping, and consciousness, exciting advancements will be possible in all areas.

REFERENCES

Antonovsky, A. (1987). *Unraveling the mystery of health: How people manage stress and stay well*. San Francisco: Jossey-Bass.

Becker, P., & Dhingra, P. (2001). Religious involvement and volunteering: Implication for civil society. *Sociology of Religion, 62*(3), 315–335.

Brown, S., Neese, R. M., Vonokur, A. D., & Smith, D. M. (2003). Providing social support may be more beneficial than receiving it: Results from a prospective study of mortality. *Psychological Science, 14*(4), 320–327.

Boucher, J. D., & Brandt, M. E. (1981). Judgment of emotion: American and Malay antecedents. *Journal of Cross-Cultural Psychology, 12*, 272–283.

Carstensen, L. L. (1992). Social and emotional patterns in adulthood: Support for socioemotional selectivity theory. *Psychology & Aging, 7*(3), 331–338.

Chevalier-Skolnikoff, S. (1973). Facial expression of emotion in nonhuman primates. In P. Ekman (Ed.), *Darwin and facial expression* (pp. 11–90). New York: Academic Press.

Danner, D. D., Snowdon, D. A., & Friesen, W. V. (2001). Positive emotions in early life and longevity: Findings from the Nun Study. *Journal of Personality and Social Psychology, 80*, 804–813.

Darwin, C. R. (1872). *The expression of emotions in man and animals*. London: John Murray.

Davidson, R. J., Ekman, P., Saron, C., Senulis, R., & Friesen, W. V. (1990). Approach-withdrawal and cerebral asymmetry: Emotional expression and brain physiology. *Journal of Personality and Social Psychology, 58*, 330–341.

Desai, R. A., Maciejewski, P. K., Dause, D. J., Caldarone, B. J., & Potenza, M. N. (2004). Health correlates of recreational gambling in older adults. *American Journal of Psychiatry, 161*, 1672–1679.

Ekman, P., Friesen, W. V., O'Sullivan, M., Chan, A., Diacoyanni-Tarlatzis, I., Heider, K., Krause, R., Lecompte, W. A., Pitcairn, T., Ricci-Bitti, P. E., Scherer, K. R., Tomita, M., & Tzavaras, A. (1987). Universals and cultural difference in the judgments of facial expressions of emotion. *Journal of Personality and Social Psychology, 53*, 712–717.

Fredrickson, B. L., & Levenson, R. W. (1998). Positive emotions speed recovery from the cardiovascular sequelae of negative emotions. *Cognition and Emotion, 12*(2), 191–220.

Herzog, A. R., & Morgan, J. N. (1993). Formal volunteer work among older Americans. In S. A. Bass, F. G. Caro, & Y.-P. Chen (Eds.), *Achieving a productive aging society* (pp. 119–142). Westport, CT: Auburn House.

Isen, A. M., Daubman, K. A., & Nowicki, G. P. (1987). Positive affect facilitates creative problem solving. *Journal of Personality and Social Psychology, 52*, 1122–1131.

Izard, C. E., Libero, D. Z., Putnam, P., & Haynes, O. M. (1993). Stability of emotion experiences and their relations to traits of personality. *Journal of Personality and Social Psychology, 64,* 847–860.

Levenson, R. W., Ekman, P., & Friesen, W. V. (1990). Voluntary action generates emotion-specific autonomic nervous system activity. *Psychophysiology, 27,* 363–384.

Musick, M., Herzog, A. R., & House J. S. (1999). Volunteerism and mortality among older adults: Findings from a national sample. *Journals of Gerontology: Social Sciences, 54B,* S173–S180.

Oman, D., Tooresen, C. E., & McMahon, K. (1999). Volunteerism and mortality among the community-dwelling elderly. *Journal of Health Psychology, 4*(3), 301–316.

Omoto, A., & Snyder, M. (1995). Sustained helping without obligation: Motivation, longevity of service, and perceived attitude change among AIDS volunteers. *Journal of Personality and Social Psychology, 68,* 671–687.

Panchanathan, K., & Boyd, R. (2004). Indirect reciprocity can stabilize cooperation without the second-order free rider problem. *Nature, 432*(7016), 499–502.

Penner, L. A. (2004). Volunteerism and social problems: Making things better or worse? *Journal of Social Issues, 60*(3), 645–666.

Scherer, K. R., Summerfield, A. B., & Walbott, H. G. (1983). Cross-national research on antecedents and components of emotion: A progress report. *Social Sciences Information, 22,* 355–385.

Tomkins, S. S. (1962). *Affect, imagery, consciousness: Vol. 1. The positive affects.* New York: Springer.

Tomkins, S. S. (1963). *Affect, imagery, consciousness: Vol. 2. The negative affects.* New York: Springer.

Woodworth, R. S., & Schlosberg, H. S. (1954). *Experimental psychology.* New York: Holt.

14 Forgiveness and Health: A Review and Theoretical Exploration of Emotion Pathways

Charlotte V. O. Witvliet
Michael E. McCullough

Our purpose in this chapter is to address the possible health connections of forgiveness, which we view as one way of expressing altruism (see Post, 2003). Because attempts to forgive may not always be born out of purely altruistic concerns, and definitions of forgiveness vary, it is important to present our view of forgiveness and to distinguish it from what it is not. Links with health are likely to hinge on a view of forgiveness that distinguishes it from pseudoforgiveness. For example, it is important not to confuse granting forgiveness with forbearing (McCullough, Fincham, & Tsang, 2003), denying, ignoring, minimizing, tolerating, condoning, excusing, forgetting the offense, suppressing one's emotions about it, or reconciling (see Baskin & Enright, 2004; Enright & Human Development Study Group, 1991).

Forgiveness is an unusual embodiment of altruism because it is an expression of love that can only emerge when the giver has first suffered harm or an offense from a person or people perceived to be blameworthy. Granting forgiveness thus is predicated on the perception that one has been the victim of a moral violation and has perhaps suffered other psychological, physical, or material losses (e.g., loss of self-esteem or damaged property, relationships, opportunities, or health). A forgiving response that is born out of other-regarding love may still call for holding the offender accountable and may require justice-oriented interventions. Indeed, a genuine motivation of concern, compassion, and love of others may pursue justice as one part of striving to ensure effective vindication and resolution for the victim, the community, and the offender (see also Govier, 2002; Lamb & Murphy, 2002; Murphy, 2002, for various views on justice and forgiveness). Against this backdrop—and sensitive to ensuring the victim's emotional, physical, and spiritual safety—forgiveness is a moral response from a victim that seeks to overcome injustice with goodness. Forgiveness involves cultivating positive prosocial responses (e.g., empathy, compassion, and desiring genuine and ultimate good) toward the offender so that they eventually edge out the hurt and bitter emotional responses characterized as unforgiveness (see Worthington, 2003).

This view of forgiveness differs from other approaches that define forgiveness primarily in terms of letting go or distancing oneself from negative responses (e.g., Luskin, 2002) or accepting the occurrence of bad things—whether interpersonal transgressions, illness, accidents, or natural disasters (e.g., Thompson et al., in press). While we see the value of these approaches for coping with various life experiences, we view altruistic forgiveness as an act of gift giving to an undeserving and blameworthy transgressor. Given this view, one can see why narcissism—that is, self-absorption, entitlement, and preoccupation with self-protection—has emerged as a barrier to forgiveness in multiple studies (Exline et al., 2004). The gift of forgiveness—in psychological terms—comprises prosocial and positive thoughts, motivations, emotions, and behaviors toward the offending person(s) so that these embodiments of love supplant the hurt-filled, bitter, negative activation that often occurs in the wake of hurtful injustice.

A MULTIFACETED VIEW OF FORGIVENESS: EMOTION THEORY AS THE LENS

Forgiveness involves a variety of psychological changes, including affective, motivational, behavioral, cognitive, social, spiritual, and physiological ones. So to think about the connections between forgiveness and health, we situate unforgiveness, forgiveness, and justice within a broad view of emotion that emphasizes active physiological response elements and that integrates affective, attentional, and motivational functions. This approach is sympathetic to Lang's (1995) bioinformational theory, which emphasizes that verbal/cognitive, behavioral, and physiological responses are integral aspects of emotion, and to Thayer and Lane's (2000) dynamical systems neurovisceral integration model, which further integrates affective, attentional, motivational, and physiological functions. Furthermore, we take seriously research highlighting the importance of two dimensions of emotion that organize verbal/cognitive and physiological expressions in response to a broad range of stimuli (Faith & Thayer, 2001). These affective dimensions are *valence* (extending from negative to positive) and *arousal* (ranging from deactivated to highly activated). Within this two-dimensional space, a variety of emotion categories can be situated, recognizing that even within categories, shifts in valence and arousal may occur from time to time. To illustrate, both fear and anger (and unforgiveness) may be situated in a nega-

tive and activated part of the valence × arousal space, whereas pleasant relaxation and peace (and forgiveness) might be situated in a positive and calmer
part of the state-space, although shifts in their precise valence and arousal qualities may vary across particular experiences within each emotion, anticipations
of them, and ruminations about them. Considering the valence and arousal
qualities of emotions can allow us to be aware of the importance of categorical
emotions that often occur in response to hurtful injustice (e.g., anger, fear, sadness), and this view enables us to hypothesize about and synthesize psychophysiological findings on forgiveness-related emotional changes that are less well studied
and that only recently have been considered from an emotion perspective.

A multifaceted view of forgiveness—involving attention, motivation, subjective emotional experience, physiology, and behavior—is supported by Thayer
and Lane's (2000) neurovisceral integration model. In this model, a variety of
physiological systems underlies and integrates attention, motivation, and emotion. From a dynamical systems perspective, these systems rely on feedback and
feed-forward circuits essential to efficient functioning and self-regulation, a
process that we believe underlies forgiveness. The neurovisceral integration
model emphasizes the significance of *inhibition*. Inhibitory processes are negative feedback circuits that enable an organism to interrupt behavior and to re-
allocate attention and responses to another task. In our view, this process would
be involved in letting go of rumination or grudge holding as one attempts to
cultivate an empathetic and forgiving response. As Thayer and Lane (2000)
detail, when these inhibitory processes fail, or when negative feedback mechanisms are ineffective, the resulting *disinhibition* leads to positive feedback loops
that perpetuate behaviors in a feed-forward fashion. We posit that a disinhibition process operates when people persist in ruminating about a past injustice
or getting revenge. When emotion is disordered, such as in anxiety disorders
(with the most evidence accrued for generalized anxiety disorder), and—for our
purposes here—when people cannot stop transgression-related ruminations or
grudges, people have an emotional system that prevents them from shifting to
process other information and from generating responses that would be more
personally beneficial or culturally appropriate. This state of being emotionally
"stuck" or "inflexible" not only reflects difficulty in shifting to a more appropriate response but also—and more likely—involves *being unable to inhibit the inappropriate response* (Thayer & Lane, 2000).[1]

People in these types of unforgiving states seem unable to shift their attention to information that could promote empathy or forgiveness, and instead they
seem compelled to ruminate about past hurts, embellish these narratives with
bitter adjectives and adverbs that stir up contempt, exhibit avoidance and revenge motivations, focus attention upon the negative features of the offender
and the offense, and rehearse a repertoire of grudge and revenge plots that—
even if never enacted in overt behavior—perpetuate a feed-forward circuit
subserved by attentional, motivational, physiological, and behavioral subsystems

of emotion. Thayer and Lane (2000) further propose that this kind of ineffi-
ciency in affective information processing results in affective dysregulation and
can ultimately lead to such problems as a hostile personality, anxiety and depressive disorders, hypertension, and coronary heart disease. As will be described
later in this chapter, forgiveness as an altruistic act and forgivingness as an altruistic personality disposition may help to remedy these problems.

FORGIVENESS AND HEALTH: EMOTION REGULATION PATHWAYS

We propose that insofar as forgiveness is associated with health, it is at least in
part because genuine forgiveness inhibits inappropriate responses and facilitates
beneficial emotion regulation processes. The connections implied here among
forgiveness, emotions, and health are not simply the net effect of decreasing
negative emotions and increasing positive emotions, however. Rather, as Ryff
and Singer (2003) observe:

> [I]t is *how* negative emotion is expressed and responded to that arbitrates
> its deleterious or beneficial effects. Positive emotion is deeply entangled in
> such processes, both as an antidote to negative feelings and as a consequence
> of working through (frequently with significant others) difficult emotions.
> Thus, it is the nature of how positive and negative emotion are entwined
> that is critical for future health research. (pp. 1098–1099)

Forgiveness as an Antidote to Potentially Destructive Post-Offense Responses

In the wake of an offense, people often ruminate about the hurt, experience
and express hostility toward the perpetrator, use harmful strategies to cope with
stress responses, and attempt to suppress their negative emotions and feelings
of vulnerability. We propose that genuine forgiveness works against hostility,
stress and related negative coping behaviors, rumination, and suppression. As a
result, genuine forgiveness may have a positive effect on health, in part by interrupting maladaptive patterns of emotion regulation.

Hostility

Forgiveness may buffer health in part because it counters revenge, anger, and
hostility. Thoughts of revenge are among the strongest elicitors of angry affect
(DiGiuseppe & Froh, 2002), which has adverse ramifications not only for physi-

ology and interpersonal relations, but also for task performance (Herrald & Tomaka, 2002). Hostility is a potent risk factor for cardiovascular difficulties (Miller, Smith, Turner, Guijarro, & Hallet, 1996; Smith, Gallo, & Ruiz, 2003). But, hostility can be quelled, and cardiovascular risks can be reduced. Friedman et al. (1986) found that Type A patients who were at risk for recurring heart attacks and were randomly assigned to a behavioral modification program (versus standard treatment from a cardiologist) showed a greater reduction in hostile behavior and in heart problems than those who received standard care only. In his analysis of this efficacious intervention, Kaplan (1992) identified forgiveness as an important antidote to hostility.

Stress and Negative Coping Behaviors

Forgiveness also mitigates against the stress that victims experience as a result of hurtful offenses and may then also reduce the use of coping behaviors that further heighten health risks (e.g., smoking, substance use, overeating). Eysenck (2000) amassed data highlighting the interaction of stress and smoking for significantly inflating the risk of mortality by coronary heart disease and cancer. If forgiveness can both reduce the stress response stimulated by an offense and decrease the use of negative coping behaviors, such as smoking, forgiveness may play an important role in buffering against negative health effects.

Rumination

Rumination is the disinhibited process of repeatedly rehearsing experiences and emotions, generally those with negative affective features. In a role critical to health, rumination has been identified as a moderating variable between anger and blood pressure (see Hogan & Linden, 2004). Rumination deters forgiveness (McCullough, Bono, & Root, 2004), and it is probably also the case that forgiveness deters rumination. When people work through the process of forgiving, they engage the hurt, interpret its significance, and reshape their response to the offender in a way that integrates the hurtful offense with a larger view of reality. This refocuses victims' attentional, motivational, and emotional processing so that they can cultivate more merciful, positive, prosocial responses to the offender. This feature highlights the importance of our definition of forgiveness. If forgiveness were merely a process in which the victim tried not to think about the offender, the offense, or the hurtful consequences of the offense, an ironic process would likely ensue in which thoughts about the offense and offender became more rather than less intrusive and more rather than less influential on other aspects of thought, emotion, and behavior (Wegner, 1997). Insofar as forgiveness involves active (even if automatic) attempts to reappraise the transgression and the transgressor rather than an attempt to control rumination effortfully, reductions in rumination can result.

Suppression

In contrast to rumination, suppression is a process whereby a person attempts to minimize awareness and expression of negative emotions, whether to make others feel better or to conceal the expression of one's inner emotional experience (Gross, 1998). Suppression is considered to have a negative health role, with links to the Type C cancer-prone personality (see Giese-Davis & Spiegel, 2003), and is associated with increased psychiatric and physical symptoms, viral replication, and medical visits (Ryff & Singer, 2003). Interpersonally, suppression also reduces intimacy and interrupts honest engagement and nurturing displays in relationships. It thereby reduces the quality and extent of one's social network, with the net effect of decreasing the beneficial and buffering effects of social support.

Gross and colleagues have found that emotion suppression has an array of other costs, including increased sympathetic nervous system responding (Gross & Levenson, 1997), heightened blood pressure in suppressors and their conversation partners, impaired relationship formation (Butler et al., 2003), and impaired incidental memory for information presented during emotionally suppressive behavior (Richards & Gross, 1999). Gross and colleagues explain that there are circumstances in which it may be wise to conceal one's emotions—to inhibit violent and aggressive behavior, for example—but that suppression is unlikely to alleviate one's own emotions (Gross & Levenson, 1997) and has its own physiological, social, and cognitive costs. In line with Gross and colleagues' work, we propose that if victims of injustice suppress their expressions of negative emotions, this has the apparent benefit of limiting aggressive behavior; however, such suppression holds potential costs for the victim as it may fail to alleviate one's hurt, angry, and bitter feelings, may heighten one's sympathetic nervous system responding, may tax one's social encounters, and may impair one's ability to remember the incident and associated information accurately. If so, people may not incorporate disconfirming or additional information that could challenge their operating assumptions, views, and affect. Gross and colleagues propose another, better way: reappraisal.

Forgiveness Promotes Positive Responding

Reappraisal

In Gross's (1998) articulation, reappraisal is an emotional down-regulation strategy in which a person thinks about an experience in a fresh way to decrease its emotional impact. This stands in contrast to the emotion-concealing approach of suppression. In contrast to suppression, reappraisal more effectively decreases emotional experience and behavioral expression, with no demonstrable memory effects. In a series of five studies, Gross and John (2003) found that people who showed a tendency to reappraise experienced subjectively and expressed outwardly more positive emotion and less negative emotion. By contrast, suppressors experienced and expressed more negative and less positive emotions. Furthermore, those who used reappraisal strategies had better interpersonal functioning and well-being, whereas the opposite occurred for those using suppression strategies.

In our view, forgiveness works against suppression and is more akin to a reappraisal process. As we articulated earlier, genuine forgiveness (in contrast to pseudoforgiveness) does not seek to deny or conceal negative emotions related to the inciting injustice and its costs, although it does involve inhibiting retaliatory behavioral expressions, which would magnify the negative effects of the initial harm. Forgiveness begins with an honest appraisal in which the victim blames the offender for the offense and its hurtful consequences. From there, forgiveness involves reappraisal of the events, their implications, and one's feelings and thoughts about them. In many cases, this will involve an explicit acknowledgment of the humanity of the offender—an empathetic response found to be at the heart of forgiveness (e.g., McCullough et al., 1997)—although for many effective forgivers, the reappraisal process is automatic and not available to consciousness. Although reappraisal may be most effective when engaged immediately (as may occur when a person has a compassionate and forgiving personality), we nevertheless hypothesize that reappraisal may have a longer time window of effectiveness. In our view, a forgiving, empathetic, or virtue-oriented reappraisal could be launched even if one has previously enacted a vengeful response to injustice (e.g., see Boehm, 1987) and could still be more effective than suppression in decreasing one's negative emotions and increasing one's positive emotions (to broaden and build, as addressed below).

Positive Emotions

To the extent that forgiveness engages positive and prosocial emotional responses toward one's offender, forgiveness may engender the benefits associated with positive emotions. Furthermore, because the positive emotions of forgiveness are concerned with other-regarding love, they inhibit the negative emotions (and associated health risks) that may otherwise flourish when people remain preoccupied with the self (Anderson, 2003). Positive emotions have been identified as inhibiting the cardiovascular after-effects of negative emotions (Fredrickson & Levenson, 1998), and they function to broaden the individual's cognitive and behavioral repertoire and to build or extend the person's cognitive, physical, and social resources (Fredrickson, 1998).

FORGIVENESS, EMOTION, MENTAL HEALTH, AND PHYSICAL HEALTH

Forgiveness (a) may provide an alternative to stress, hostility, rumination, and suppression, which tend to have negative implications for health and well-being; and (b) may engage reappraisal and positive emotion responses, which tend to have positive implications for health and well-being. As a result, it is likely that forgiveness promotes health and psychological well-being among people who have experienced an interpersonal transgression. Most of the data on the associations of forgiveness with mental health, physiology, and physical health tend to support this notion. Presently, we will review some of these findings with an emphasis on articulating the emotional processes that might lead to the associations of forgiveness with mental health and physical health.

Mental Health and Forgiveness: Correlational Research

There is good evidence that forgiving leads to reductions in psychopathology and to improved psychological well-being. Studies show correlations between self-report measures of forgiveness and measures of psychological well-being and depressive symptoms (Brown, 2003; Maltby, Macaskill, & Day, 2001; Seybold, Hill, Neumann, & Chi, 2001). In a study of combat veterans with PTSD, both depression and PTSD symptom severity were significantly correlated with difficulty in forgiving oneself and others, even after controlling for combat exposure, socioeconomic status, ethnicity, and hostility levels (Witvliet, Phipps, Feldman, & Beckham, 2004). Bono and McCullough (2004) also found on a within-persons level that when people are more benevolent, less avoidant, and less vengeful toward a specific transgressor than is typical for them (i.e., when they are more forgiving than usual), they also report higher levels of positive mood, more satisfaction with life, lower levels of negative mood, and fewer illness-related symptoms than is typical for them.

In addition, epidemiological research shows that people who tend to feel vengeful after they have been harmed by someone have an elevated risk for being diagnosed with major depression, generalized anxiety disorder, phobia, and panic disorder (Kendler et al., 2003), whereas people who score high in measures of forgiveness as a personality trait have a lower risk for nicotine dependence and drug abuse/dependence (Kendler et al., 2003) . Taken together, these findings suggest that effective self-regulation of vengeful impulses, perhaps specifically via forgiveness, could reduce people's risk for mental disorders and improve their psychological well-being.

Mental Health and Granting Forgiveness:
The Efficacy of Interventions

Moreover, forgiveness interventions reduce anxiety and depressive symptoms and increase self-esteem and hope. In a meta-analytic review of experimental studies that evaluated the efficacy of interventions for promoting forgiveness, Baskin and Enright (2004) assessed the efficacy of nine forgiveness intervention studies versus control group studies for prompting forgiveness and influencing emotion variables. Baskin and Enright concluded that interventions that seek to help people forgive exclusively by persuading them to make a decision to forgive are ineffective at producing forgiveness or facilitating positive emotional outcomes. However, forgiveness interventions administered as psychoeducational groups that were specifically designed to help people engage in processes that have been hypothesized to be active ingredients for helping people forgive (e.g., engaging love, compassion, and empathy for someone who has caused harm) are considerably more helpful: The average person in these process-oriented forgiveness groups forgave as much or more than 75% of those in the control groups ($d = 0.82$), and they scored as having as good or better emotional health on the variables assessed as 65% of those in the control groups ($d = 0.59$). The most potent interventions for facilitating forgiveness and thereby improving mental health, however, are individually administered process-oriented interventions. For example, Freedman and Enright (1996) studied survivors of incest (occurring at least 2 years prior to therapy) who completed their therapy, and assessed their hope, state and trait anxiety, self-esteem, and depression in comparison to a wait-listed control group. Overall, Baskin and Enright's (2004) meta-analysis indicated that average members of the individual process-oriented forgiveness intervention forgave as much or more than 95% of those in the control group ($d = 1.66$), and their scores indicated as good or better emotional health on the variables assessed than 92% of those in the control group ($d = 1.42$).

Forgiveness in Relation to Autobiographical
Experiences, Psychophysiology, and Physical Health

Granting Forgiveness: State Effects in Victims

Based on emotion and psychophysiology research linking the valence and arousal of emotional imagery to patterns of facial electromyography, skin conductance, and heart rate, Witvliet, Ludwig, and Vander Laan (2001) tested hypotheses about the psychophysiology of forgiveness and unforgiveness. They measured continuous physiological response patterns as 71 (36 male, 35 female) college students each adopted two states of unforgiveness (rumination about the transgression, nursing a grudge toward the offender) versus two states of forgiveness (cultivating empathy for the offender, forgiving the offender by finding a way to genuinely wish him or her well while releasing hurt and angry emotions) toward a particular real-life offender. This study used a within-subjects design in which each participant imagined each of the four types of imagery eight times (32 trials total with continuous physiology), counterbalancing condition orders. For each measure, physiological reactivity during each imagery trial and recovery patterns during the subsequent relaxation period were assessed (compared to that same trial's pretrial baseline data).

As predicted, the unforgiving imagery evoked higher arousal and more negative valence ratings compared to the forgiving imagery. Consistent with the high arousal ratings, unforgiving imagery was associated with higher levels of tonic eye muscle tension (orbicularis oculi EMG) during imagery and higher heart rate and skin conductance level scores (indicating sympathetic nervous system activation) during both imagery and recovery. Consistent with the negative valence of unforgiving imagery (versus the positive valence of forgiving imagery), participants showed more brow muscle tension (corrugator EMG) during imagery and recovery periods. Although blood pressure has not been specifically measured in reference to valence and arousal, heightened blood pressure has been linked to state and trait anger, which may be characterized as aroused and negatively valent. Witvliet et al. (2001) found that systolic blood pressure (SBP; during the middle of imagery), diastolic blood pressure (DBP), and mean arterial pressure (MAP) were all significantly higher during unforgiving versus forgiving imagery.

These data patterns were replicated in a subsequent study of the associations of justice and forgiveness with effects on continuous measures of physiological functioning (Witvliet, Root, Sato, & Ludwig, 2003). When 56 (27 male, 29 female) college students imagined not granting (versus granting) forgiveness to a fictitious burglar in this scenario-based study, they reported more aroused and negatively valent emotion. Consistent with lower arousal levels for forgiveness imagery, orbicularis oculi EMG was lower during imagery (as long as the no-justice outcome occurred), and heart rate scores were lower during both imagery and recovery periods. Consistent with the more positive valence of forgiving imagery, corrugator brow tension levels were lower during imagery.

State and Trait Effects of Granting Forgiveness

These data converge with findings from Lawler et al.'s (2003, in press) and Toussaint and Williams's (2003) psychophysiology research using combined between- and within-subjects designs and interview paradigms. Lawler et al. (2003) found cardiovascular benefits of both trait and state forgiving in 108 (44 male, 64 female) college students. Higher trait forgivingness was associated with lower SBP, DBP, and MAP (when values for each measure were averaged across baseline, three time periods during the parent conflict and peer/partner conflict interviews, and two time periods during recovery from each type of interview). Lower state unforgivingness and higher state forgivingness for both parent and peer/partner were associated with lower SBP, DBP, MAP, heart rate, and rate pressure product (SBP × heart rate/100, an indicator of myocardial oxygen demand and stress). Additionally, Lawler et al. (2003) assessed the interaction of trait and state forgivingness variables on physiology during the two types of conflict interviews and the subsequent recovery periods, covarying baseline values. In response to an interview about a salient memory of conflict with a parent or primary caregiver, Lawler et al. (2003) found that high trait forgivers showed the least reactivity and best recovery patterns for SBP, DBP, and MAP, rate pressure product, and forehead EMG, whereas low trait forgivers in unforgiving states showed the highest levels of cardiovascular reactivity and poorest recovery patterns. When these same participants were interviewed about a conflict with a friend or partner, the only significant effect was that high state forgiving women showed smaller increases in rate pressure products than did the low state forgiving women. In the subsequent recovery period, high trait forgivingness was associated with lower blood pressure for DBP and MAP.

In subsequent research with a community sample of 27- to 72-year-olds who prepared in advance to be interviewed about an experience with betrayal, Lawler et al. (in press) found that trait forgivingness was associated with lower levels of rate pressure product reactivity—but not mean arterial pressure—in the first part of the interviews. Lawler et al. propose that follow-up psychophysiological research should recruit participants in ways that will lead to a greater heterogeneity of offenses and severities, given that the differences in college students emerged in the context of widely varying offenses and degrees of forgiveness.

Lawler and colleagues also conducted path analyses. Lawler et al. (2003) found that trait forgivingness predicted state forgiveness, and higher state forgiveness and lower hostility predicted lower stress levels, which in turn predicted lower self-reported illness. Assessing the link between forgiveness and physical health symptoms, Lawler et al. (in press) found that reduced negative affect was the strongest mediator, followed by reduced stress. Spirituality and social skills were also mediators.

In another interview study, Toussaint and Williams (2003) measured blood pressure in a diverse sample of 100 midwestern community residents, with 25 in each cell: 2 SES (high, low) × 2 race (Black, White), and participant sex almost evenly divided across cells. Across participants, higher levels of total forgiveness (i.e., forgiveness of others and self and feeling forgiven by God) were associated with lower resting DBP. Among White participants of high socioeconomic status, total forgiveness and forgiveness of self were associated with lower resting DBP. By contrast, among Black participants with low socioeconomic status, forgiveness of others was associated with lower resting DBP, and forgiveness of others, total forgiveness, and perceived divine forgiveness were associated with lower resting cortisol levels. When assessing raw blood pressure values for all participants at baseline, at two points during a 10-minute interview about "a time when you were treated unfairly" and a 5-minute recovery period, being forgiving toward others and feeling God's forgiveness were each associated with lower blood pressure during the interview.

Collectively, the findings of Lawler et al. (2003, in press), Toussaint and Williams (2003), and Witvliet et al. (2001, 2003) suggest that chronic unforgiving responses (e.g., rumination about the hurt and its implications, harboring grudges) could contribute to adverse health by perpetuating stress beyond the duration of the original stressor; heightening cardiovascular reactivity during recall, imagery, and conversations about the hurt; and impairing cardiovascular recovery even when people try to focus on something else. By contrast, forgiving responses may buffer health by quelling these responses and by nurturing positive emotional responses in their place.

The Motivation to Forgive Matters in Victims

Pertinent to our interest in forgiveness that is altruistic, Huang and Enright (2000) compared the effects of forgiving out of moral love versus obligation in 22 matched pairs of male and female Taiwanese community members. When interviewed about a typical day, the groups did not differ in their BP. When interviewed about a past experience with conflict, the groups did not differ on self-reported anger. However, those who forgave out of obligation-oriented versus unconditional love motives cast down their eyes and showed more masking smiles, which the authors interpreted as signs of hidden anger. These facial patterns are also consistent with the idea that the obligatory forgivers were engaging in suppression of negative emotions rather than in forgiveness as defined earlier in this chapter. In line with this view, the obligatory forgivers had significantly higher blood pressure values than the moral love forgivers on 3 of 12 raw blood pressure comparisons. Obligatory forgivers had higher raw SBP at the beginning of the interview, and higher raw SBP and DBP 1 minute into the interview.

Scenario-Based Victim Research

Granting Forgiveness in Response to an Apology and Restitution

Examining interpersonal forgiveness, empathy, and unforgiveness as dependent variables, Witvliet, Worthington, and Wade (2002) conducted a within-subjects study of college students' ($N = 61$, 29 female, 32 male) psychophysiology in response to an imagined burglary and four different outcomes: the offender later apologized, made restitution, both, or neither in a 2 apology × 2 restitution design. Participants' unforgiveness decreased and their empathy and forgiveness levels increased when imagining that the transgressor in these situations offered a strong apology (in which the offender specifically named the offense, clearly accepted responsibility, expressed sincere regret and remorse, and promised that it was a one-time-only offense) or made restitution (by returning the stolen goods and some money for damages). Apology and restitution also benefited an array of emotion self-reports—including less arousal and more positive valent emotion —and mitigated corrugator (brow) EMG reactivity. The apology alone had a broader array of physical effects than did restitution, reliably ameliorating or-bicularis oculi (eye) EMG and heart rate reactivity—consistent with lower arousal—and improving both rate pressure product reactivity and recovery pat-terns. These results suggest that while restitution offers a tangible means of re-storing what a victim lost, a strong apology (an effort to recognize and respond to the hurts of the victim through a verbally conveyed social exchange) has sa-lient effects on recipients' emotion systems.

EFFECTS IN THE RECIPIENTS OF FORGIVENESS

While the focus of this book and chapter is on altruism from the perspective of the giver (or forgiver), one may wonder about the effects of forgiveness on those who receive it. This was examined in a within-subjects psychophysiology imag-ery study with 40 (20 female, 20 male) college students who reflected on a par-ticular transgression they committed against someone else (Witvliet, Ludwig, & Bauer, 2002). Part of this study compared imagery of receiving (1) an unforgiv-ing response from one's victim with imagery of receiving (2) forgiveness and (3) reconciliation. Forgiveness and reconciliation imagery each prompted improve-ments in basic emotions (e.g., sadness, anger) and moral emotions (e.g., guilt, shame, gratitude, hope). Receiving forgiveness and reconciliation each also prompted less furrowing of the brow muscle (corrugator EMG), associated with negative emotion, and more smiling activity (zygomatic EMG). Autonomic ner-vous system measures were largely unaffected by imagery, although skin conduc-tance data suggested greater emotional engagement when transgressors imagined reconciling with their victims. When considered in combination with the studies of forgiveness in victims, these data suggest that when it comes to forgiveness and psychophysiology, it is even better to give than to receive forgiveness.

REVIEW SUMMARY

In order for laboratory studies of cardiovascular reactivity to generalize well to real life, they must employ tasks that mirror daily life, aggregate repeated measures across tasks, and measure physiology before, during, and after the conditions of interest (Schwartz et al., 2003). Considering the forgiveness and physiology studies, those with designs closest to Schwartz et al.'s (2003) ideals show cardiovascular reactivity patterns that reliably distinguish unforgiving responses toward others (as a state or trait) as generating more reactivity and prolonged activation than forgiving responses toward others (and they also link facial EMG patterns with the negative aroused emotion of unforgiveness). Exploratory studies that seek to correlate single resting physiology measures with forgiving personality variables do not show these patterns (Brenneis, 2001; Seybold et al., 2001). Nevertheless, it is important to keep in mind that it is sustained elevations in blood pressure that predict end-organ damage, and the impact of brief peaks in BP, such as those measured in the forgiveness studies, is unclear (see Schwartz et al., 2003). Hence, the extant data speak only to immediate, short-term patterns. As we interpret the autonomic and cardiovascular effects, it is also important to keep in mind that they may reflect not only heightened sympathetic nervous system arousal, but also impaired parasympathetically mediated responding.

Forgiveness has been shown to be beneficial in reducing victims' unforgiveness, which is associated with prolonged physiological activation and is theorized to have more cardiovascular health implications than short-term stress reactivity (Brosschot & Thayer, 2003). Forgiveness research suggests that it also promotes positive and prosocial emotions for victims and offenders, calming physiological indicators of negative and aroused emotions. To the extent that forgiveness may eclipse or reduce anger, sympathetic nervous system activation may be mitigated (McCraty et al., 1995). To the degree that forgiveness involves positive and calm emotions, the parasympathetic nervous system may exert better control (see McCraty et al., 1995).

CONCLUSION

In the present chapter, we have proposed that forgiveness of transgressors represents an extraordinary form of love: Forgiveness is love directed toward those who have done us harm—people whose behavior typically has elicited within us a variety of negative feelings, such as sadness, fear, and anger.

Such negative emotions as these, the rumination that perpetuates them, and efforts to suppress them can have a variety of negative effects on health, well-being, and human performance. Conversely, forgiveness appears to be quite consistently related to better mental health, reduced risk for psychopathology, and healthier autonomic and cardiovascular responses to stress. Insofar as forgiveness has positive implications for health and well-being, it might be because forgiveness provides an alternative to ruminative and suppressive ways of regulating negative emotions—perhaps by employing reappraisal and positive emotion processes found to yield largely positive effects on health and psychological well-being.

Correspondence concerning this article should be addressed to Charlotte vanOyen Witvliet, Ph.D., Associate Professor, Psychology Department, Hope College, Holland, Michigan 49422–9000. E-mail: witvliet@hope.edu. This research was supported in part by a grant from the Hope College Faith and Learning Fund to the first author and a grant from the Campaign for Forgiveness Research to the second author.

NOTE

1. A comment about cultural differences is useful here. In cultures in which revenge is condoned as a problem-solving strategy (see Ericksen & Horton, 1992), limited inhibitory control over grudges and vengeful behavior may be viewed not as a *failure* of emotion regulation per se but rather as a normal and acceptable feature of human nature (Boehm, 1987). Cultural differences in the acceptability of grudges and revenge-seeking behavior notwithstanding, inhibitory failure may describe quite aptly what happens when people cannot or will not forgive (see Witvliet et al., 2001; Worthington, 2003).

REFERENCES

Anderson, N. B. (2003). *Emotional longevity: What really determines how long you live*. New York: Viking.

Baskin, T. W., & Enright, R. D. (2004). Intervention studies on forgiveness: A meta-analysis. *Journal of Counseling and Development, 82*, 79–90.

Boehm, C. (1987). *Blood revenge: The enactment and management of conflict in Montenegro and other tribal societies* (2nd ed.). Philadelphia: University of Pennsylvania Press.

Bono, G., & McCullough, M. E. (2004). *Forgiveness and well-being*. Coral Gables, FL: University of Miami.

Brenneis, M. J. (2001). The relationship between forgiveness and physical health indicators in recovering members of the clergy. *Journal of Ministry in Addiction and Recovery, 7*, 43–59.

Brosschot, J. F., & Thayer, J. F. (2003). Heart rate response is longer after negative emotions than after positive emotions. *International Journal of Psychophysiology, 50*, 181–187.

Brown, R. P. (2003). Measuring individual differences in the tendency to forgive: Construct validity and links with depression. *Personality and Social Psychology Bulletin, 29*, 759–771.

Butler, E. A., Egloff, B., Wilhelm, F. H., Smith, N. C., Erickson, E. A., & Gross, J. A. (2003). The social consequences of expressive suppression. *Emotion, 3*, 48–67.

DiGiuseppe, R., & Froh, J. J. (2002). What cognitions predict state anger? *Journal of Rational-Emotive & Cognitive Behavior Therapy, 20*, 133–150.

Enright, R. D., & Human Development Study Group. (1991). The moral development of forgiveness. In W. Kurtines & J. Gewirtz (Eds.), *Moral behavior and development* (Vol. 1, pp. 123–152). Hillsdale, NJ: Erlbaum.

Ericksen, K. P., & Horton, H. (1992). "Blood feuds": Cross-cultural variations in kin group vengeance. *Behavior Science Research, 26,* 57–85.

Exline, J. J., Baumeister, R. F., Bushman, B. J., Campbell, W. K., & Finkel, E. J. (2004). Too proud to let go: Narcissistic entitlement as a barrier to forgiveness. *Journal of Personality and Social Psychology, 87,* 894–912.

Eysenck, H. J. (2000). Personality as a risk factor in cancer and coronary heart disease. In D. T. Kenny & J. G. Carlson (Eds.), *Stress and health: Research and clinical applications* (pp. 291–318). Amsterdam, Netherlands: Harwood Academic.

Faith, M., & Thayer, J. F. (2001). A dynamical systems interpretation of a dimensional model of emotion. *Scandinavian Journal of Psychology, 42,* 121–133.

Fredrickson, B. L. (1998). What good are positive emotions? *Review of General Psychology, 2,* 300–319.

Fredrickson, B. L., & Levenson, R. W. (1998). Positive emotions speed recovery from the cardiovascular sequelae of negative emotions. *Cognition and Emotion, 12,* 191–220.

Freedman, S. R., & Enright, R. D. (1996). Forgiveness as an intervention goal with incest survivors. *Journal of Consulting & Clinical Psychology, 64,* 983–992.

Friedman, M., Thoresen, C. E., Gill, J., Ulmer, D., Powell, L. H., Price, V. A., Brown, B., Thompson, L., Rabin, D. D., Breall, W. S., Bourg, W., Levy, R., & Dixon, T. (1986). Alteration of Type A behavior and its effect on cardiac recurrences in post myocardial infarction patients: Summary results of the Recurrent Coronary Prevention Project. *American Heart Journal, 112,* 653–665.

Giese-Davis, J., & Spiegel, D. (2003). Emotional expression and cancer progression. In R. J. Davidson, K. R. Scherer, & H. H. Goldsmith (Eds.), *Handbook of affective sciences* (pp. 1053–1082). New York: Oxford University Press.

Gross, J. J. (1998). Antecedent- and response-focused emotion regulation: Divergent consequences for experience, expression, and physiology. *Journal of Personality & Social Psychology, 74,* 224–237.

Gross, J. J., & John, O. P. (2003). Individual differences in two emotion regulation processes: Implications for affect, relationships, and well-being. *Journal of Personality & Social Psychology, 85,* 348–362.

Gross, J. J., & Levenson, R. W. (1997). Hiding feelings: The acute effects of inhibition negative and positive emotion. *Journal of Abnormal Psychology, 106,* 95–103.

Govier, T. (2002). *Forgiveness and revenge.* London: Routledge.

Herrald, M. M., & Tomaka, J. (2002). Patterns of emotion-specific appraisal, coping, and cardiovascular reactivity during an ongoing emotional episode. *Journal of Personality & Social Psychology, 83,* 434–450.

Hogan, B. E., & Linden, W. (2004). Anger response styles and blood pressure: At least don't ruminate about it! *Annals of Behavioral Medicine, 27,* 38–49.

Huang, S.-T. T., & Enright, R. D. (2000). Forgiveness and anger-related emotions in Taiwan: Implications for therapy. *Psychotherapy: Theory, Research, Practice, Training, 37,* 71–79.

Kaplan, B. H. (1992). Social health and the forgiving heart: The Type B story. *Journal of Behavioral Medicine, 15*, 3–14.

Kendler, K. S., Liu, X., Gardner, C. O., McCullough, M. E., Larson, D. B., & Prescott, C. A. (2003). Dimensions of religiosity and their relationship to lifetime psychiatric and substance use disorders. *American Journal of Psychiatry, 160*(3), 496–503.

Lamb, S., & Murphy, J. (2002). *Before forgiving: Cautionary views of forgiveness in psychotherapy*. Oxford: Oxford University Press.

Lang, P. J. (1995). The emotion probe: Studies of motivation and attention. *American Psychologist, 50*, 372–385.

Lawler, K. A., Younger, J. W., Piferi, R. L., Billington, E., Jobe, R., Edmondson, K., & Jones, W. H. (2003). A change of heart: Cardiovascular correlates of forgiveness in response to interpersonal conflict. *Journal of Behavioral Medicine, 26*, 373–393.

Lawler, K. A., Younger, J. W., Piferi, R. L., Jobe, R. L., Edmondson, K. A., & Jones, W. H. (in press). *The unique effects of forgiveness on health: An exploration of pathways*.

Luskin, F. M. (2002). *Forgive for good*. New York: HarperCollins.

Maltby, J., Macaskill, A., & Day, L. (2001). Failure to forgive self and others: A replication and extension of the relationship between forgiveness, personality, social desirability and general health. *Personality and Individual Differences, 30*, 881–885.

McCraty, R., Atkinson, M., Riller, W. A., Rein, G., & Watkins, A. D. (1995). The effects of emotion on short-term power spectrum analysis of heart rate variability. *The American Journal of Cardiology, 76*, 1089–1093.

McCullough, M. E., Bono, G., & Root, L. M. (2004). *Rumination, affect, and forgiveness*. Unpublished manuscript.

McCullough, M. E., Fincham, F. D., & Tsang, J. (2003). Forgiveness, forbearance, and time: The temporal unfolding of transgression-related interpersonal motivations. *Journal of Personality & Social Psychology, 84*, 540–557.

McCullough, M. E., Sandage, S. J., & Worthington, J. L., Jr. (1997). *To forgive is human: How to put your past in the past*. Downers Grove, IL: InterVarsity.

Miller, T. Q., Smith, T. W., Turner, C. W., Guijarro, M. L., & Hallet, A. J. (1996). Meta-analytic review of research on hostility and physical health. *Psychological Bulletin, 108*, 322–348.

Murphy, J. (2002). *Getting even: Forgiveness and its limits*. Oxford: Oxford University Press.

Post, S. G. (2003). *Unlimited love: Altruism, compassion, and service*. Radnor, PA: Templeton Foundation Press.

Richards, J. M., & Gross, J. J. (1999). Compose at any cost? The cognitive consequences of emotion suppression. *Personality & Social Psychology Bulletin, 25*, 1033–1044.

Ryff, C. D., & Singer, B. H. (2003). The role of emotion on pathways to positive health. In R. J. Davidson, K. R. Scherer, & H. H. Goldsmith (Eds.), *Handbook of affective sciences* (pp. 1083–1104). New York: Oxford University Press.

Schwartz, A. R., Gerin, W., Davidson, K. W., Pickering, T. G., Brosschot, J. F.,

Thayer, J. F., Christenfeld, N., & Linden, W. (2003). Toward a causal model of cardiovascular responses to stress and the development of cardiovascular disease. *Psychosomatic Medicine, 65,* 22–35.

Seybold, K. S., Hill, P. C., Neumann, J. K., & Chi, D. S. (2001). Physiological and psychological correlates of forgiveness. *Journal of Psychology and Christianity, 20,* 250–259.

Smith, T. W., Gallo, L. C., & Ruiz, J. M. (2003). Toward a social psychophysiology of cardiovascular reactivity: Interpersonal concepts and methods in the study of stress and coronary disease. In J. Suls & K. A. Wallston (Eds.), *Social psychological foundations of health and illness* (pp. 335–366). Malden, MA: Blackwell.

Thayer, M. F., & Lane, R. D. (2000). A model of neurovisceral integration in emotion regulation and dysregulation. *Journal of Affective Disorders, 61,* 201–216.

Thompson, L. Y., Snyder, C. R., Hoffman, L., Michael, S. R., Rasmussen, H. N. Billings, L. S., Heinze, L., Neufeld, J. E., Shorey, H. S., Roberts, J. C., & Roberts, D. E. (in press). Dispositional forgiveness of self, others, and situations. *Journal of Personality.*

Toussaint, L. L., & Williams, D. R. (2003, October). *Physiological correlates of forgiveness: Findings from a racially and socio-economically diverse sample of community residents.* Paper presented at Campaign for Forgiveness Research Conference, Atlanta, GA.

Wegner, D. M. (1997). Why the mind wanders. In J. D. Cohen and J. W. Schooler (Eds.), *Scientific approaches to consciousness* (pp. 295–315). England: Lawrence Erlbaum.

Witvliet, C. V. O., Ludwig, T. E., & Bauer, D. (2002). Please forgive me: Transgressors' emotions and physiology during imagery of seeking forgiveness and victim responses. *Journal of Psychology and Christianity, 21,* 219–233.

Witvliet, C. V. O., Ludwig, T., & Vander Laan, K. (2001). Granting forgiveness or harboring grudges: Implications for emotion, physiology, and health. *Psychological Science, 12,* 117–123.

Witvliet, C. V. O., Phipps, K. A., Feldman, M. E., & Beckham, J. C. (2004). Posttraumatic mental and physical health correlates of forgiveness and religious coping in military veterans. *Journal of Traumatic Stress, 17,* 269–273.

Witvliet, C. V. O., Root, L., Sato, A., & Ludwig, T. E. (2003). Justice and forgiveness: Psychophysiological effects for victims. *Psychophysiology, 40*(Suppl.), 87.

Witvliet, C. V. O., Worthington, E. L., & Wade, N. G. (2002). Victims' heart rate and facial EMG responses to receiving an apology and restitution. *Psychophysiology, 39*(Suppl.), S88.

Worthington, E. L., Jr. (2003). *Forgiving and reconciling: Bridges to wholeness and hope.* Downers Grove, IL: InterVarsity.

15 Befriending Man's Best Friends: Does Altruism Toward Animals Promote Psychological and Physical Health?

Marivic Dizon
Lisa D. Butler
Cheryl Koopman

Animals have contributed to human welfare since the beginning. In the wild, they provided food, clothing, and building materials, and many were revered as sacred symbols of our deepest spiritual and cultural values. Since their domestication, the contributions of animals to our well-being have continued to be invaluable and have become even more varied. We still use animals as primary food sources and materials for clothing and decoration, and their likenesses are employed as cultural emblems, but they have also become beasts of burden; working partners (e.g., for herding, search and rescue, and protection); sporting champions; sources of recreation; specialists in assisting the disabled (and recently in the detection of diseases); and biological surrogates in the development of drugs, medical procedures and devices, and cosmetic products; and, of course, for many humans, animals are integrated into our families and have become companions in our daily lives.

The fond term "man's best friend" has been applied to animals in reference to these valuable services, specifically in the case of domesticated dogs, yet it is an apt label for pets generally because for many individuals, a pet is a best friend, a caring companion, and a loyal partner. Although humans certainly gain such benefits from other humans, there is something distinctive about the love and companionship of a pet and the bond that can develop between the person and the animal. For one thing, many of the biases and value judgments that people learn as they navigate through life are not of concern to animals. Companion animals do not discriminate or judge based on race, class, gender, age, or disability, but instead appear to have unconditional and unwavering love for and devotion to their human partners.

In recent decades, researchers in the health and social science fields have begun investigating the psychological and physical health benefits of the human-animal bond, which can be described as a "dynamic relationship between people and animals in that each influences the psychological and physiological state of the other" (Center for the Human-Animal Bond, 2004, p. 1). As we discuss in the following, the strength of the human-animal bond and its positive effects on health and wellness have been demonstrated in a variety of populations, including children, adolescents, the elderly, and the physically and mentally ill (Hart, 2000; Melson, 2003). In this chapter, we discuss animal-directed altruism and the origins of the human-animal bond, and we provide a brief review of the literature on the effects of pet ownership and attachment and how befriending animals can promote health and wellness for individuals across the developmental lifespan.

ALTRUISM AND ANIMALS

Two considerable literatures exist documenting human altruism directed at other humans (reviewed in Batson, Ahmad, Lishner, & Tsang, 2002; Post, Underwood, Schloss, & Hurlbut, 2002) and apparently altruistic behaviors manifested by animals that either benefit their kin (Hamilton, 1964) or demonstrate compassion to unrelated others (e.g., Masson & McCarthy, 1995). In fact, Masson and McCarthy have gathered anecdotal accounts of apparent cross-species altruism among nonhuman animals. In one such case, an elephant, upon hearing the distress calls of a rhino calf trapped in deep viscous mud, left its group and approached the baby. After running its trunk over the juvenile, the elephant knelt, inserted its tusks under the calf, and started to lift. The mother rhino, who had been foraging in a forest nearby, charged the elephant, forcing it to retreat. The elephant's attempts to extricate the calf continued for several hours, each being rebuffed by the charging protective mother. Finally, the elephants moved on (and the calf pried itself free the next morning). Although unsuccessful, why did the elephant repeatedly risk injury to help an unrelated juvenile? As Masson and McCarthy put it, "Perhaps it recognized the youth of the rhino and its predicament and felt a generous impulse to help" (1995, p. 155). Reports of animal altruism toward humans have also been recorded (e.g., von Kreisler, 1997).

But what is it for a human to act altruistically toward an animal? Kagan (2002) has observed that human altruism involves actions intended to benefit another that flow from an awareness of need in the other. The requirements of intention and awareness distinguish such behaviors from others that may incidentally result in benefits and also from altruistic behaviors documented among

(nonhuman) animals that are defined by the benefit or survival advantage con-
ferred, rather than by inference of a particular cognitive or affective state.

Kagan (2002) notes that altruistic behaviors are motivated in two general
ways. In one case, the human agent acts in conformity with a personal moral
standard, either to experience the positive feelings that accompany virtue-
consistent behavior or to avoid the aversive feelings that accompany failures to
act under such circumstances. In the other case, love motivates altruism; altruistic actions are spurred by feelings of gratitude for past pleasures associated with
the target of the altruism or by the anticipated vicarious positive experience that
the altruistic actor will enjoy from the pleasure the target experiences from being
helped.

Given these definitions, it is not difficult to see animal-directed altruism in
many of the acts of humans. Throughout history, human beings have demonstrated their compassion for and devotion to animals in both impressive and
humble ways. When a human becomes a dedicated vegan, or fights for animal
rights in the political and social arena, or rescues abandoned or injured animals,
or volunteers for or financially supports animal welfare organizations and shel-
ters, his or her animal-benefiting conduct is being determined by a personal
ethical standard, the recognition of a need for such actions, and an intention to
meet that need.

However, even more common than activities that benefit animals who are
strangers to the actor are the acts of compassion and kindness seen when a human
befriends an animal that becomes a cherished companion and (is viewed as) a
member of the family. In 2003–2004, 40.6 million American households owned
dogs and 35.4 million households owned cats (American Pet Products Manufacturers Association, 2002), and an earlier survey found that almost three quar-
ters of U.S. households with children also have pets (American Veterinary
Medical Association, 1997, cited in Melson, 2003, p. 31). Interestingly, animal-
directed ethical precepts and affection may go together. Research suggests that
individuals who cared for pets during childhood report views that are more
humane toward animals and show more concern about animal welfare (Paul &
Serpell, 1993, cited in Melson, 2003).

In sum, acts of kindness and compassion directed at stranger animals in need
or at a beloved pet are properly classified as altruistic. Although there is a history
of debate in the literature on human-to-human altruism (Batson et al., 2002) with
regard to establishing whether actions meet the standard of altruism if the agent
ultimately benefits from them (even if the future benefit was not the motivation
for the action), in the case of kindnesses directed toward animals, the authentic-
ity of the altruism is perhaps more stark. There are few benefits to be derived
from such actions other than the satisfaction of acting in accord with one's values
or the animal's possible reciprocation of love. This unique relationship between
people and animals and the evidence of the apparent, yet only recently investigated benefits of that association for humans are the focus of this chapter.

POSSIBLE ORIGINS
OF THE HUMAN-ANIMAL BOND

> The wish to keep an animal usually arises from a general long-
> ing for a bond with nature. . . . This bond is analogous with
> those human functions that go hand in hand with the emo-
> tions of love and friendship in the purest and noblest forms.
> —Konrad Lorenz

Several theoretical models shed light on the possible sources or mechanisms of the human-animal bond (HAB). To account for the origins of a general and generally positive orientation to animals, it has been theorized (Wilson, 1984, cited in Beck & Katcher, 2003) that the tendency to pay attention to animals in the environ-ment developed because of the critical importance of animals as a source of food for humans and/or as guides to other nutrition sources. The *biophilia hypothesis*, as this view is termed, suggests that evolution selected for a human predisposition to orient to animals and the natural world. Although this model does not imply that humans have an innate predisposition to bond with or take care of animals (Beck & Katcher, 2003), it may account for some early human-animal contacts and the recognition of animals as a potential resource to enhance human welfare by pro-viding labor, domesticated food production, and perhaps companionship.

Although the salience and utility of animals to humans may be a necessary precondition to human-animal contact and interdependence, it is not sufficient to account for the development of the HAB. A key factor in the human–companion animal relationship that may contribute to its widespread prevalence and appeal is the unconditional, nonjudgmental love and acceptance that is offered by a companion animal or pet (Hart, 2000; Levinson, 1972). In a re-cent survey of more than a 1,000 pet owners (American Animal Hospital Asso-ciation, 1995), 80% of the sample indicated that companionship was the major reason for acquiring the pet, and 72% endorsed affection as the pet's most en-dearing quality. It seems reasonable to suggest, therefore, that human models of attachment and social support may be applied to understanding the HAB. As we review in the following, both psychosocial and physical health benefits accrue to humans who associate with animals, and many of these may flow, at least in part, from their recapitulation of the powerful and widely demonstrated benefits of social support for human psychological and physical health.

HUMAN–COMPANION ANIMAL ATTACHMENT

Researchers seeking to understand the human-animal bond have looked to the mother-child attachment model as a framework for understanding the attach-ment that occurs between people and pets (Melson, 2001; Triebenbacher, 1998).

The term *attachment*, as defined by scholars Ainsworth and Bowlby, describes a lasting emotional bond or tie between an individual and the object of attachment, which is founded upon an innate need for social interaction (Triebenbacher, 1998). Just as a child may seek out his or her mother for comfort and security, it appears that a child may seek out animals for a similar purpose, as research has found evidence of attachment behavior between people and pets from the first year of life (Kidd & Kidd, 1987, reviewed in Melson, 2003). In a study of young children and their interactions with live versus toy animals, children (aged 6 to 30 months) displayed more attachment behaviors (e.g., holding, following, vocalizing to, and/or smiling at the animal) with live pets than with toy animals (Kidd & Kidd, 1987, reviewed in Melson, 2003).

In another study of young children and pets, children were found to view their pets as a source of social interaction, affection, and emotional support (Triebenbacher, 1998). It was concluded that pets act as transitional objects (e.g., security blankets, toys) for children, promoting safety and comfort by providing a familiar connection between themselves and the outside world. By helping to establish a general sense of safety and security, pets may help to lessen anxiety for children and adolescents as they navigate through normal developmental tasks (Blue, 1986). It therefore appears that human-animal attachment may help to facilitate healthy social and emotional development and serve as a source of social support.

Psychosocial Health Benefits for Children and Adults

Social Support

Beck and Katcher (2003) have noted, "Animals are demonstrably a source of social support, as indicated by the number of Americans who say that the pet is 'a member of the family,' talk to their pet as they would a person, or consider their pet a confidant" (p. 80; see also Cain, 1983; Katcher, 1981). The literature on human social support addresses the centrality of relationships to humans and their effects on physical health and psychological stress (Hart, 2000). It is possible that positive relationships with animals have the same effects through the same means. In the previously mentioned study that explored the role of pets in the emotional development of young children, the children considered their pets as friends and family members, and 88% said that their pets knew when they were sick, sad, and/or upset (Triebenbacher, 1998). Children also typically rank pets among the most important individuals in their lives (Bryant, 1985, reviewed in Melson, 2003) and are as likely to share their sad, angry, happy, and secret experiences with their pets as with their siblings (Bryant, 1985).

Similar results have been found among adolescents. In interviews with Michigan adolescents aged 10–14, about 75% said that they turned to their pets when they were upset (Covert, Whiren, Keith, & Nelson, 1985, reviewed in Melson, 2003). In an exploratory study on self-esteem factors for early adolescents, aged 12 to 14, subjects ranked pets above the adults in their lives, with the exception of their parents, as something that made them feel satisfied and good about themselves (Juhasz, 1983, reviewed in Davis & Juhasz, 1985). It appears to be the unconditional love and acceptance of pets that may help to foster the emotional connection and bond between people and their pets (Hart, 2000).

Like close family members and friends, pets are a form of social support that might be used to help combat loneliness and depression (Hart, 2000). In a study of loneliness and pet ownership among single women, pet ownership appeared to decrease loneliness for women living alone (Zasloff & Kidd, 1994, reviewed in Hart, 2000). Among the bereaved elderly, depression levels were lower for those who owned pets compared to those who did not (Garrity, Stallones, Marx, & Johnson, 1989, reviewed in Baun & McCabe, 2000). Notably, it was the strength of the attachment, rather than simply pet ownership, that predicted lower depression.

Increasing Social Contact

Pets may also enhance social support for people by facilitating contact and communication with other human beings. This has particular significance for sometimes marginalized populations, including the elderly and the mentally or physically disabled. Mugford and M'Comisky (1975) demonstrated this effect in their study of elderly participants who were given either a parakeet or a begonia plant or received no intervention. Five months later, the group members who received the parakeets reported improved mental health and happiness, compared to the other groups in the study, with the birds becoming a central topic of conversation among friends, family, and neighbors who visited (reviewed in Messent, 1983). Messent (1983) observed this socializing effect in his study of dog owners in public parks. Owners who were accompanied by their pets engaged in more social interactions than when they walked alone. Social support appears, therefore, to underpin the HAB and may be one of the primary psychosocial benefits of animal companionship to humans.

Empathy

The human-animal bond may not just benefit the individual in the relationship; it may foster empathy and concern for other animals, nature, and human beings. Through caring for pets, it is possible that children begin to develop altruistic tendencies. By learning to nurture animals, children may develop a sense of social competence and empathetic understanding (Blue, 1986; Melson, 2003). More important, caring for pets also appears to have positive benefits for both male and female children, as it is perceived to be a gender-neutral activity, unlike child care, which is considered more female-oriented by young children (Melson & Fogel, 1989, reviewed in Melson, 2003). But is there a direct link between concern and care for the welfare of pets and other animals and concern for the welfare of human beings?

Among studies conducted with children, a positive association has been found between the strength of the child-pet bond and child-oriented empathy, and empathy with pets was associated with greater empathy with other children (Poresky & Hendrix, 1990; Poresky, 1990, reviewed in Paul, 2000). Similar results have been found among adults where pet ownership and attachment were positively associated with human-directed empathy (Hyde, Kurdek, & Larson, 1983, reviewed in Paul, 2000). Ascione and Weber (1996) sought to demonstrate the link between animal-directed and human-directed empathy through investigating whether a school-based intervention to enhance children's attitudes toward animals would generalize to greater empathy for human beings. The results showed that fourth- and fifth-grade children who underwent a 40-hour school-based humane education program had increased levels of empathy directed toward human beings, both at the end of the program and then 1 year later. Although the effect size was small, students who had more positive relationships with their pets had higher humane attitude scores, underscoring the importance of the relational element.

Evidence of this association between empathy for animals and empathy for humans has been inconsistent, however. In a study of university students, caring for pets during childhood was only associated with more humane attitudes toward animals and concern for animal welfare (Paul & Serpell, 1993, reviewed in Melson, 2003), not human welfare. Further research is clearly needed to elucidate the factors that determine concern for animals and concern for humans, and how these may develop together in the same individual.

Using Animals as Psychological Interventions

There are some interventions/programs that are demonstrating how altruism toward animals can be reciprocal and mutually beneficial. Animal-assisted activities (AAA) are goal-directed activities that can improve an individual's quality of life by utilizing the strength of the human-animal bond (Granger & Kogan, 2000).

AAA has been found to be effective with children and adults in a variety of settings, including hospitals, schools, counseling settings, nursing homes, geriatric wards, prisons, and residential treatment centers (Granger & Kogan, 2000). Prison inmate–animal interaction programs are one form of AAA that has demonstrated positive benefits for both the inmates and the animals involved (Strimple, 2003). One such program at a women's correctional facility in Washington involved a dog-training program where dogs were rescued from a local humane society and then were trained by female inmates to help people with special needs. The benefits to the women included increased self-esteem, gaining marketable skills, and earning college credit. The dogs benefited as well: They were rescued from potential death and subsequently trained and adopted.

Project Pooch was another program that worked with the prison population, and it was one of the first programs to connect incarcerated youth with dogs who were abused and abandoned (Strimple, 2003). In this program, the juveniles learned practical skills, including dog grooming and training, and they studied the health needs of the animals. An evaluation of the program found that the youth reported improvements in both behavior (e.g., respect for authority, social action, and leadership) and social competency (e.g., honesty, empathy, nurturing, social growth, etc.) (Merriam-Arduini, 2000, reviewed in Strimple, 2003). It is noteworthy that the employment of animals for their mental health–promoting effects has shown relatively consistent positive results with a variety of populations.

In summary, a growing body of research suggests that both children and adults can reap psychological benefits from having prosocial relationships with companion animals. In the following, we review evidence for the physical health benefits of caring for animals.

Physical Health Benefits for Children and Adults

Pet Presence and Attachment

Among both children and adults, researchers have found positive short-term physiological health effects of being in the presence of a familiar or unfamiliar pet (Friedmann, Thomas, & Eddy, 2000). Just as companion animals appear to reduce anxiety and stress by acting as a form of social support, there is also physiological evidence that pet presence and interaction can lower stress, induce relaxation, and create a calming effect by affecting blood pressure and heart rate.

The literature on the relationship between pets and physical health has centered on cardiovascular health. Heart disease was one of the first chronic diseases for which it was established that psychological and social factors played significant roles (Jenkins, 1976, cited in Friedmann et al., 2000). Being in the presence of and/or observing animals that appear to be nonthreatening seem to directly lower blood pressure and heart rate by drawing attention outward and interrupting any private internal dialogue or worries (Friedmann et al., 2000). The calming effect of animals has been demonstrated in one experiment with children, aged 9 to 15, in which children were asked to sit silently or read a story aloud, with a dog either present or absent in the room. The children's blood pressure was found to be significantly lower when the dog was present, and those children who saw the dog when they first entered the room had lower blood pressure than those who saw the dog enter later (Friedmann, Katcher, Thomas, Lynch, & Messent, 1983, reviewed in Friedmann et al., 2000). It is possible that the presence of the dog was viewed by children as a signal that they were in a safe situation, or it made them feel less alone.

The presence of a companion animal has also been found to moderate or buffer the effect of stress. In a study that examined the extent to which close friends and pets are perceived as evaluative during a stressful task performance, women who had their pet present displayed less physiological reactivity than women in the friend and control conditions (Allen, Blascovich, Tomaka, & Kelsey, 1991, reviewed in Friedmann et al., 2000). Similarly, in a study that involved an unfamiliar pet, dog owners and nonowners indicated lower state anxiety on a psychological checklist and behaved less anxiously in a high-stress environment when the experimenter was accompanied by her dog (Sebkova, 1977, reviewed in Friedmann et al., 2000). One factor of the human-animal bond which may help to explain the lower physiological response in human–companion animal interactions is that the animal is considered nonthreatening because of its nonjudgmental nature when compared with human-human interactions, which may be perceived as stressful or more threatening (Friedmann et al., 2000). Other factors that may also contribute to the moderating effect of animals on the stress response include the type of stressor, type and familiarity of setting, perception of the animal, and relationship with the animal (Friedmann et al., 2000). The topic merits further investigation, however, as some studies have failed to find these stress-buffering effects (Grossberg, Alf, & Vormbrock, 1988; Rajack, 1997, both cited in Friedmann et al., 2000).

Pet Interaction

Companion animals also appear to lower stress and create a sense of calm through "touch-talk dialogue," or touch combined with gentle talk that creates a feeling of intimacy and closeness (Beck & Katcher, 1996). Additionally, dialogue with pets helps to establish connection and create companionship, and it may be through this relationship that dialogue has an effect on health (Beck & Katcher, 1996). In a study of dog owners who were recruited from a veterinary clinic waiting room, results showed that their blood pressure did not increase when interacting with their pets, but increased significantly when reading aloud without their pets present in the room (Katcher, 1981, reviewed in Friedmann et al., 2000).

Pet Ownership and Companionship

Research has sought to establish the long-term effects of pet ownership on a person's physical health and well-being. The ground-breaking study by Friedmann, Katcher, Lynch, and Thomas (1980) was the first to establish the beneficial effect of pets on human health in their survey of 92 cardiac patients (reviewed in Friedmann, 2000). Their results showed that 1 year after being discharged from a coronary care unit, 28.2% of patients who did not own pets had died, compared to only 5.7% of patients with pets. Pet ownership was, therefore, found to be a significant factor in cardiac disease survival, and this relationship was independent of previous health status, the type of pet owned, access to social support, and severity of the disease. One possible competing explanation for the results, however, was the differences in personality that might distinguish pet owners from nonowners. Therefore, it is important that additional studies followed that also demonstrated health benefits from positive relationships with animals.

A longitudinal study that examined the impact of pet ownership on health found that adopting a pet was associated with almost immediately improved physical health and emotional well-being (Serpell, 1991, reviewed in Friedmann, 2000). A significant decrease in minor health problems was reported just 1 month after the adoption of a pet, and this health effect was maintained for dog owners, but not cat owners, during the 10–month period of the study. Dog owners who walked more at baseline reported a significant increase in physical exercise at 10 months in the number and duration of walks. Evidence was also present for improved psychological well-being during the first 6 months of the study and was maintained through all 10 months of the study (Serpell, 1991). Some studies, however, have not found an association between pet ownership and health status (e.g., Ory & Goldberg, 1983; Robb & Stegman, 1983, both cited in Siegel, 1990). Such mixed findings indicate the need for developing further theory and research to provide a greater base of understanding of the nature and consequences of the human-animal bond.

IMPLICATIONS, FUTURE RESEARCH, AND CONCLUDING COMMENTS

The research to date provides a good foundation for further inquiry. The totality of the evidence indicates that humans' altruistic behavior toward animals can yield psychological and physical health benefits. However, further empirical research is needed in this area to address unresolved questions and to build a more unified theory in this field.

One question concerns how we can integrate our microlevel understanding of the HAB benefits with analysis of this issue on the macrolevel. The HAB that has been documented on the individual level may have wider ramifications for how we treat and respect other animals, nature and the environment, and our fellow human beings. Rosak (1992), in *The Voice of the Earth: An Exploration of Ecopsychology*, argues that a lack of the experience of connection to nature results in an "epistemological loneliness," which characterizes much of modern urban life. He views compulsive, never-ending consumerism as a futile attempt to fill this void, which fails not only at the individual level but also contributes to the destruction of the natural world upon which humanity depends. Rosak's recommendation is that we revive both our awareness of and appreciation for nature in all of its manifestations and thereby increase our sense of responsibility for the natural world. Failure to do this, he argues, is likely to lead to cataclysmic environmental conditions that will pose grave threats to humanity.

Rosak's (1992) argument cannot be directly addressed by the kinds of studies reviewed here. Consideration of the consequences of humanity's treatment of nature for our ecology and cultural milieu are relevant to understanding the impact of human-animal relationships on our own psychological and physical well-being. Reflecting on the large-scale consequences for humanity of this lack of connection may tax our imaginations and challenge our tolerance for uncertainty and change—not to mention our research methods—but such deliberations clearly merit further discussion and study. At the same time, the burgeoning research on the health benefits to humans of relationships with animals is consistent on the microlevel with Rosak's notion of the essential interdependency between humanity and the natural world. Both levels of thinking recognize the benefits to humans of appreciating and nurturing animals. Therefore, these kinds of analyses and research endeavors may help to expand the paradigm in psychology and psychiatry that has underemphasized the importance of the psyche's connection to nature, in contrast to the emphasis placed upon the intrapsychic and interpersonal human realms.

To improve future research, the choice of research design should be carefully considered (Friedmann et al., 2000). A variety of research designs has been used, making it a challenge to compare and interpret findings across studies. Adding to this difficulty is the fact that the area of inquiry is complex due to the many possible pathways connecting differences in sociodemographic and cultural factors, conditions of pet ownership, kinds of social support, and aspects of physical and mental health. Consequently, Friedmann and colleagues recommend using a cross-over research design—one that evaluates the responses of each subject to the stressor with and without the animal present—because it takes into account within-subject variability. Such a design has the potential to strengthen the causal argument between the human-animal connection and health benefits beyond what can be deduced from correlational studies, which cannot specify causal relations.

Additionally, further research is needed to determine whether there are interspecies differences in the kinds and degree of social support and health benefits that can be derived. For example, Bonas, McNicholas, and Collis (2000) found that human-human relationships provide significantly more support than human-pet relationships overall, but that dogs, in particular, were a source of support comparable to human-human relationships. This suggests that there may be specific characteristics of dogs (compared to other animals) or of the quality of relationships that we develop with them that enhance their potential to provide significant emotional support. Future research could examine this by systematically examining the interactions of humans with dogs versus other types of companion animals to isolate the differences in the nature of these relationships.

Another gap in our knowledge concerns the impact of negative animal treatment on the human perpetrator, including the effects of pet neglect and cruelty, and this issue is of particular relevance to Rosak's concerns. Although we certainly do not advocate an experimental examination of this topic, a quasi-experimental research design (i.e., studying the predictors and consequences of naturally occurring instances) could expand the range of our understanding of the effects of human behavior toward animals on humans themselves.

In conclusion, an increasing body of research now documents a range of physical and mental health benefits associated with pet companionship and the human-animal bond. Although both the research and theoretical bases of this area of investigation are still evolving, and much more work is needed in both, it appears that significant benefits accrue to humans who form prosocial bonds with animals and that such benefits are experienced across the lifespan. In short, altruism toward animals appears to be good for all concerned.

We wish to acknowledge the Institute for Research on Unlimited Love and its director, Stephen G. Post, for the grant support and encouragement provided for our research on altruism. We also wish to thank Robert Garlan for his thoughtful improvements to this manuscript and John D. Krumboltz for his contributions to our thinking.

REFERENCES

Allen, K. M., Blascovich, J., Tomaka, J., & Kelsey, R. M. (1991). Presence of human friends and pet dogs as moderators of autonomic responses to stress in women. *Journal of Personality and Social Psychology, 61*(4), 582–589.

American Animal Hospital Association. (1995). *Pet Owner Survey.* Retrieved January 11, 2005, from http://www.cyberpet.com/cyberdog/articles/general/crawford.htm.

American Pet Products Manufacturers Association. (2002). *National Pet Owners Survey 2001–02.* Retrieved January 5, 2004, from http://www.chesterfieldhumane.org/page6.html.

American Veterinary Medical Association (AVMA) (1997). *Veterinary economic statistics.* Schaumburg, IL: Center for Information Management.

Ascione, F., & Weber, C. V. (1996). Children's attitudes about the humane treatment of animals and empathy: One-year follow up of a school-based intervention. *Anthrozoos, 9*(4), 188–195.

Batson, C. D., Ahmad, N., Lishner, D. A., & Tsang, J. A. (2002). Empathy and altruism. In C. R. Snyder & S. J. Lopez (Eds.), *Handbook of positive psychology* (pp. 485–498). Oxford: Oxford University Press.

Beck, A., & Katcher, A. (1996). *Between pets and people: The importance of animal companionship.* West Lafayette, IN: Purdue University Press.

Beck, A. M., & Katcher, A. H. (2003). Future directions in human-animal bond research. *American Behavioral Scientist, 47*(1), 79–93.

Baun, M. M., & McCabe, B. W. (2000). The role animals play in enhancing quality of life for the elderly. In A. Fine (Ed.), *Handbook on animal-assisted therapy: Theoretical foundations and guidelines for practice* (pp. 237–251). San Diego, CA: Academic.

Blue, G. F. (1986). The value of pets in children's lives. *Childhood Education, 63,* 85–90.

Bonas, S., McNicholas, J., & Collis, G. M. (2000). Pets in the network of family relationships: an empirical study. In A. L. Podberscek, E. S. Paul, & J. A. Serpell (Eds.), *Companion animals and us: Exploring the relationships between people and pets* (pp. 209–236). Cambridge: Cambridge University Press.

Bryant, B. (1985). The neighborhood walk: Sources of support in middle childhood. *Monographs of the Society for Research in Child Development, 50*(3), 34–44. Chicago, IL: University of Chicago Press.

Cain, A. (1983). A study of pets in the family system. In A. Katcher & A. Beck (Eds.), *New perspectives on our lives with companion animals* (pp. 72–81). Philadelphia, PA: University of Pennsylvania Press.

Center for the Human-Animal Bond. Purdue University School of Veterinary Medicine. (2004). Retrieved January 5, 2004, from http://www.vet.purdue.edu/chap/history.htm.

Covert, A. M., Whiren, A. P., Keith, J., & Nelson, C. (1985). Pets, early adolescents, and families. *Marriage and Family Review, 8,* 95–108.

Davis, J. H., & Juhasz, A. M. (1985). The preadolescent pet bond and psychological development. *Marriage and Family Review, 8,* 79–94.

Friedmann, E. (2000). The animal-human bond: Health and wellness. In A. Fine (Ed.), *Handbook on animal-assisted therapy: Theoretical foundations and guidelines for practice* (pp. 41–58). San Diego, CA: Academic.

Friedmann, E., Katcher, A. H., Lynch, J. J., and Thomas, S. A. (1980). Animal companions and one-year survival of patients after discharge from a coronary unit. *Public Health Reports, 95,* 307–312.

Friedmann, E., Katcher, A. H., Thomas, S. A., Lynch, J. J. & Messent, P. R. (1983). Social interaction and blood pressure: Influence of animal companions. *Journal of Nervous and Mental Disease, 171*(8), 461–465.

Friedmann, E., Thomas, S. A., & Eddy, T. J. (2000). Companion animals and human health: physical and cardiovascular influences. In A. L. Podberscek, E. S. Paul, & J. A. Serpell (Eds.), *Companion animals & us: Exploring the relationships between people & pets* (pp. 125–142). Cambridge: Cambridge University Press.

Garrity, T. F., Stallones, L., Marx, M. B., & Johnson, T. P. (1989). Pet ownership and attachment as supportive factors in the health of the elderly. *Anthrozoos, 3*(1), 35–44.

Granger, B. P., & Kogan, L. (2000). Animal-assisted therapy in specialized settings. In A. Fine (Ed.), *Handbook on animal-assisted therapy: Theoretical foundations and guidelines for practice* (pp. 213–236). San Diego, CA: Academic.

Grossberg, J. M., Alf, Jr., E. F., & Vormbrock, J. K. (1988). Does pet dog presence reduce human cardiovascular responses to stress? *Anthrozoos, 2*, 38–44.

Hamilton, W. D. (1964). The genetical evolution of social behaviour II. *Journal of Theoretical Biology, 7*(1), 17–52.

Hart, L. A. (2000). Psychosocial benefits of animal companionship. In A. H. Fine (Ed.), *Handbook on animal-assisted therapy: Theoretical foundations and guidelines for practice* (pp. 59–78). San Diego, CA: Academic.

Hines, L. M. (2003). Historical perspectives on the human-animal bond. *American Behavioral Scientist, 47*(1), 7–15.

Hyde, K. R., Kurdek, L., & Larson, P. C. (1983). Relationships between pet ownership and self-esteem, social sensitivity, and interpersonal trust. *Psychological Reports, 52*(1), 110.

Jenkins, C. D. (1976). Recent evidence supporting psychological and social risk factors for coronary disease. *New England Journal of Medicine, 294*(19), 1033–1038.

Juhasz, A. M. (1983). *Problems in measuring self-esteem in early adolescents.* Unpublished manuscript, Loyola University of Chicago.

Kagan, J. (2002). Morality, altruism, and love. In S. G. Post, L. G. Underwood, J. P. Schloss, & W. B. Hurlbut (Eds.), *Altruism and altruistic love: Science, philosophy, and religion in dialogue* (pp. 40–50). New York: Oxford University Press.

Katcher, A. H. (1981). Interactions between people and their pets: Form and function. In B. Fogle (Ed.), *Interrelations between people and pets* (pp. 41–67). Springfield, IL: Thomas.

Kidd, A. H., & Kidd, R. M. (1987). Reactions of infants and toddlers to live and toy animals. *Psychological Reports, 61*, 455–464.

Levinson, B. M. (1972). *Pets and human development.* Springfield, IL: Thomas.

Masson, J. M., & McCarthy, S. (1995). *When elephants weep: The emotional lives of animals.* New York: Delacorte.

Merriam-Arduini, S. (2000). *Evaluation of an experimental program designed to have a positive effect on adjudicated violent, incarcerated male juveniles age 12–25 in the state of Oregon.* Unpublished doctoral dissertation, Pepperdine University.

Melson, G. F. (2000). Companion animals and the development of children: Implications of the biophilia hypothesis. In A. Fine (Ed.), *Handbook on animal-assisted therapy: Theoretical foundations and guidelines for practice* (pp. 375–383). San Diego, CA: Academic.

Melson, G. F. (2001). *Why the wild things are: Animals in the lives of children.* Cambridge, MA: Harvard University Press.

Melson, G. F. (2003). Child development and the human-companion animal bond. *American Behavioral Scientist, 47*(1), 31–39.

Melson, G. F. & Fogel, A. (1989). Children's ideas about animal young and their care: A reassessment of gender differences in the development of nurturance. *Anthrozoos, 2,* 265–273.

Messent, P. R. (1983). Social facilitation of contact with other people by pet dogs. In A. H. Katcher & A. M. Beck (Eds.), *New perspectives on our lives with companion animals* (pp. 37–46). Philadelphia, PA: University of Pennsylvania Press.

Mugford, R. A., & M'Comisky, J. G. (1975). Some recent work on the psychotherapeutic value of caged birds with old people. In R. S. Anderson (Ed.), *Pet animals and society* (pp. 54–65). London: Balliere-Tindall.

Ory, M. G., & Goldberg, E. L. (1983). Pet possession and life satisfaction in elderly women. In A. H. Katcher & A. M. Beck (Eds.), *New perspectives on our lives with companion animals* (pp. 303–317). Philadelphia: University of Pennsylvania Press.

Paul, E. S. (2000). Love of pets and love of people. In A. L. Podberscek, E. S. Paul, & J. A. Serpell (Eds.), *Companion animals & us: Exploring the relationships between people & pets* (pp. 168–86). Cambridge: Cambridge University Press.

Paul, E. S., & Serpell, J. A. (1993). Childhood pet keeping and humane attitudes in young adulthood. *Animal Welfare, 2,* 321–337.

Poresky, R. H. (1990). The young children's empathy measure: reliability, validity and effects of companion animal bonding. *Psychological Reports, 66,* 931–936.

Poresky, R. H., & Hendrix, C. (1990). Differential effects of pet presence and pet-bonding on young children. *Psychological Reports, 67,* 51–54.

Post, S. G., Underwood, L. G., Schloss, J. P., & Hurlbut, W. B. (2002). *Altruism and altruistic love: Science, philosophy, and religion in dialogue.* Oxford: Oxford University Press.

Rajack, L. S. (1997). Pets and human health: The influence of pets on cardiovascular and other aspects of owners' health. Doctoral dissertation, University of Cambridge, UK.

Robb, S. S., & Stegman, C. E. (1983). Companion animals and elderly people: A challenge for evaluators of social support. *Gerontologist, 23*(3), 277–282.

Rosak, T. (1992). *The voice of the earth: An exploration of ecopsychology.* New York: Touchstone.

Sebkova, J. (1977). *Anxiety levels as affected by the presence of a dog.* Unpublished thesis, Department of Psychology, University of Lancaster, UK.

Serpell, J. A. (1991). Children's ideas about animal young and their care on some aspects of human health and behaviour. *Journal of the Royal Society of Medicine, 84,* 717–720.

Siegel, J. M. (1990). Stressful life events and use of physician services among the elderly: The moderating role of pet ownership. *Journal of Personality and Social Psychology, 58*(6), 1081–1086.

Strimple, E. O. (2003). A history of prison inmate-animal interaction programs. *American Behavioral Scientist, 47*(1), 70–78.

Triebenbacher, S. L. (1998). Pets as transitional objects: Their role in children's emotional development. *Psychological Reports, 82,* 191–200.

von Kreisler, K. (1997). *The compassion of animals.* New York: Three Rivers.

Wilson, E. O. (1984). *Biophilia.* Cambridge, MA: Harvard University Press.

Zasloff, R. L., & Kidd, A. H. (1994). Loneliness and pet ownership among single women. *Psychological Reports, 75,* 747–752.

PART III

*Evolutionary Models
of Altruism and Health*

Introduction

Stephen G. Post
Brie Zeltner

Let us assume that altruistic actions and emotions have some association with health. If so, how did this association emerge evolutionarily? What models of evolution can help us to make sense of this?

Stephanie L. Brown, R. Michael Brown, Ashley Schiavone, and Dylan M. Smith, in "Close Relationships and Health Through the Lens of Selective Investment Theory," bring an evolutionary perspective to bear. We know that social contact is beneficial to human health, longevity, and happiness, but there is little evidence to explain how this relationship works, and why. Traditional studies of close relationships have focused on the importance of support received from a friend, child, or spouse to explain the mental and physical health benefits, but results in this area are mixed. The authors believe that giving support may account for the health benefits of social contact, and they explore this possibility with several studies using a new evolutionary theory called selective investment theory (SIT). SIT explains the existence of costly long-term investment by suggesting that this investment evolved between individuals whose fitness was intertwined, encouraging selfless behavior by dampening egoistic tendencies and allocating resources to the relationship partner. Viewed through the lens of SIT, sacrifice is no longer pathological (as has been suggested by most of evolutionary theory); it becomes a key characteristic of healthy close relationships. The authors cite several current studies that provide results consistent with SIT, including the important Changing Lives of Older Couples Study, which provides evidence that giving, not receiving, support reduces mortality risk, and giving may increase resiliency in the face of spousal loss. The authors also formulated their own study to examine the effects of caregiver burnout and showed that when the act of caregiving to a severely ill loved one is disentangled from the detrimental effects of witnessing that person's decline and suffering, there are actually benefits to giving this kind of care when compared to those who were simply married to an ill partner. In conclusion, the authors offer several questions for future research that will further examine the relationship between giving and health. Because SIT recasts the nature of social relationships, the authors believe it has significant potential to solve anomalies in the relationship literature, generate interesting new testable predictions, and enhance our understanding of the relationship between social contact and health.

David Sloan Wilson and Mihaly Csikszentmihalyi, in "Health and the Ecology of Altruism," test an ecological and evolutionary hypothesis of the fitness of altruists, using the Sloan Study of Youth and Social Development, which includes information on a large sample of American adolescents gathered through questionnaires and the experience sampling method. Wilson and Csikszentmihalyi's hypothesis places altruism in its ecological context as a human behavioral strategy that will be advantageous in some environments (stable ones where altruism thrives) and that may cause stress in others (where altruism is unreciprocated or unappreciated). In order to test this hypothesis, Wilson used a 17-item questionnaire measuring prosocial behavior within the Sloan Study, and found that the highly prosocial teens tended to inhabit positive, stable, and encouraging environments while low-prosocial teens experienced more events typical of harsh social environments (i.e., fighting and teen pregnancy). Wilson and Csikszentmihalyi believe that transplanting these altruistic and selfish teens would cause stress to both groups, and this is supported by the fact that the highly prosocial teens are less able to cope with the stresses typical of the low-prosocial environment. Wilson and Csikszentmihalyi gain further support for their hypothesis from the predominantly male sample of narcissists (low-prosocial teens with high self-esteem and plans for the future) within the study who had extremely good mental health, much like the highly prosocial individuals within supportive environments. Wilson also found that religiousness is highly correlated to prosocial behavior, and religions appear to be very effective at creating social environments or niches where altruism flourishes. In conclusion, the Sloan Study offers evidence that highly prosocial individuals do tend to thrive as individuals, but not in all environments. Last, Wilson and Csikszentmihalyi stress the importance of avoiding normative bias in studies of altruism, pointing out that selfish behavior, while frowned upon, is just as often the more successful and "healthy" strategy. If we, as a society, wish to increase the prevalence of altruism, we need to create niches in which it can safely thrive.

Christopher Boehm, in "A Short Natural History of Altruism and Healing," explores the deep evolutionary roots of altruism and healing. Boehm discusses medical practices among the apes, as well as their medical helping behaviors. He then moves to a focus on the role of the shaman as an altruistic healer and the salutary aspects of reduced stress in the agent of altruism. Boehm finds that the roots of genetic altruism that affect health are ancient and heavily involved with our evolved human nature. He understands humans to have evolved to be altruistic in various ways and concludes that "our altruism impinges significantly on our own health and that of others."

Gregory Fricchione, in "Altruistic Love, Resiliency, Health, and the Role of Medicine," reflects on the relationships among attachment, resiliency, altruism, and health within the background of brain evolution and allostasis. Fricchione begins by speaking of the disconnected relationship between doctor and patient that has arisen in our culture due to our preoccupation with evidence-based medicine and the doctor's disregard of the important psychological and social concerns that accompany human disease. He uses the separation-attachment dialectic to advocate an attachment solution to this separation challenge in which the doctor and patient are reconnected through the healing power of compassionate love. To explain why love is healing, the author takes us through the evolution of the brain as it finds attachment solutions to separation challenges (the most basic of these being separation from food or energy sources) and becomes the higher mammalian brain capable of planning and executing attachment solutions. This evolution also leads to the psychological development of secure base attachment, in which offspring are effectively and responsively nurtured by caregivers who provide a secure base from which to explore the world. Individuals with a secure base attachment are more resilient and have lower stress levels. Stress occurs when an external separation challenge is presented which necessitates an internal homeostatic alteration, i.e., the fight-or-flight response. Although stress is designed to be helpful, prolonged exposure to stress or an overwhelming stressor can be health eroding, as is the case in depressive and anxiety disorders. There are several ways to reduce allostatic loading and the negative effects of the stress response, including the relaxation response, cognitive-behavioral therapy, effective social support, and belief and conscious expectation. All of these increase resiliency and reduce stress reactivity, as do maternal nurturance and, potentially, altruistic prosocial behavior. Further, those with a secure base attachment have more resources available to devote to other-regarding behavior, which may further improve their health. The author concludes by advocating resiliency-building techniques to prevent disease and to encourage altruistic behavior in the human population and the importance of compassionate love to the healing of the doctor-patient relationship.

C. Sue Carter, in "Monogamy, Motherhood, and Health," discusses her recent research with prairie voles, rodents that live in a state of social monogamy similar to that of human beings. Knowledge of the relatively simple brains and neurohormonal processes of these animals is helping to explain the origins of the human tendency to form strong, long-lasting social bonds and the emotions that accompany them. The author uses the term "social monogamy" to distinguish the concept from that of sexual fidelity, which genetic testing has revealed to be exceedingly rare even in the apparently devoted prairie vole. Carter argues that while lifelong sexual fidelity is extremely rare in humans and rodents alike, monogamy is a social system based on more than just sex. Social monogamy refers to a way of living that promotes (but does not guarantee) sexual fidelity, shared parental care, and the reinforcement of social and emotional bonds. Despite its frequent failure, monogamy is the most accepted marriage pattern for human beings around the world and most likely evolved as a way for fathers to ensure the paternity of their offspring and to increase the number of individuals available to care for them. Monogamy also promotes paternal care and defense of the mate and offspring and, as recent studies show, is not simply a cultural construct. Carter's research with prairie voles has identified two hormones, oxytocin and vasopressin, that appear to form the neural underpinnings of the social monogamy system. Interestingly, the physiological and emotional processes involved in social bonding and parental care are very similar to those that ensure wellness and survival (both hormones are important to healthy responses to stress and general coping). Carter believes that increased knowledge of the "social nervous system" of prairie voles will help us to understand why social support is so critical to human health and longevity. It may also explain why love and benevolence, which she sees as emotional reinforcements of social bonding, have healing powers.

16 Close Relationships and Health Through the Lens of Selective Investment Theory

Stephanie L. Brown
R. Michael Brown
Ashley Schiavone
Dylan M. Smith

In this chapter, we review a program of research that was designed to explore the health benefits of helping or giving support to others. This work was inspired by a new evolutionary theory of altruism, selective investment theory (SIT), which recasts the functional significance of social bonds as designed by natural selection to promote adaptive instances of giving (S. L. Brown, 1999; S. L. Brown & Brown, 2006). SIT assumes that social bonds enable individuals to suppress self-interest so that they can reliably prioritize and promote the well-being of an other, even at a cost to the self. In this way, the social bond resolves the motivational conflict inherent in deciding whether to promote self versus other interests.

SIT represents a departure from prevailing social psychological theories, which assume that individuals maintain their close relationships in order to get more rewards and benefits than they could get by going it alone. As applied to mental and physical health, the view of close relationships generated by SIT raises the possibility that the health benefits of social contact reside in the contribution made to relationship partners. We will describe the results of four studies that demonstrate the health benefits of helping others, including (a) decreased mortality risk, (b) recovery from depressive symptoms following spousal loss, and (c) relief from cardiovascular stress. We will conclude with a discussion of promising new directions for future research in this area.

CLOSE RELATIONSHIPS AND HEALTH

People in close relationships are happier and healthier and live longer than individuals who are socially isolated (House, Landis, & Umberson, 1988). Despite the robust effect of social contact on health and well-being, we know very little about *how* close relationships influence our health. That is, researchers have assumed that the benefits of social contact are due to support that is received from others (House et al., 1988), yet tests of this assumption have produced contradictory findings. A meta-analysis of the link between receiving support and health outcomes, for example, demonstrated that the health benefit of receiving support was surprisingly small (Smith, Fernengel, Holcroft, Gerald, & Marien, 1994). Based on their work, Smith and his colleagues concluded that the "amounts of shared variance [between social support and health] may not be considered significant nor generalizable" (p. 352).

So, why have researchers failed to confirm the receiving-support hypothesis? One possibility is that support received is confounded with a variety of undesired consequences that are harmful to health, such as dependence or feeling like a burden to others. Dependence has been associated with increased anxiety (Lu & Argyle, 1992), and burdensome feelings have been linked to increased depression and suicidal thinking (R. M. Brown, Dahlen, Mills, Rick, & Biblarz, 1999; de Catanzaro, 1986). Another possibility is that there are additional aspects of close relationships that are beneficial for health, beyond what individuals receive from their partners. Recently, Brown and her colleagues (2003) suggested that *providing support to others*—as opposed to receiving support—would be beneficial for health. This hypothesis was inspired by evolutionary theories of altruism that note the considerable importance of making a contribution to others. Before describing evidence in favor of a link between altruism and health, we first review evolutionary theories of altruism, including selective investment theory, that highlight the adaptive significance of helping others.

EVOLUTIONARY THEORIES OF ALTRUISM

Evolutionary biologists have characterized altruism as any act that benefits other individuals at a cost to the altruist. Altruism is seen as a central problem for evolution theory, recognized as such by Darwin (1859). How can a behavior that advances the survival and reproduction of other individuals (personal or classical fitness) at the expense of one's own survival and reproduction be selected for? If a "selfish" (uncooperative, exploitative) mutant suddenly appeared in a population of altruists, with successive generations altruism would disappear. But clearly, altruism is evident in many animal groups and appears to have the design features that would qualify it as an evolved characteristic. The by now familiar resolution of the paradox is that the costs entailed in being altruistic can be offset by helping genetic relatives to reproduce (they carry copies of the altruist's genes)—the theory of *kin selection* (Hamilton, 1964); or by helping genetically unrelated individuals, who then reciprocate the help at some future time—the theory of *reciprocal altruism* (Trivers, 1971).

Because reciprocation from genetically unrelated altruistic recipients is not always reasonable to assume, alternatives to reciprocal altruism theory have been offered, specifically, the theories of indirect reciprocity (Alexander, 1987; Nowak & Sigmund, 1998), strong reciprocity (Fehr & Fischbacher, 2003; Fehr & Gächter, 2002; Gintis, 2000; Gintis, Bowles, Boyd, & Fehr, 2003), and costly signaling (Dessalles, 1999; Gintis, Smith, & Bowles, 2001; Zahavi, 1995, 1997). According to these theories, for altruism among unrelated individuals to evolve, individuals in a population must be able to (a) identify altruists (directly or through reputation) and cooperate selectively with them (indirect reciprocity), (b) punish those who do not cooperate with altruists (strong reciprocity), or (c) be attracted to and mate selectively with individuals who can afford to advertise costly traits such as altruism (costly signaling).

Although each of these theories, beginning with kin selection, specifies conditions under which altruism *could* have evolved, none of them details proximate cognitive and motivational mechanisms that would have made this possible in humans and other social mammals (Brosnan & de Waal, 2002; Korchmaros & Kenny, 2001). Evolutionary psychologists have attempted to remedy this situation by invoking perceptual kin recognition devices (Porter, 1987), social exchange reasoning mechanisms that function to identify cheaters (Cosmides, 1989; Cosmides & Tooby, 1992), fitness-enhancing friends (Cosmides & Tooby, 1992; Tooby & Cosmides, 1996), and altruists (W. M. Brown & Moore, 2000).

The clear emphasis in these and other evolutionary accounts of kin recognition and social exchange mechanisms has been on identifying and reducing the *costs* of altruism. There has been considerably less emphasis on identifying the benefits of giving (but see Tooby & Cosmides, 1996) and, until recently, almost no interest in addressing a pivotal question related to giving, the question of *motivation*. What drives an individual to set short-term selfish (survival) interests aside and allocate valuable resources to others, on a sustained basis and in ways that do not compromise the altruist's inclusive fitness?[1] Recently, we formulated an evolutionary theory that addresses this question and that provides the foundation for our investigations of the health consequences of giving, described later in this chapter. We call our formulation *selective investment theory* (Brown & Brown, 2006).

SELECTIVE INVESTMENT THEORY

We formulated selective investment theory to help explain, from an evolutionary perspective, the motivational basis for a particular form of altruism that we call *costly long-term investment* (CLI). Examples of CLI include expending considerable time and energy to raise children, forgoing favorite activities and/ or social opportunities to spend months by the bedside of a terminally ill mate, compromising one's own health and well-being to provide continuous care to an elderly or sick relative or friend, risking injury and death on a daily basis to protect comrades in times of war. Considering its ubiquity, its centrality in close relationships, and its significant benefits to others (in some cases, the preservation of life) and costs to self (in some cases, death), it is surprising that CLI has received little theoretical or empirical attention from psychologists, who have preferred instead to focus their attention on low-cost giving in the context of short-term (or nonexistent) relationships. From an evolutionary perspective, CLI is a most intriguing phenomenon because of the adaptive problem it posed for our ancestors: how to inhibit self-centered impulses and give to others in ways that do not compromise reproductive success.

Selective investment theory presents arguments that address the problem of CLI, arguments that we think have important implications for the study of close relationships. In particular, we suggest that *social bonds*—the glue of close relationships—evolved primarily to motivate allocating valuable resources to relationship partners. A key component of our argument is that (a) if social bonds evolved to motivate CLI, then (b) the formation of social bonds must have occurred only between individuals who were dependent upon one another for reproductive success, a condition we call *fitness interdependence*.

Selective investment theory tethers CLI to close relationships. We think that a critical foundation piece for CLI is an evolved motivational circuitry that functions to (a) effect a neurohormonal affinity between individuals whose reproductive needs are intertwined, (b) reliably suppress egoistic impulses that interfere with giving to such individuals, and (c) direct the allocation of resources to such individuals. The interpersonal affinity, and its cognitive and emotional correlates, are commonly referred to as a "social bond."

Evidence for Selective Investment Theory

There are considerable data, from both nonhuman and human species, that are consistent with the central tenets of selective investment theory.

Neuroendocrine studies show that oxytocin (and other hormones, especially vasopressin and endogenous opioids) may help to structure social bonds in socially monogamous species under conditions of fitness interdependence (Carter, 1998). Neuroendocrine data and at least one model of the neurophysiology of stress are also consistent with selective investment theory's claim that the social bond may function to override self-preservation motivation (Carter, 1998; Henry & Wang, 1998).

Data from ethology and animal behavioral ecology reveal correlations among indicators of fitness interdependence, social bonds, and CLI in a variety of social species, especially socially monogamous birds, social carnivores, and non-human primates (e.g., Black, 2001; Mitani, Watts, & Muller, 2002).

Findings from human relationship studies show links between indicators of fitness interdependence and social bonds (Korchmaros & Kenny, 2001; Neyer & Lang, 2003), fitness interdependence and helping (e.g., Korchmaros & Kenny, 2001; Rossi & Rossi, 1990), and social bonds and helping (e.g., Feeney & Collins, 2003; Korchmaros & Kenny, 2001). There is also evidence to suggest that bonds *mediate* between fitness interdependence and the willingness to render costly help to family members (Korchmaros & Kenny, 2001), consistent with a central prediction of selective investment theory. A similar mediational relationship is suggested by anecdotal reports of soldiers' willingness to help buddies in wartime conditions (e.g., Wong, Kolditz, Millen, & Potter, 2003).

Finally, direct tests of selective investment theory have shown that the constructs of interdependence, bond, and investment are psychometrically distinct and that bonds mediate between various measures of interdependence and willingness to provide costly help across different types of relationships—biological relatives, friends, romantic partners—as predicted (S. L. Brown, 1999).

Selective Investment Theory and Traditional Relationship Theories

Selective investment theory contrasts markedly with traditional self-interest theories of close relationships. While SIT emphasizes the importance of relationships for *giving*, self-interest relationship theories emphasize the importance of *receiving*. For example, social psychological accounts of romantic relationships (e.g., social exchange theories, attachment theory) emphasize the reward value of being in close relationships (e.g., Hazan & Shaver, 1994; Rusbult, 1980; Sprecher & Schwartz, 1994) and tend to highlight the costs of behaving altruistically toward relationship partners (e.g., Thompson, Medvene, & Freedman, 1995). Even evolution-based models of social bonds between infants and caregivers (e.g., Bowlby, 1958, 1969) and between romantic partners (e.g., Hazan & Shaver, 1994) suggest that the adaptive value (evolutionary significance) of such bonds is to promote the *receipt* of resources and protection from others.

These reward-based models of social bonds channel relationship science, both basic and applied, along predictable paths. For example, when social psychologists assess the quality of adult interpersonal relationships, they often ask whether individuals experience relationship satisfaction, receive adequate social support or security, or experience stress and burnout as a consequence of providing care to a relationship partner. They tend not to ask whether people feel able or willing to meet a partner's needs, able or willing to make contributions that satisfy a partner, or experience stress when selfish needs compromise the well-being of a partner. But if viewed from the perspective of selective investment theory, the fabric of close relationships appears different. Sacrifice becomes a characteristic feature of healthy, enduring relationships rather than aberrant, inexplicable, or diagnostic of pathology.

IMPLICATIONS OF SIT: THE HEALTH BENEFITS OF GIVING

We think SIT's central propositions have broad and important implications for existing psychological approaches to understanding the link between close relationships and health. Because SIT shifts the emphasis to the giving side of the social support equation, it raises the possibility that there are fitness-related benefits (e.g., improved health and well-being) associated with helping a relationship partner. As described above, individuals incur fitness benefits when they help relatives or others with whom they are interdependent for fitness. Those who could act to promote their own health and fight to stay alive would have been able to prolong the amount of time that contributions could be made to relationship partners. In this way, knowledge that one is effectively contributing may have led to a stronger will to live, increased positive health behaviors, and at a neurophysiological level may have been associated with a more restorative stress response (e.g., increased restorative hormones such as oxytocin that contribute to cell growth and repair and that down-regulate cortisol).

As described earlier, the possibility that there are health benefits of giving has been overlooked due to a preoccupation with the presumed benefits of *receiving* support from a relationship partner. Below, we describe empirical research that has confirmed an association between giving and health and well-being.

Giving and Mortality Risk

Data from the Changing Lives of Older Couples (CLOC) Study was used to (a) test the hypothesis that reports of giving support would be associated with a reduced risk of mortality and (b) clarify the unique influence of support received on mortality risk (Brown, Nesse, Vinokur, & Smith, 2003). The CLOC Study included reports of giving and receiving support from 423 older married couples, followed over 5 years, and was designed to investigate psychological issues surrounding bereavement. Several factors made the CLOC Study an ideal choice for assessing the health benefits of giving. For example, it contained identically worded measures of giving and receiving support, enabling direct comparisons of the health benefits of each. The CLOC Study also contained multiple measures of physical health, health behaviors, mental health, and personality. These measures enabled us to evaluate the alternative possibility that any beneficial effect of giving on mortality risk is due instead to enhanced mental or physical robustness on the part of the giver. Finally, the CLOC data contained responses from married couples, so we were able to evaluate alternative relationship dynamics that might account for a benefit of giving, such as perceived equity (the perception that one receives the same amount as one provides to the relationship partner).

Results of this study demonstrated that individuals who reported providing tangible forms of help to friends, relatives, and neighbors reduced their risk of dying by about one half, compared to individuals who reported providing no help to others (Brown et al., 2003). In addition, people who reported giving high amounts of emotional support to their spouses (e.g., being willing to listen when a spouse needs to talk) also had a reduced risk of mortality by about one third, compared to people who reported providing lower amounts of emotional support. Measures of receiving support either had no association with mortality or were associated with an increased risk of mortality.

These beneficial effects of giving remained after controlling for a variety of other factors that are typically associated with mortality risk: age, gender, socioeconomic status, race, self-rated health, functional health, smoking, drinking, exercise, depression, anxiety, subjective well-being, social contact, dependence on one's partner, and individual differences such as extroversion, agreeableness, openness, locus of control, self-esteem, and emotional stability. This pattern of findings increases our confidence that our results are not due to an enhanced physical or mental robustness on the part of the giver. Moreover, our findings are not attributable to perceived equity—the equal give and take of support. Nevertheless, it is premature to conclude from this study alone that receiving support will not be beneficial and that giving support accounts for the benefits of social contact. As far as we know, this was the first study to advance the hypothesis that giving support would account for the traditional effects of receiving support found in the literature. Thus, future studies are needed to replicate and extend these findings. We need answers to questions such as: Do the benefits of giving extend to other outcomes, beyond mortality risk? Are the benefits of giving restricted to certain populations or certain individuals? What is the mechanism by which giving exerts a health benefit? Are there circumstances in which giving becomes too costly to yield a health benefit—as in the case of caregiver burnout? Below, we briefly summarize the results from subsequent work that has begun to address these and other questions.

Giving and Depression

The CLOC data were also used to determine whether the benefits of giving social support to others extend to coping with spousal loss, as indicated by faster recovery from depressive symptoms following bereavement (Brown, House,

Brown, & Smith, 2004). To test this hypothesis, we assessed the extent to which widowed respondents' reports of giving tangible support to others 6 months after spousal loss (Wave 1) predicted changes in depressive symptoms from Wave 1 to Wave 2 (18 months after spousal loss). Results showed an interaction between giving and grief. For respondents experiencing high grief, reports of giving were significantly associated with faster recovery from depressive symptoms. The benefit of giving was not found for individuals experiencing low levels of grief after spousal loss. Importantly, measures of *receiving* support did not account for this pattern of results and did not predict recovery from depressive symptoms. Furthermore, the main and interactive effects of health, demographics, relationship, and personality variables could not account for the interaction between giving and grief, raising the possibility that giving buffers the effect of bereavement on depressive symptoms.

Giving and Stress

If giving buffers against stress, as our study of bereavement seems to suggest, then the next question is: how? One possibility is that giving activates neurohormonal processes that regulate harmful aspects of the human stress response. Neurophysiologists have proposed that the physiological system underlying social bonds and giving behavior—"species preservation"—is distinct from (and can suppress) potentially harmful neuroendocrine responses associated with the fight-or-flight self-preservation system (Henry & Wang, 1998). Specifically, Henry and Wang provide evidence that the hormone oxytocin, which is restorative and health promoting, not only induces giving behavior in nonhuman mammals (Carter, 1998; Insel, 1993), but it also regulates the cortisol stress response, shortening the length of time individuals are exposed to harmful levels of cortisol. Thus, it is possible that giving benefits health and longevity because it is causally linked to restorative hormones that promote faster recovery from the fight-or-flight stress response.

We examined this possibility using 20 undergraduates (Brown, Johnson, Fredrickson, Figa, Gupta, & Cohn, 2006). The physiological arousal of all participants was measured by monitoring cardiovascular reactivity (e.g., heart rate and blood pressure) both before and after exposure to a stressor (i.e., preparation of a public speech). Participants were randomly assigned to help or not to help a confederate, and results showed that participants who attempted to help a confederate (successfully or unsuccessfully) returned to their baseline levels of arousal faster than participants who were never given the opportunity to help the confederate. These results offer support for the possibility that helping produces benefits by engaging a more healthful and restorative stress response system—a type of social regulation of the stress response.

The Costs of Giving: The Case of Caregiver Burnout

The health benefits of giving that we have discovered stand in stark contrast to the health costs of providing care to another person who is disabled or suffering from illness. The caregiving literature underscores the serious costs of helping others who are handicapped or seriously or terminally ill (e.g., Figley, 1998; Rainer, 2000). For example, Rainer (2000) suggests that caregiving creates withdrawal and isolation, the loss of pleasure, and a sense of being overwhelmed and pressured. And Cummins (2001) concludes that primary caregivers risk having substantial amounts of stress and depression and unusually low levels of life quality. Long-term caregiving has been linked to poorer immune functioning in old age (Robinson-Whelen, Kiecolt-Glaser, & Glaser, 2000) and even to increased risk of mortality (Schulz & Beach, 1999).

But previous research that purports to demonstrate caregiver burnout and other adverse caregiver effects is limited in at least two important ways. First, it is not clear from such research that undesirable caregiver effects are actually consequences of providing care. Typically uncontrolled in caregiver studies are the effects of observing and interacting with a loved one who is experiencing cognitive or physical decline. It is conceivable that repeated exposure to a suffering family member, spouse, partner, or friend is sufficient to drive caregiver distress, independent of the support provided by the caregiver. A second limitation of this work is that most studies have been conducted on relatively small samples in extreme caregiving circumstances—for example, providing care to a person with dementia—which may be considerably more taxing and stressful than caring for others whose needs are not as demanding.

In an effort to shed light on these issues, we conducted a study in which we examined the association between caregiver status and mortality risk in a sample of older adults (Brown, Smith, et al., 2006). We used data from the Health Retirement Survey (HRS), a national sample of older adults making the transition to retirement. The goals of this study were twofold. First, we wanted to investigate the relationship between caregiving and mortality, using a more inclusive definition of caregiving, with a larger, more representative sample. Second, we wanted to disentangle the hours spent caregiving from the distress related to having a loved one suffer from cognitive impairment. Caregiver status was determined based on whether help was provided in at least one activity of daily living and the number of hours per week that such help was provided. We used Cox proportional hazard models to examine the simultaneous relationship of both caregiver status and recipient cognitive impairment to mortality risk over a period of 7 years. In total, data from 4,121 married respondents were examined.

Results of these analyses demonstrated that caregiving was associated with a *decreased* risk of mortality, whereas simply being married to a partner suffering from cognitive impairment was associated with an increased risk of mortality.

Even after controlling for the health status and depressive symptoms of the caregiver, there was still a decreased risk of mortality for caregivers providing more than 14 hours of care. These results suggest that it may be a mistake to presume that caregiving will always be harmful to health. Moreover, the results offer further support for the possible health benefits of helping others.

CONVERGING EVIDENCE

The results of our research are consistent with findings from other investigations that have discovered the health benefits of helping others. For example, there is mounting evidence that volunteering can produce benefits to health and well-being (Omoto & Snyder, 1995; Wilson & Musick, 1999), including reduced mortality risk (Musick, Herzog, & House, 1999; Oman, Thoresen, & McMahon, 1999). Among elderly populations, providing support to others improves physical functioning, after controlling for health status (Avlund, Damsgaard, & Holstein, 1998; Hays, Saunders, Flint, Kaplan, & Blazer, 1997). And dialysis patients who provide support to their friends and family also have a lower risk of mortality (McClellan, Stanwyck, & Anson, 1993). Finally, emotions and personality styles that may be associated with giving—such as a sense of meaning, purpose, belonging, mattering, self-efficacy, and self-esteem—have also been linked to happiness and reduced depression (Baumeister, 1991; Taylor & Turner, 2001). These results, as well as our own, suggest that giving may be a more important determinant of well-being than receiving (see also Schwartz, this volume; Schwartz, Meisenhelder, Ma, & Reed, 2003; Schwartz & Sendor, 2000), and they also highlight promising new directions for understanding the ways in which social contact improves health and well-being.

If the results of subsequent studies replicate and extend these findings, then we may need to rethink the way we care for our loved ones: It may be that the best way to support another person is to provide them with an opportunity to feel useful.

DIRECTIONS FOR FUTURE RESEARCH

There are several unanswered questions that await future research. For example, is the benefit of giving different depending on the nature of the relationship between two people (or relationships that are interdependent versus one-sided)? How much helping is optimal (and can too much be harmful)? Are some types of helping more beneficial than others? Are there instances where receiving support is more beneficial?

We also need to know more about the precise mechanisms through which helping others benefits health. For example, how does giving protect against the negative effects of stress hormones? Conceivably, giving also creates positive emotions, which have been shown to speed the recovery from cardiovascular stress (Fredrickson, Mancuso, Branigan, & Tugade, 2000). Consequently, giving may benefit health via its association with positive emotions.

FINAL THOUGHTS

Through the lens of SIT, with its emphasis on the essential prosocial nature of close relationships, we have begun to enhance our understanding of the links between social contact and physical health and emotional well-being. SIT has led to novel predictions in this area, potentially resolved some anomalies in the literature, and generated interesting new predictions. Because SIT recasts the central function of close relationships, we believe it has the potential to make similar contributions in many other areas of relationship science.

Preparation of this chapter was supported by a career grant from the National Institute of Mental Health (K01-MH065423). Its contents are solely the responsibility of the authors and do not necessarily represent the official views of NIMH.

NOTE

1. The term "inclusive fitness" refers to the number of genes an individual transmits to subsequent generations through sexual reproduction and through helping relatives (who carry copies of the individual's genes) reproduce, weighted by degree of genetic relatedness.

REFERENCES

Alexander, R. D. (1987). *Biology of moral systems.* New York: de Gruyter.

Avlund, K., Damsgaard, M., & Holstein, B. (1998). Social relations and mortality: An eleven-year follow-up study of 70-year-old men and women in Denmark. *Social Science & Medicine, 47*(5), 635–643.

Baumeister, R. F. (1991). *Meanings of life.* New York: Guilford.

Black, J. M. (2001). Fitness consequences of long-term pair bonds in barnacle geese: Monogamy in the extreme. *Behavioral Ecology, 12,* 640–645.

Bowlby, J. (1958). The nature of a child's tie to his mother. *International Journal of Psycho-Analysis, 39,* 350–373.

Bowlby, J. (1969). *Attachment and loss: Vol. 1. Attachment.* New York: Basic.

Brosnan, S. F., & de Waal, F. B. M. (2002). A proximate perspective on reciprocal altruism. *Human Nature, 13,* 129–152.

Brown, R. M., Dahlen, E., Mills, C., Rick, J., & Biblarz, A. (1999). Evaluation of an evolutionary model of self-preservation and self-destruction. *Suicide and Life-Threatening Behavior, 29*(1), 58–71.

Brown, S. L. (1999). The origins of investment: A theory of close relationships. *Dissertation Abstracts International, 60*(11-B), 5830. (UMI No. 9950232)

Brown, S. L., & Brown, R. M. (2006). Selective investment theory: Recasting the functional significance of close relationships. *Psychological Inquiry, 17,* 1–29.

Brown, S. L., Johnson, K., Fredrickson, B. L., Cohn, M., Figa, B., & Gupta M. (Submitted). Helping behavior accelerates recovery from cardiovascular stress.

Brown, S. L., House, R. M., Brown, R. M., & Smith, D. M. (2006). *Coping with spousal loss: The buffering effects of giving social support to others.* Manuscript submitted for publication.

Brown, S. L., Nesse, R., Vinokur, A. D., & Smith, D. M. (2003). Providing support may be more beneficial than receiving it: Results from a prospective study of mortality. *Psychological Science, 14,* 320–327.

Brown, S. L., Smith, D. M., Schulz, R., et al. (Submitted). Caregiving and decreased mortality in a national sample of older adults.

Brown, W. M., & Moore, C. (2000). Is prospective altruist-detection an evolved solution to the adaptive problem of subtle cheating in cooperative ventures? Supportive evidence using the Wason selection task. *Evolution & Human Behavior, 21,* 25–37.

Carr, D., House, J. S., Kessler, R. C., Nesse, R. M., Sonnega, J., & Wortman, C. (2000). Marital quality and psychological adjustment to widowhood among older adults: A longitudinal analysis. *Journal of Gerontology, 55B*(4), S197–S207.

Carter, C. S. (1998). Neuroendocrine perspectives on social attachment and love. *Psychoneuroendocrinology, 23,* 779–818.

Cialdini, R. B., Darby, B. K., & Vincent, J. E. (1973). Transgression and altruism: A case for hedonism. *Journal of Experimental Social Psychology, 9,* 502–516.

Cialdini, R. B., & Kenrick, D. T. (1976). Altruism as hedonism: A social development perspective on the relationship of negative mood state and helping. *Journal of Personality & Social Psychology, 34,* 907–914.

Cosmides, L. (1989). The logic of social exchange: Has natural selection shaped how humans reason? Studies with the Wason selection task. *Cognition, 31,* 187–276.

Cosmides, L., & Tooby, J. (1992). Cognitive adaptations for social exchange. In J. H. Barkow, L. Cosmides, & J. Tooby (Eds.), *The adapted mind: Evolutionary psychology and the generation of culture* (pp. 163–228). New York: Oxford University Press.

Cummins, R. A. (2001). The subjective well-being of people caring for a family member with a severe disability at home: A review. *Journal of Intellectual & Developmental Disability: Special Issue, 26*(Pt. 2), 83–100.

Darwin, C. (1859). *On the origin of species by means of natural selection; or, the preservation of favoured races in the struggle for life.* London: John Murray.

de Catanzaro, D. (1986). A mathematical model of evolutionary pressures regulating self-preservation and self-destruction. *Suicide and Life-Threatening Behavior, 16,* 166–181.

Dessalles, J.-L. (1999). Coalition factor in the evolution of non-kin altruism. *Advances in Complex Systems, 2,* 143–172.

de Waal, F. (1996), *Good natured: The origins of right and wrong in humans and other animals*. Cambridge, MA: Harvard University Press.

Feeney, B. C., & Collins, N. L. (2003). Motivations for caregiving in adult intimate relationships: Influences on caregiving behavior and relationship functioning. *Personality and Social Psychology Bulletin, 29*, 950–968.

Fehr, E., & Fischbacher, U. (2003). The nature of human altruism. *Nature, 425*, 785–791.

Fehr, E., & Gächter, S. (2002). Altruistic punishment in humans. *Nature, 415*, 137–140.

Figley, C. R. (1998). *Burnout in families: The systemic costs of caring*. Boca Raton, FL: CRC Press.

Fredrickson, B., Mancuso, R., Branigan, C., & Tugade, M. (2000). The undoing effect of positive emotions. *Motivation and Emotion, 24*, 237–258.

Gintis, H. (2000). Strong reciprocity and human sociality. *Journal of Theoretical Biology, 206*, 169–179.

Gintis, H., Bowles, S., Boyd, R., & Fehr, E. (2003). Explaining altruistic behavior in humans. *Evolution and Human Behavior, 24*, 153–172.

Gintis, H., Smith, E. H., & Bowles, S. (2001). Costly signaling and cooperation. *Journal of Theoretical Biology, 213*, 103–119.

Hamilton, W. D. (1964). The genetic evolution of social behavior: I and II. *Journal of Theoretical Biology, 7*, 1–52.

Hays, J., Saunders, W., Flint, E., Kaplan, B., & Blazer, D. (1997). Social support and depression as risk factors for loss of physical function in late life. *Aging & Mental Health, 1*(3), 209–220.

Hazan, C., & Shaver, P. R. (1994). Attachment as an organizational framework for research on close relationships. *Psychological Inquiry, 5*, 1–22.

Henry, J., & Wang, S. (1998). Effects of early stress on adult affiliative behavior. *Psychoneuroendocrinology, 23*, 863–875.

House, J. S., Landis, K. R., & Umberson, D. (1988). Social relationships and health. *Science, 241*, 540–545.

Insel, T. R. (1993). Oxytocin and the neuroendocrine basis of affiliation. In J. Schulkin (Ed.), *Hormonally induced changes in mind and brain* (pp. 225–251). San Diego, CA: Academic.

Korchmaros, J. D., & Kenny, D. A. (2001). Emotional closeness as a mediator of the effect of genetic relatedness on altruism. *Psychological Science, 12*, 262–265.

Lu, L., & Argyle, M. (1992). Receiving and giving support: Effects on relationships and well-being. *Counseling Psychology Quarterly, 5*, 123–133.

McClellan, W. M., Stanwyck, D. J., & Anson, C. A. (1993). Social support and subsequent mortality among patients with end-stage renal disease. *Journal of American Society of Nephrology, 4*, 1028–1034.

Mitani, J. C., Watts, D. P., & Muller, M. N. (2002). Recent developments in the study of wild chimpanzee behavior. *Evolutionary Anthropology, 11*, 9–25.

Musick, M. A., Herzog, A. R., & House, J. S. (1999). Volunteering and mortality among older adults: Findings from a national sample. *Journals of Gerontology, 54B*, S173–S180.

Neyer, F. J., & Lang, F. R. (2003). Blood is thicker than water: Kinship orientation across adulthood. *Journal of Personality and Social Psychology, 84,* 310–321.

Nowak, M., & Sigmund, K. (1998). Evolution of indirect reciprocity by image scoring. *Nature, 393,* 573–576.

Oman, D., Thoresen, C. E., & McMahon, K. (1999). Volunteering and mortality among the community-dwelling elderly, *Journal of Health Psychology, 4,* 301–316.

Omoto, A. M., & Snyder, M. (1995). Sustained helping without obligation: Motivation, longevity of service, and perceived attitude change among AIDS volunteers. *Journal of Personality and Social Psychology, 16,* 152–166.

Porter, R. H. (1987). Kin recognition: Functions and mediating mechanisms. In C. Crawford, M. Smith, & D. Krebs (Eds.), *Sociobiology and psychology: Ideas, issues, and applications* (pp. 175–203). Hillsdale, NJ: Erlbaum.

Rainer, J. P. (2000). Compassion fatigue: When caregiving begins to hurt. In L. Vandecreek & T.^sL. Jackson (Eds.), *Innovations in clinical practice: A source book* (Vol. 18, pp. 441–453). Sarasota, FL: Professional Resource Press.

Robinson-Whelen, S., Kiecolt-Glaser, J., & Glaser, R. (2000). Effects of chronic stress on immune function and health in the elderly. In S. Manuck (Ed.), *Behavior, health, and aging* (pp. 69–82). Mahwah, NJ: Erlbaum.

Rossi, A. S., & Rossi, P. H. (1990). *Of human bonding: Parent-child relations across the life course.* New York: de Gruyter.

Rusbult, C. (1980). Commitment and satisfaction in romantic associations: A test of the investment model. *Journal of Experimental Social Psychology, 16*(2), 172–186.

Schulz, R., & Beach, S. (1999). Caregiving as a risk factor for mortality: The Caregiver Health Effects Study. *Journal of the American Medical Association, 282,* 2215–2219.

Schwartz, C., Meisenhelder, J. B., Ma, J., & Reed, G. (2003). Altruistic social interest behaviors are associated with better mental health, *Psychosomatic Medicine, 65,* 778–785.

Schwartz, C., & Sendor, M. (2000). Helping others helps oneself: Response shift effects in peer support. In C. Schwartz & M. Sprangers (Eds.), *Adaptation to changing health: Response shift in quality-of-life research* (pp. 175–188). Washington, DC: American Psychological Association.

Smith, C. E., Fernengel, K., Holcroft, C., Gerald, K., & Marien, L. (1994). Meta-analysis of the associations between social support and health outcomes. *Annals of Behavioral Medicine, 16,* 352–362.

Sprecher, S., & Schwartz, P. (1994). Equity and balance in the exchange of contributions in close relationships. In M. J. Lerner (Ed.), *Entitlement and the affectional bond: Justice in close relationships* (pp. 11–41). New York: Plenum.

Taylor, J., & Turner, J. (2001). A longitudinal study of the role and significance of mattering to others for depressive symptoms. *Journal of Health and Social Behavior, 42,* 310–325.

Thompson, S. C., Medvene, L. J., & Freedman, D. (1995). Caregiving in the close relationships of cardiac patients: Exchange, power, and attributional perspectives on caregiver resentment. *Personal Relationships, 2,* 125–142.

Tooby, J., & Cosmides, L. (1996). Friendship and the banker's paradox: Other pathways to the evolution of adaptations for altruism. *Proceedings of the British Academy, 88,* 119–143.

Trivers, R. L. (1971). The evolution of reciprocal altruism. *Quarterly Review of Biology, 46,* 35–57.

Wilson, J., & Musick, M. (1999). The effects of volunteering on the volunteer. *Law and Contemporary Problems, 62,* 141–168.

Wong, L., Kolditz, T. A., Millen, R. A., & Potter, T. M. (2003). *Why they fight: Combat motivation in the Iraq war.* Carlisle Barracks, PA: Strategic Studies Institute.

Zahavi, A. (1995). Mate selection—a selection for handicap. *Journal of Theoretical Biology, 53,* 205–214.

Zahavi, A. (1997). *The handicap principle: A missing piece of Darwin's puzzle.* New York: Oxford University Press.

17 Health and the Ecology of Altruism

David Sloan Wilson
Mihaly Csikszentmihalyi

Biological communities are diverse in part because there are many ways to survive and reproduce. Any given species thrives in some environments and becomes stressed in others, ultimately to the point of failing to persist.

Human behavioral diversity can potentially be explained in the same way as biological diversity. A particular behavioral strategy, such as risk avoidance, conscientiousness, or cooperation, is advantageous in some situations but not others. Individuals who employ the wrong strategy in a given situation become stressed, ultimately to the point of changing their behavior, removing themselves from the situation, or suffering the physical and psychological consequences of maladaptive behavior. Because there is no single best strategy for all situations, a mix of strategies will be maintained in the population through a number of proximate mechanisms, including short-term individual flexibility (e.g., becoming cautious in dangerous situations), developmental processes (e.g., becoming temperamentally cautious as a result of childhood experiences), and long-term evolutionary processes (e.g., being innately cautious).

This ecological perspective has important implications for the study of altruism and health. Other-regarding behavioral strategies have coexisted with more self-regarding strategies throughout human history. Clearly, both must be advantageous in some situations and disadvantageous in others to be maintained over such long periods of time. Altruism should have beneficial health consequences primarily when it thrives as a behavioral strategy. Otherwise it should become stressful, which is why it is abandoned. The same goes for self-regarding behaviors.

These predictions seem inevitable because they apply to any behavioral strategy that thrives in some niches but not others. However, the situation is more complicated for altruism and selfishness than for other behavioral strategies because selfishness is often morally objectionable and the niche for altruism is often of our own making. We don't counsel people to be selfish—for their health or any other reason—because that would impair the health and well-being of others. We do counsel people to be altruistic because altruism thrives in the company of other altruists. By encouraging altruism and discouraging selfishness, we create the niche for altruism (Sober & Wilson, 1998; Wilson 2002).

Given the complications that are specific to altruism and selfishness, along with the basic predictions that apply to any behavioral strategy, it is essential to appreciate the importance of context in the study of altruism and health. Altruism can be highly gratifying (and therefore healthful) in some situations, especially when it involves working with others who reciprocate or express gratitude. Altruism practiced in face-to-face interactions might be especially healthful because the psychological mechanisms that make altruism personally rewarding evolved in the context of face-to-face interactions. On the other hand, altruism can be stressful in other situations, especially when it is unreciprocated, unappreciated, or fails to trigger appropriate proximate mechanisms. Selfish behavioral strategies might be unhealthful in some situations, especially when they result in social isolation in the long run despite their short-term benefits, but in other situations they might yield health benefits in addition to other benefits, much as we might wish otherwise. Finally, we might expect individual differences based on past experiences and (conceivably) genetic factors. People who are currently practicing different behavioral strategies will not necessarily experience the same health consequences of altruism in a given situation.

TESTING ECOLOGICAL PREDICTIONS

Testing ecologically informed predictions such as these requires a database that provides information about behavioral differences and their consequences in everyday life. One such database is the Sloan Study of Youth and Social Development, conducted by a team of scientists headed by psychologist Mihaly Csikszentmihalyi and sociologist Barbara Schneider, which examined how adolescents make the transition from school to the workforce (Csikszentmihalyi & Schneider, 2000). Twelve geographical locations in the United States were chosen to represent rural, urban, and suburban environments and different racial and ethnic compositions, labor force characteristics, and economic stability. Within each geographical location, a number of middle schools and high schools participated, resulting in 33 schools for the entire study. More than 1,000 students were followed for a period of 5 years. Information gathered at biyearly intervals included a battery of questionnaires totaling more than 400 items and a week of the experience sampling method (ESM), which involves being signaled eight times a day and recording basic information about external circumstances (where you are, what you are doing, and who you are with) along with 33 variables measuring psychological experience (e.g., anger, happiness, cooperation, concentration) on numerical scales. In addition to these "focal" students, a subset of information was gathered on more than 3,000 classmates of the focal students (termed "cohort" students).

The information gathered by the Sloan Study can be used for many purposes in addition to its original focus. In collaboration with Csikszentmihalyi and Schneider, David Sloan Wilson used 17 questionnaire items to construct a scale that measures individual differences in prosociality (a term that includes all forms of other-oriented behavior). Items on the PRO scale include questions such as "For the job you expect to have in the future, how important is helping people?" and "How often do you spend time volunteering or performing community service outside of school?" that clearly relate to other-oriented attitudes and behavior. Construction and validation of the PRO scale will be reported in more detail elsewhere. In this chapter, we use the scale to show that prosociality can be either good or bad for one's health, depending upon the context.

Altruism's Niche

A broad look at the ecology of altruism is provided by the multiple regression analysis shown in Table 17.1. Fourteen items from the database account for almost 40% of the variance in the PRO scale. The items fall into the following categories:

> *Gender*: Females on average score higher than males, independent of the other variables.
>
> *Social support*: The items "How many teachers care," "Neighbors will help," and "Family avoids hurting feelings" suggest that prosocial *individuals* tend to inhabit prosocial *environments*, receiving benefits in addition to bestowing them.
>
> *Personal efficacy*: The items "Feels hopeful about the future," "Energetically pursues goals," and "Feels like a person of worth" suggest that highly prosocial individuals are also highly efficacious *as* individuals.
>
> *Long-term goals*: The items "Time spent on homework out of school," "Importance of having children," "Importance of giving own children opportunities," "Expects to encounter obstacles," and "The importance of partying among friends" (negative correlation) suggest that highly prosocial individuals are more likely to work toward long-term goals. They have a long temporal horizon in addition to a wide social horizon.
>
> *Religious participation*: The items "Religion affects decisions" and "Importance of religion among friends" indicate the role of religion in promoting prosociality, independent of the other factors.

Table 17.1. Items Retained in a Stepwise Multiple Regression Analysis Explaining 39.3% of the Variance in the PRO Scale

Item #	Item	Coeff.	SE	t Ratio	Probability
1	Gender	4.49	0.59	7.56	****
2	How many teachers care	1.61	0.30	5.39	****
3	Neighbors will help	0.85	0.32	2.67	**
4	Family avoids hurting feelings	1.52	0.60	2.54	**
5	Feels hopeful about future	2.01	0.34	6.00	****
6	Energetically pursues goals	2.59	0.52	5.03	****
7	Feels like a person of worth	1.34	0.45	2.98	**
8	Time on homework out of school	0.73	0.15	4.74	****
9	Importance of having children	1.91	0.44	4.39	****
10	Importance of giving own kids opportunities	2.29	0.56	4.08	****
11	Expects to encounter obstacles	1.62	0.45	3.58	***
12	Importance of partying among friends	−1.37	0.39	−3.48	***
13	Religion affects decisions	1.25	0.24	5.16	****
14	Importance of religion among friends	2.05	0.47	4.38	****

Note: *p < .05; **p < .01; ***p < .001; **p < .0001.

Taken together, these items suggest that highly prosocial individuals tend to inhabit stable, nurturing environments that enable them to thrive as individuals and to work toward long-term goals. Broadly speaking, this can be said to be the niche for altruism. Needless to say, it is a picture of health at both the individual and societal levels. It is also exactly what we would expect from a theoretical perspective, since altruism and other forms of prosociality can only persist over the long term if those who produce benefits for others also receive them.

As we leave the niche for altruism and enter less stable and less nurturing environments, individuals become less prosocial on average. This could be caused by a variety of proximate mechanisms. Perhaps individuals are flexible enough to change their prosociality in response to environmental change. Perhaps they are not so flexible, but their stable dispositions cause them to sort into different environments. Either way, a high-PRO individual inhabiting a low-PRO environment is like a fish out of water and should find the experience stressful.

When Bad Things Happen to Good People

Participants of the Sloan Study were asked whether a number of important and potentially stressful events had occurred during the previous 2 years, ranging from moving to a new home to being assaulted. During year 5, they were also asked how stressed they were by the events. Some of the events were rare, but the sample sizes were so large that out of 1,779 participants who responded to the question "Were you shot at?" for example, 165 answered yes. Table 17.2 shows a very consistent pattern: Low-PRO individuals are more likely to experience events characteristic of harsh social environments, such as physical conflict and teenage pregnancy (negative coefficient values in the "likelihood of occurrence" section of Table 17.2). When these events are experienced, however, the degree of stress correlates *positively* with prosociality (positive coefficient values in the "stress upon occurrence" section of Table 17.2). Low-PROs are apparently better able to cope with these events, either because they are more familiar or because they are less upsetting whenever they occur. Either way, these results provide a convincing demonstration of the fish-out-of-water phenomenon. Altruism is not a successful behavioral strategy in all environments and should not be expected to have beneficial health consequences, such as stress reduction, in all environments. People who freely give should be highly stressed in situations that involve aggressive or manipulative taking, for the same reason that they protectively change their behavior, attempt to change the situation, or attempt to leave the situation.

When Good Things Happen to Bad People

On average, low-PRO individuals suffer from low self-esteem, are pessimistic about the future, and believe that luck is more important than hard work. They score significantly higher on the items "I usually feel stressed," "I usually feel sick," and "I usually feel tired" (ANOVAs: $N = 1653, 1648, 1651$; $df = 4$; $F = 2.9, 4.69, 4.92$; $p = .020, .0009, .0006$, respectively). Nevertheless, this unhealthy portrait based on averages obscures differences that exist among low-PRO individuals. In particular, it does not fit the image of the narcissist who cares only about himself and treats others as a means to personal ends. Such a person might easily have high self-esteem, be optimistic about his own future, and exult in his ability to manipulate people without leaving anything to luck. This is the standard image of a selfish person in popular culture, "cheating" strategies in models of social behavior (Gintis et al., 2005; Hammerstein, 2003; Sober & Wilson, 1998), Machiavellianism in the psychological literature (Wilson et al., 1996), and psychopathology (Mealey, 1995). Why isn't this kind of low-PRO individual more conspicuous in our data?

The answer is that this kind of low-PRO *does* exist in our sample population but is obscured in the multiple regression analysis by other individuals whose lack of prosociality appears due to various forms of stress. To distinguish these two profiles, we performed a cluster analysis on the lower 30% of the PRO score distribution using nine items that we predicted would discriminate the two types of low-PRO individuals (indicated by the asterisks in the second column of Table 17.3). Two distinct clusters emerged, as shown in the top graph of Figure 17.1,

Table 17.2. Single-Factor Regression Analysis With PRO Scale as the Dependent Variable and a Number of Stress Factors as the Independent Variables

Did this event happen in last 2 years?	Likelihood of Occurrence			Stress Upon Occurrence		
	Coeff.	R^2	p	Coeff.	R^2	p
Moved to new home	−1.55	0.10				
Parent got married						
Parent got divorced						
Mother lost job						
Father lost job						
Mother started work						
Father started work						
Family member sent to jail						
Had baby	−5.13	0.60	****	2.33	3.40	*
Became seriously ill						
Father died						
Mother died	−4.63	0.20	**			
Close relative died				1.72	2.20	****
Family member ill	2.25	0.40	**			
Family went into counseling						
Family member victim of crime				1.93	3.00	***
Had something stolen				0.91	0.90	*
Someone offered to sell drugs	−3.49	1.50	****			
Someone threatened to hurt	−2.83	0.70	****			
Got into a physical fight	−5.86	2.00	****			
Hit or beaten up	−3.00	0.70	***	1.35	2.10	**
Shot at	−6.11	0.02	****	2.02	0.04	**
Witnessed a violent crime	−3.60	1.20	****	2.23	5.30	****
Self or someone known assaulted	−1.42	0.20	*	2.02	4.70	

Note: $^*p < .05$; $^{**}p < .01$; $^{***}p < .001$; $^{**}p < .0001$.

which were used as groups in an analysis of variance for other items from the database. Significant differences were found for the variables shown in Table 17.3, which have been normalized to a 0–1 scale and reversed as necessary so that higher values indicate agreement with the item. Mean values are provided for the entire sample population in addition to the two types of low-PRO individuals for comparative purposes.

To interpret Table 17.3, we can begin by noting that almost 80% of the narcissistic low-PROs (designated "low-PRO-A") are male, in contrast to an even sex ratio for the other low-PROs (designated "low-PRO-B") and the general sample. Proceeding to the religious items, the A group scores higher than the B group, but both are below the general sample average. For the remaining items, the most important pattern to note is that *the two low-PRO groups usually straddle the population mean*. For items likely to contribute to health, such as self-esteem and control, the A group scores not only higher than the B group but also higher

Table 17.3. Significant Differences (Based on ANOVA) Between Two Types of Low-PROs, Whose Mean Values Sometime Straddle the Average for the Total Sample Population

Category	Item	Low-PRO-A	Low-PRO-B	Total Average	Probability
Basic Variables	Gender (Male = 0, Female = 1)	0.21	0.55	0.53	**
Religion	How often attended services?	0.13	0.06	0.44	*
	Thinks is a religious person	0.41	0.20	0.43	**
	Among friends, importance of religious activity	0.21	0.04	0.33	**
	How much religion affects decisions	0.31	0.15	0.46	**
Self-Esteem	R feels good about self*	0.83	0.60	0.73	***
	R feels s/he is a person of worth*	0.83	0.56	0.73	***
	R able to do things as well as others*	0.80	0.63	0.74	***
	On the whole, R is satisfied with self*	0.86	0.53	0.70	***
	Feels useless at times	0.40	0.55	0.45	**
	At times thinks s/he is no good at all	0.30	0.47	0.41	**
	Does not have much to be proud of	0.22	0.40	0.34	***
	R usually feels emotionally empty	0.27	0.42	0.34	*
	Feels empty about the future	0.14	0.27	0.25	*
Control	Should have baby only after marriage	0.77	0.65	0.65	*
	I energetically pursue my goals*	0.79	0.69	0.73	**

Lots of ways around any problem*	0.76	0.65	0.69	**
I know I can solve problems*	0.74	0.59	0.67	***
I meet the goals I set for myself*	0.71	0.57	0.65	***
Prepared for the future*	0.73	0.44	0.64	***
Parents check about homework	0.45	0.24	0.45	**
Good luck more important than hard work	0.28	0.40	0.32	*
Others stop R from getting ahead	0.35	0.46	0.40	*
Plans hardly ever work out	0.29	0.47	0.37	**
When makes plans R is certain they will work	0.73	0.51	0.64	***
Many ways to get important things in life	0.78	0.67	0.70	**
Things do not go as planned	0.40	0.54	0.56	*
Confident about the future	0.76	0.60	0.71	**
Worried about the future	0.45	0.60	0.56	*
Powerful about the future	0.57	0.43	0.57	*
Hopeful about the future	0.80	0.65	0.77	**
Trust				
Misbehaving students often get away with it	0.62	0.49	0.53	*
How many teachers listen to R's problems	0.56	0.34	0.47	**
R thinks others see R as trustworthy	0.84	0.71	0.75	*
Stress				
Got into a physical fight in school	0.00	0.12	0.11	*
R feels stressed	0.42	0.59	0.52	*
R feels tired	0.54	0.69	0.55	*
R feels relaxed	0.63	0.46	0.56	**

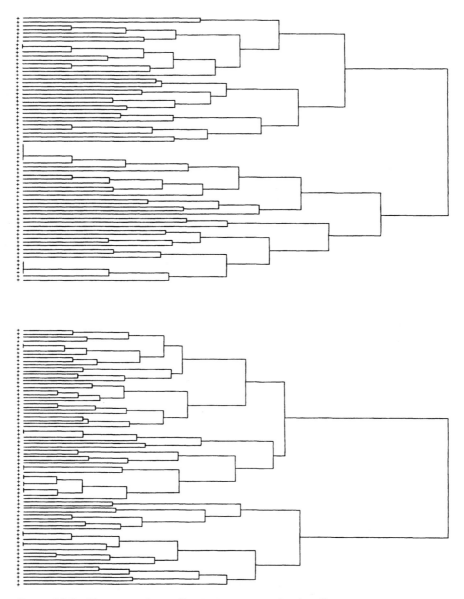

Figure 17.1. Cluster analyses discriminating two kinds of low-PRO (*top*) and high-PRO (*bottom*) individuals.

than the general sample average. Similarly, for items likely to detract from health, such as emotional emptiness, stress, and fatigue, the A group scores not only below the B group but below the general sample average. In short, *low-PRO-A individuals appear to be a picture of mental health, more like high-PRO individuals than low-PRO-B individuals.* They are not maladaptive as individuals, although their behaviors may well be maladaptive to others.

Different Ways to Be Good

Individual differences are also likely to exist among high-PROs, with potential health consequences. In particular, religion is an important correlate of pro-sociality in the general sample, but not all high-PROs are religious. To examine differences between religious and nonreligious high-PROs, a cluster analysis was performed on the upper 30% of the PRO score distribution using six religious items (indicated by asterisks in Table 17.4). Two distinct clusters were identified (bottom graph of Figure 17.1), which served as groups in an analysis of variance for other items, as with our analysis of low-PROs. Significant differences were found for the items listed in Table 17.4. Differences for the religious variables were expected, because they served as the basis for discrimination in the cluster analysis. More interesting is the fact that nonreligious high-PROs (labeled "high-PRO-A") are *highly* nonreligious, scoring not only below the religious high-PROs but considerably below the mean for the general sample. Proceeding to the other variables, religious high-PROs (labeled "high-PRO-B") reported higher self-esteem, self-confidence, and faith in the future than did nonreligious high-PROs. They were subject to more parental control but resented it less. Finally, they were more likely to be known by their neighbors than were nonreligious high-PROs. In short, religious high-PROs present a more robust picture of mental health than do nonreligious high-PROs, who even score worse than the average for the general sample on some items. Altruism can be stress relieving or stress inducing, depending upon how it is conceived and carried out.

Altruism, Health, and Immediate Experience

So far, our analysis has been based on questionnaire items that were answered on a one-time basis, but the most important part of the Sloan Study database is the experience sampling method, which involves recording thoughts and feelings as they are being experienced at roughly 2-2-hour intervals for a week. Table 17.5 shows that individual differences measured by the PRO scale were amply reflected in everyday experience. On average, high-PROs were able to concentrate, felt that they were living up to the expectations of others, and enjoyed themselves more than low-PROs. They felt more happy, active, sociable, in-

Table 17.4. Significant Differences (Based on ANOVA) Between Nonreligious (A) Religious (B) High-PROs, Whose Mean Values Sometimes Straddle the Average for the Total Sample Population

Category	Item	High-PRO-A	High-PRO-B	Total Average	Probability
Religion	How often attended services?*	0.37	0.83	0.44	***
	Thinks is a religious person*	0.35	0.80	0.43	***
	Among friends, importance of religious activity*	0.18	0.58	0.33	***
	How much religion affects decisions*	0.33	0.87	0.46	***
	How much religion affects future job*	0.13	0.80,	0.38	***
	Depend on science too much vs. faith*	0.35	0.75	0.48	***
Self-Esteem	Feels useless at times	0.54	0.35	0.45	**
	At times thinks s/he is no good at all	0.46	0.25	0.41	**
	R usually feels emotionally empty	0.29	0.15	0.34	*
Control	Tries as hard as possible in math	0.75	0.88	0.76	*
	Parents assign household chores	0.72	0.88	0.72	*
	Parents limit TV watching/video game time	0.22	0.42	0.27	*
	R does not have enough control over life	0.31	0.16	0.37	*
	I energetically pursue my goals	0.78	0.88	0.73	**'
	I know I can solve problems	0.68	0.79	0.67	*
	Worried about the future	0.62	0.48	0.56	*
	Prepared for the future	2.41	0.76	0.64	**
Support	Neighbors know who R is	0.59	0.76	0.60	**

volved, and excited. They felt more challenged and engaged by their activities, which were perceived as more important with respect to future goals. As with the regression analysis presented in Table 17.1 on the basis of one-time questionnaire items, this is a picture of health at both the societal and individual levels.

The last two columns of Table 17.5 compare the different types of low-PROs and high-PROs that were analyzed in Tables 17.3 and 17.4, respectively. Apart from the single item "Did you feel good about yourself?" the differences between A and B low-PROs do not appear to be strongly reflected in daily experience. However, numerous differences exist between the high-PRO groups, indicating substantial emotional benefits for religious prosociality (B) compared to nonreligious prosociality (A) at a day-to-day level.

THE ECOLOGICAL PARADIGM

This chapter makes three contributions to the study of altruism and health. First, we provide evidence that other-oriented individuals tend to flourish *as* individuals. Science works best when it uses a combination of methods, from naturalistic observations to controlled experiments. The Sloan Study and especially its use of the experience sampling method provides a superb source of naturalistic information, acting as an invisible observer perched on the shoulders of people as they go about their daily rounds of life. It is gratifying that the benefits of altruism can be demonstrated at such an intimate and noninvasive level for a representative sample of American youth.

Second, we provide evidence that other-oriented individuals do not *invariably* flourish as individuals. It can be unhealthy to be altruistic and healthy to be selfish. Some forms of altruism appear to be healthier than others. Studying the health consequences of altruism requires a sophisticated understanding of context.

Third, we provide a theoretical framework for predicting *when* altruism flourishes or fails to flourish. The framework was briefly presented at the beginning of the chapter and will be elaborated below to provide a guide for future research.

Avoiding Normative Bias

Altruism is good for others and society, almost by definition (although its virtue is occasionally challenged by thinkers such as Rand, 1961). People have a passion for promoting altruism, in others if not always in themselves. One way to do this is by calling altruism "natural," "healthy," and "mature" while branding selfishness as "unnatural," "sick," and "immature." These labels might help

Table 17.5. Experience Sampling Method Items Answered at Roughly 2-Hour Intervals for a Period of a Week

Item #	Item	PROcorr	Sig	Low-PRO	High-PRO
1	How well were you concentrating?	0.225	****		
2	Were you living up to the expectations of others?	0.262	****		
3	Was it hard to concentrate?	-0.023			
4	Did you feel self-conscious or embarrassed?	0.025			
5	Did you feel good about yourself?	0.111	*	A>B*	
6	Did you enjoy what you were doing?	-0.091			B>A**
7	Were you living up to your expectations?	0.179	***		B>A**
8	Did you feel in control of the situation?	0.051			
9	Did you expect to get what you want easily?	0.071			

Describe your feelings as you were beeped on scale from

10	Sad-Happy	0.149	**		B>A**
11	Weak-Strong	0.105			B>A***
12	Passive-Active	0.114	*		B>A**
13	Lonely-Sociable	0.194	***		B>A*
14	Ashamed-Proud	0.094			B>A*
15	Detached-Involved	0.179	***		
16	Bored-Excited	0.159	**		B>A*
17	Confused-Clear	0.053			B>**

		PROcorr	Sig	
18	Worried-Relaxed	-0.014		B>A**
19	Competitive-Cooperative	0.105		
20	Discouraged-Hopeful	0.098		
21	Tired-Alert	0.097		

Indicate how you felt about the main activity

		PROcorr	Sig	
22	Challenges of the activity	0.146	**	
23	Skills in the activity	0.065		
24	Was this activity important to you?	9.229	****	
25	How difficult did you find this activity?	0.127	*	
26	Were you succeeding at what you were doing?	0.085		
27	Did you wish you had been doing something else?	-0.092		
28	Was this activity interesting?	0.151	**	
29	How important was it to your future goals?	0.146	**	
30	How angry did you feel?	-0.023		
31	Were you making the best possible use of your time?	0.229	****	
32	What did the people you were with think of you?	0.122	*	
33	Did you feel any physical pain or discomfort?	-0.076		

Notes: The PROcorr and Sig columns give correlation coefficients and statistical significance values for single-factor regressions. Items 2, 13, 24, and 27 are retained in a stepwise multiple regression analysis, accounting for 12.2% of the variance in the PRO scale. The low-PRO and high-PRO columns show the results of ANOVAs comparing the two groups of low-PROs and high-PROS.

to promote altruism, but they are questionable as statements of fact. How can selfishness be called "unnatural" when it is displayed by other species and has existed throughout human history? In what sense are people who profit from exploiting others "sick" in terms of their individual health? How can such people —who might be 80 years old—be called "immature," as if they are more like children than adults? It might seem that sophisticated thinkers would not commit these errors, but intellectual history proves otherwise, from Rousseau's noble savage, to Kohlberg's stages of moral development (Kohlberg, 1984; Krebs, 1998), to fear and trembling that evolutionary theory might show something considered immoral to be "natural" and therefore somehow acceptable. Given such a widespread tendency for normative goals to influence interpretations of reality, it is important for the modern scientific study of altruism and health to distinguish itself from the kind of moral encouragement so common in everyday life, which takes the form of the claim "if you behave altruistically, then you will also be happier, healthier, and wealthier." Scientists who study altruism might well have the practical goal of making the world a better place (we certainly do), but as scientists they have an additional burden of telling a story about altruism that is factually correct.

It's a Darwinian World

One purely scientific approach is to imagine a world inhabited by beings who employ any feasible behavioral strategy, for example, from pristine altruism to wanton selfishness. The individuals compete, and some emerge victorious in terms of raw survival and reproduction. If the strategies are inherited in some sense (more on that below), then the winners will inherit the earth and the losers will pass out of existence. We call this approach "purely scientific" because it does not have any normative commitment. The victorious strategies could be altruistic, selfish, or a mixture of both. We simply endow the world with certain properties, add the individuals with their behavioral strategies, and let the chips fall where they may.

It might seem that altruists are certain to lose such a Darwinian contest. One reason that Darwin's theory provokes such an allergic reaction is because it seems so good at explaining selfishness and so bad at explaining altruism. However, Darwin had a key insight that has been confirmed by modern evolutionary theory. Altruists are indeed vulnerable to nonaltruists in their immediate vicinity, but groups of altruists robustly outcompete groups of nonaltruists. Whenever altruists can interact primarily with each other, they can thrive even in a strictly Darwinian world.

The behavioral strategies that emerge from evolutionary models of social behavior (which formalize the thought experiment of the previous paragraph) bear an uncanny resemblance to human social behaviors, including altruism, selfishness, retaliation, forgiveness, contrition, punishment, revenge, and arbitrary social conventions (norms). The particular strategies that emerge victorious depend upon the parameters of the model, which define properties of the particular "world" that is being imagined. The real world is a mosaic of the parameters that make up the model worlds, so each behavioral strategy is expected to have a distribution and abundance, much like species in a multispecies community. The fact that altruism and other forms of prosociality can flourish at least some of the time in a Darwinian world provides a theoretical framework for studying their distribution, abundance, and health consequences, as we have tried to show in this chapter.

MATERIAL AND PSYCHOLOGICAL BENEFITS OF ALTRUISM

The benefits of altruism can be divided into those with an obvious material basis (such as food, shelter, and medicine) and those with a more subtle psychological basis (such as comfort, respect, and forgiveness). A woman who helps disaster victims is obviously increasing *their* health; the striking result is that she might also be increasing *her* health.

Evolutionary theory can help to clarify the relationship between these two kinds of health benefits. All adaptations have both an ultimate (their effect on survival and reproduction) and proximate (the particular mechanism that causes them to be expressed) explanation. Flowers bloom in spring because those that bloomed earlier were nipped by frost and those that bloomed later failed to mature their fruits (the ultimate explanation). Flowers also bloom in spring because of a physiological mechanism that is sensitive to day length (the proximate explanation).

In addition to orchestrating the behaviors that obviously influence fitness, proximate mechanisms can have fitness consequences of their own. *In general, the mechanistic and behavioral consequences are expected to parallel each other.* Zebras are not stressed in the absence of lions. When a lion suddenly appears, zebras are briefly stressed in a way that clearly enhances their survival behaviorally without causing them to suffer unduly from the stress response per se. If zebras were placed in a cage next to a lion, they would suffer from chronic stress that would become debilitating in its own right (Sapolsky, 1998). Most people are unstressed in the company of friends, become stressed in isolation in a way that causes them to remedy the situation without suffering from their stress response per se, but can suffer health-damaging stress in permanent isolation. In both of these examples, the proximate mechanisms are most healthful in their own right when they successfully enhance survival and reproduction behaviorally, as they were designed to do.

It follows that the psychological benefits of altruism can be maximized by providing the kind of social environment that enables altruism to flourish in behavioral terms. It should also be important to provide the cues that reliably indicate such environments, especially in the context of small face-to-face groups. To be known, liked, respected, needed, and in the company of others are powerful psychological motivators because they consistently led to prosocial groupings in our evolutionary past. As proximate mechanisms, they are satisfying (and healthful) in their own right even when they don't lead to material benefits.

BUT AREN'T HUMANS DIFFERENT?

Humans are profoundly different from other animals in their use of language, their cognitive abilities, and their capacity for culture. These differences are often used to argue that evolutionary theory has little to say about humans, however relevant it might be to the rest of life. Ironically, our unique attributes might enable us to play the evolutionary game *better* than other species, especially when it comes to sophisticated behavioral strategies, altruistic or otherwise (Gintis et al., 2005; Hammerstein, 2003; Richerson & Boyd, 2004). The concept of inheritance in the Darwinian contest needs to be interpreted broadly. Any process that causes the most successful strategies to increase in frequency counts as an inheritance mechanism, including learning and imitation in addition to genetic inheritance. Nongenetic inheritance mechanisms enable humans to adapt rapidly to their environments, vastly accelerating the pace of evolution. Moreover, humans are like beavers in their ability to change their environments, especially when it comes to the parameters relevant to altruism. We have derived ways to create prosocial groups and to solve the problem of exploitation within groups in ways that are completely beyond the abilities of other species. These unique human attributes are better explained in terms of evolutionary theory than as a mysterious exception to the theory. Human uniqueness cannot be used to argue against the relevance of the evolutionary perspective.

EXPANDING ALTRUISM'S NICHE

Earlier, we stressed the need to distinguish the scientific study of altruism and health from the kind of moral encouragement, so common in everyday life, that altruism is good for the altruist. As an unconditional statement, this one is clearly false from an ecological and evolutionary perspective. However, it can be true as a conditional statement. *Given the right conditions*, altruism can be very good for the altruist, as our results show. Once we think of altruism as like a species, with a distribution and abundance, we can attempt to modify the environment to expand altruism's niche. This is not a new enterprise, and religions appear to be especially effective at creating environmental conditions favorable for altruism, at least among their own members. Scientists interested in altruism have much to learn from religion (see also Wilson, 2002, 2005). It will be interesting to see if the scientific study of altruism from an ecological perspective can expand altruism's niche still further.

We thank Jack Berry, Anne Clark, Katherine Laws, Lynn O'Conner, Stephen Post, Jeffrey Schloss, Elliott Sober, and Binghamton University's Evolutionary Studies Program for their considerable intellectual and logistic help. This research was supported by a grant from the Institute for Research on Unlimited Love.

REFERENCES

Csikszentmihalyi, M., & Schneider, B. (2000). *Becoming adult: How teenagers prepare for the world of work*. New York: Basic.

Gintis, H., et al. (Eds.). (2005). *Moral sentiments and material interests: The foundations of cooperation in economic life*. Cambridge, MA: MIT Press.

Hammerstein, P. (Ed.). (2003). *Genetic and cultural evolution of cooperation*. Cambridge, MA: MIT Press.

Kohlberg, L. (1984). *Essays on moral development: Vol. 2. The psychology of moral development*. San Francisco: Harper and Row.

Krebs, D. L. (1998). The evolution of moral behaviors. In C. Crawford and D. L. Krebs (Eds.), *Handbook of evolutionary psychology*, 337–368. Mahwah, NJ: Erlbaum.

Mealey, L. (1995). The sociobiology of sociopathy. *Behavioral and Brain Sciences*, *18*, 523–599.

Rand, A. (1961). *The virtue of selfishness*. New York: Signet.

Richerson, P. J., & Boyd, R. (2004). *Not by genes alone: How culture transformed human evolution*. Chicago: University of Chicago Press.

Sapolsky, R. M. (1998). *Why zebras don't get ulcers*. New York: Freeman.

Sober, E., & Wilson, D. S. (1998). *Unto others: The evolution and psychology of unselfish behavior*. Cambridge, MA: Harvard University Press.

Wilson, D. S. (2002). *Darwin's cathedral: Evolution, religion, and the nature of society*. Chicago: University of Chicago Press.

Wilson, D. S. (2005). Testing major evolutionary hypotheses about religion with a random sample. *Human Nature, 16*, 382–409.

Wilson, D. S., et al. (1996). Machiavellianism: A synthesis of the evolutionary and psychological literatures. *Psychological Bulletin, 199*, 285–299.

18 A Short Natural History
of Altruism and Healing

Christopher Boehm

The connections between altruism and health surely have deep evolutionary roots, and they appear to be many-faceted and complex. Here, we will examine, first, altruism in the form of medical practice and, later, altruism in the form of conflict management to determine the effect of such behaviors on the health of altruists and recipients alike.

In this chapter, the goal is to provide a basic evolutionary background for the various other studies in this book and also to experiment with alternative ways of explaining altruistic behavior. Painting with a rather large brush, I shall begin by exploring the natural history of healing, including altruistic healing.

MODELING OUR HUMAN ANCESTOR

What did the apes from which we descended do about needs for healing? Before the discovery of the double helix, all we could do was to speculate wildly about the behaviors of our distant ape ancestors in Africa, or of hominids and early humans. However, once DNA studies were made, it became clear that the four African great ape species (humans, bonobos, chimpanzees, and gorillas) form a unique clade whose members are closely related genetically.

A molecular clock told us that the four of us share an African ancestor who lived only about 7 million years ago, and in 1987 primatologist Richard Wrangham introduced a methodology for assessing the behaviors of this ape. He called it the common ancestor (CA), and triangulation was straightforward. Because natural selection tends to be a conservative process, and because major convergences by which two species accidentally acquire the same adaptation are statistically so rare, Wrangham (1987) decided that if all four of these species shared a pattern of behavior, it could then be attributed to the CA.

Some basic social traits that Wrangham arrived at in his experimental reconstruction were as follows: The CA lived in bounded groups; males stalked members of the same species; and females transferred to new groups at breeding time. This was a great deal to know socially about a previously mysterious ancestor, but in fact Wrangham's portrait just scratched the surface.

In *Hierarchy in the Forest*, I created a more extensive social and political portrait of the CA, which included social dominance hierarchies with alpha males; formation of coalitions within groups for a variety of purposes, including to restrict the dominance of the highest ranking individuals or to guard resources from conspecifics; spontaneous reconciliations between individuals after quarrels and fights; and impartial power interventions, by which powerful third parties stopped the fights of their inferiors (Boehm, 1999).

These power interventions that resolve conflicts are altruistic insofar as they are impartial and the beneficiaries are unrelated to the peacemaker. They impinge on the health of the parties involved, because there is a reduction of the kind of extreme and often protracted stress that damages immune systems. Making such interventions is not very costly, while the benefits to others can be very large—for instance, if wounding that could lead to death is prevented, or if extreme stress is avoided.

As for the practice of medicine per se, two other candidates for behaviors can be added to the ancestral repertoire we are discussing. One is self-medication, which of course is not altruistic, and the other is ministering to the wounds of others, which can be.

MEDICAL PRACTICES OF APES

One way that plants protect themselves against predation by herbivores is to develop secondary compounds that are toxic (Kuroda, 1997), but humans have found medicinal use for some of these compounds and the same goes for African great apes. For instance, bitter plant substances are ingested by gorillas and chimpanzees living in the Ndoki Forest (Kuroda, 1997), and medicinal use is very likely. One compound is extremely bitter, and it is also used by indigenous people in curing illness; another, like the first, is eaten nonnutritionally by the two ape species with the leaves being swallowed whole instead of being chewed.

In addition, the bonobos Kuroda studied in the Wamba Forest swallow these same leaves and others, so the apparent medicinal use of similar nonnutritive plants is found in these three apes and also among humans in Africa. On this basis, we may attribute a similar pattern of self-medication to the CA. It would appear that herbal medicine has a long natural history.

Apes are by no means the only nonhuman animals to use medicinal herbs found in their environment (see Rodriguez & Wrangham, 1993). Indeed, in Africa, humans have added important items to their herbal inventories by observing animals, such as porcupines, who eat herbs when they are showing obvious symptoms of being sick (Huffman, 2001). After a diseased porcupine demonstrated to a Tanzanian medicine man that a plant considered by villagers to be poisonous was medicinally useful, he introduced it as a new medicine that became part of his village's herbal lore.

The circumstantial evidence for the three apes' self-medicating is quite good, but for chimpanzees detailed investigations have produced much firmer conclusions than for the other two species. Michael Huffman has investigated their use of plants to control parasite loads, focusing on plants that clearly are not eaten for nutrition. For instance, the chimpanzees at Gombe and Mahale national parks sometimes eat the smaller leaves of the *Aspilia* plant in limited quantities early in the morning, and this is the only type of leaf that they swallow whole (Huffman & Wrangham, 1994; Wrangham & Goodall, 1989; Wrangham & Nishida, 1983). *Aspilia* is widely used in African cultures as a medicinal herb.

We know that wild chimpanzees carry substantial parasite loads as adults and that infants and juveniles, if they suffer a major shock (i.e., loss of their mother), will quickly develop serious parasite loads that distend their stomachs and that half the time will kill them within a year (Goodall, 1986). In comparison, adult captive chimpanzees whose stomachs are parasite-free tend to have much larger bodies and significantly greater longevity than wild adults.

Huffman (2001) has evidence from the Mahale field site in Tanzania that infestation by a specific nodular worm (*Oesophagostomum stephanostomum*) is correlated with bitter-pith chewing among the apes there. And at Gombe, correlations have been made between ingesting *Vernonia amygdalina*, hypothesized to be a medicinal plant, and obvious improvements in health. Controlling all of the variables needed to verify medicinal effects obviously poses a challenge when the individuals under study are ranging free, but there is some good quantitative evidence.

Chewing the pith of this last plant has been observed at a number of field sites, and it is of interest that the chimpanzees "meticulously remove the outer bark and leaves to chew on the exposed pith, from which they extract extremely bitter juice and residual amounts of fiber" (Huffman, 2001, p. 655). Chemical analysis shows that the Mahale chimpanzees are avoiding toxic parts of the plant.

The intricacy and apparent rationality of the extraction process suggest that the practice is largely socially learned, as a tradition that is applied only when individuals feel malaise. Healthy-seeming adults in the vicinity do not eat the pith, and the assumption is that they are not feeling similar symptoms. With respect to social learning, it is of interest that infants may sample the residue when their mothers are ill and then discard part of the plant.

Eating this plant at Mahale occurs mainly during the rainy season. Markers for ill health include diarrhea, lethargy, weight loss, and other obvious signs of nematode infection. In two cases, recovery took place within a day after self-medication. In one case, fecal analysis showed that parasite eggs per gram dropped from 130 to 15 in 20 hours. However, loads of other parasites were not affected by this particular type of self-medication (Huffman, 2001; see also Huffman & Siefu, 1989).

To further support Huffman's conclusions, there are indigenous human groups in Africa that use the same plant for amoebic dysentery and for several intestinal parasites. It is also used by people to reduce parasitic infections in domesticated swine.

When great apes swallow leaves of plants whole, this practice is associated only with self-medication—as opposed to normal leaf eating, where leaves are always chewed (Huffman, 2001). When the same worms described above were found in 4% of 254 dung samples in a Mahale study group, the donors displayed symptoms of malaise and diarrhea. Over a 2-year period, 6 of 9 dung samples with worms also contained whole undigested leaves of *A. mossambicensis*, *Tremata orientalis*, or *Aneilema acquinoctiale*. This leaf-eating practice is correlated with diminution of *O. stephanostomum* loads, which becomes apparent toward the end of the rainy season.

An infected individual may engage in both bitter-pith eating and leaf-swallowing in the same day, and it seems possible that the two medicines may combine synergistically; however, they still affect only this one type of parasite (Huffman, 2001). At a Ugandan field site, Kibale, Wrangham (1995; see also Ashford et al., 2000) found that whole-leaf ingestion also increased the chances of expelling tapeworms. Wrangham hypothesized that stomach discomfort was the proximate mechanism that triggered whole-leaf swallowing and that the leaves relieved this symptomatic discomfort while also addressing the cause if susceptible parasites were involved.

It is because the hypotheses about chimpanzees are so well supported and because the nonnutritive eating of bitter pith and whole leaves is so similar in bonobos and gorillas that we may assume self-medication to have definitely been an ancestral practice. Although so far we are not dealing with altruism in this background discussion, it is clear that taking active measures involving self-medication has a deep natural history and that human nature may be oriented in the direction of active medical treatment.

We have now established that self-medication goes back 7 million years, as a nonaltruistic ancestral behavior. We now turn to the question of helping others medically, which would have to be either nepotistic or altruistic, depending on the relationship between the person in need and the helper.

MEDICALLY ORIENTED HELPING

Did the CA practice altruistic medicine? Many highly social species seem to make allowances for sickly others (see Trivers, 1971), including cetaceans (Caldwell & Caldwell, 1966) and social carnivores and great apes (Fabrega, 1997). Some typical adjustments include allowances in travel speed and food sharing.

The information available for medical helping behavior among African apes is very sparse, but one altruistic practice of wild chimpanzees is worth noting, with respect to wounds they sometimes receive in their frequent fights within the group. Chimpanzees at Gombe not only clean their own wounds but clean the wounds of others when they are in places where the injured chimpanzee can't reach them (Goodall, 1986). Because these ministrations do have slight immediate costs, in terms of energy and loss of feeding activity, they may be counted as being altruistic when nonrelatives are the recipients.

There are also some really major altruistic donations that may be classified as health related. When I was studying wild chimpanzees at Gombe in the late 1980s, the study group experienced an upper-respiratory epidemic, and several infants were orphaned. One, Mel, was co-adopted by a juvenile male, Pax, who also had been orphaned and was raised by his older brother and an adolescent male, Spindle, who had no other living kin. Their reproductively costly donations to this unrelated orphan, who was weakened by a heavy parasite load that distended his stomach and made him thin and feeble, were substantial. They lost time feeding while waiting for him to travel with them, and often they carried him on their backs. This was energetically quite costly, especially for Pax, whose own growth had been stunted due to being orphaned.

This aid was not specifically medical, in the sense that wound licking is, but it illustrates nicely the capacity of chimpanzees to understand the weakened condition of others and to help them out. The fact that both of Mel's saviors were nonrelatives makes their donations significant cases of genetic altruism, since there was no likelihood of his repaying them.

The Gombe chimpanzees are so well studied that we have several other adoption-by-a-nonrelative case histories (see Goodall, 1986). Gorillas are capable of giving similar help, as shown by the well-publicized female who took care of a human child who fell into her zoo enclosure and was knocked unconscious. In the wild, Dian Fossey (1983) reported an infant's losing both parents, one being the silverback, at age 3. A young male, who temporarily led the group, groomed the wounded orphan and also, being in control, slowed the group's travel to accommodate the orphan's weakened condition.

Kano (1992) reports neither orphans nor sick or wounded individuals in his pioneering bonobo field study. However, on the assumption that adequate study time would reveal similar helping behavior in bonobos, we may assume our CA to have been a creature who perceived the practical needs of others who were suffering disadvantages of health and who would do something about it.

ALTERNATIVES TO GROUP SELECTION

The question is, how could natural selection support such unselfish behavior when it benefits genetic competitors in the same group? As we turn to humans and to the relationship between altruism and health in our own species, we'll need to further define our terms with respect to altruistic acts and the mechanisms that might support such behavior.

The basic paradox of genetic altruism is well known in evolutionary biological circles (see E. O. Wilson, 1975), and attempts to explain helping behavior that is extended to nonrelatives (e.g., Boehm 1981, 1997; Simon, 1990; Sober & Wilson, 1998; Wilson & Sober, 1994) are now leading to some serious reconsideration of how natural selection works. The contentious issue of group selection has dominated past debate about the possibility of genetic altruism, but there are several other models that could explain self-sacrificial helping.

Group Selection

Group selection models (see Wilson & Sober, 1994) explain altruism as the result of evolutionarily efficient mechanisms, by which benefits to trait groups are sufficiently robust that the individual losses of altruists within groups are more than compensated by benefits that accrue to the groups. Elsewhere (Boehm, 1997), I have made the case that, compared to other social mammals, humans living in small egalitarian bands were unusually good candidates for group selection. This is because within bands, phenotypic variation was damped by egalitarian cultural practices, while free-riders' advantages were seriously eroded or nullified by moralistic social control that punished cheaters and thieves. This would have substantially changed the balance of power between within-group selection and between-group selection.

There's more. Whenever a small Pleistocene hunting band depended on large game for its nutrition, it had to have at least five or six active hunters if it was to make it through hard times when game intake became sporadic (see Smith, 1988; Winterhalder, 1986). A sizable cooperative hunting team was necessary to reduce week-to-week variance in the meat supply. Thus, another factor favoring group selection was the extreme interdependence of band members, for they tended to survive or starve as an entire foraging unit (Boehm, 2002).

The social and foraging policies of entire bands were bound to vary, and this variation also provided grist for the group-selection mill. A band that made better decisions about hunting would outclass one that didn't, and an egalitarian band that shared its meat evenly would outclass ones that couldn't get rid of their alpha males (Boehm, 2000). Finally, a band that assisted hunters when they were injured or ill would have a better chance of keeping a large enough hunting team in the field to keep nutritious meat coming in regularly, whereas one that didn't might experience famine, or worse.

Extending Kin Benefits to Nonkin

Independent of group selection, there is a piggybacking model (e.g., Boehm, 1981; Wright, 1994) which holds that a helping behavior which is very helpful to kin might simply "spill over" to nonkin. Take a behavior such as intervening in conflicts, which assists close kin greatly at little expense to the donor. In practice, this helping behavior readily becomes extended to nonkin, and this can be explained in terms of piggybacking (Boehm, 1981). As long as the donor is reaping greater fitness rewards from helping kin than he is losing fitness when helping nonkin, the one gene supporting both behaviors can stay in place. This model requires a further assumption, namely that, for some mechanical reason, natural selection simply is not efficient enough to get rid of the second, self-sacrificial aspect of the behavior.

Here's another example of such "slippage." Chimpanzee mothers will fiercely defend their offspring if an attack comes, and this makes perfectly good sense as a nepotistic investment. But then we have the time at Gombe that adult sterile female Gigi drew an infuriated bushpig away from adolescent male Freud (see Goodall, 1971) when the counterattacking adult bushpig was about to kill him during a pig hunt. Gigi was not related to Freud, but she had played "aunt" to many of the young of her group. It could have been her prior bonds with Freud that impelled her to this very risky and patently altruistic action.

My point is this: If the proximate mechanism through which natural selection sets up individuals to help their close kin is spatial proximity, which leads to close social bonding (see Wright, 1994), this allows for some slippage because sometimes similar bonds are formed with nonkin in the same group. The help given to kin is nepotistic, in perfect accordance with inclusive fitness. The help given to nonkin is altruistic, but group selection is not needed to explain it. It is subsidized by nepotistic gains made by the same donor.

Docility Leads to Altruism

The third model involves Herbert Simon's (1990) explanation of cultural docility, which is somewhat similar. Simon considers genes that make humans docile, in the sense that we readily learn (and internalize) the rules and values of our groups. They bring enormous individual fitness benefits, which stem from being a good citizen. However, this innate tendency to absorb rules also makes it possible for the group to send out altruistic messages which encourage individuals to sacrifice their own fitness for the welfare of the group as a whole—as in being cooperative, or making generous contributions of food to the needy. When individuals receive these messages, they often are influenced to act against their own inclusive fitness.

This, too, amounts to genetic piggybacking. The assumption is that, overall, being culturally docile brings a large net benefit to individuals because consequently they readily behave themselves. It's true that docility also can incur some modest fitness costs, but the benefits easily subsidize the costs. Again, the assumption is that natural selection simply isn't clever enough to get rid of the docility effects that lead to altruism.

A Social Control Model

There's also a fourth, cultural model, which takes social punishment into account. Boyd and Richerson (1992) point out that sometimes cooperative behavior is coerced: If you don't behave this way, your group will punish you. Such altruism is motivated by fear, not compassion, and genetically it has a deleterious effect on individual fitness at the same time that it contributes to group fitness.

An Intrinsic Reward Model

A new model, which is emerging from this book, makes any emotionally satisfying act of altruism easier to explain. The hypothesis is that behaving helpfully brings positive feelings that improve the helper's health, and thereby behaving helpfully assists fitness.

With these five theories in mind, we'll turn to the shamanistic practices of mobile foragers living today, who present us with reasonable models for what was taking place 40,000–50,000 years ago.

SHAMANS AS ALTRUISTIC HEALERS

Human hunter-gatherers experience copious problems with their health, and many bands have individuals who use supernatural connections to assist the unhealthy. The term generally used for such individuals is "shaman," and often they enter trance states as part of their medical curing practice. They also tend to deal in herbal remedies.

Fabrega (1997) has broadly discussed the natural history of healing, and I believe him to be in error in one important respect which has to do with shamans. Fabrega believes that hunter-gatherers live in "family groups" and that basically there are no specialist medical practitioners because larger social groups are not salient. In his view, every family has its own "medicine man." The problem lies in the fact that nomadic hunter-gatherers basically live in bands with numerous families, some of which are unrelated (see Kelly, 1995; Knauft, 1991).

To be certain that Fabrega (1997) is in error about the near-absence of medical specialists, I surveyed a number of Late Pleistocene–type extant hunting societies with this in mind. Among these nomads, shamanistic specializations are very widely distributed, ranging from the Arctic (e.g., Balikci, 1963; Borré, 1994; Fletcher, 1997; Hutton, 2001; Michael, 1963; Mikhailowskii, 1894; Murphy, 1964; Popov, 1968; Rasmussen, 1929; Thalbitzer, 1931; Turner, 1989; Yamada, 1997) to Aboriginal Australia (e.g., Akerman, 1979; Cawte, 1974; Elkin, 1977; Gould, 1969; Smythe, 1984; Spencer & Gillen, 1927; Warner, 1958) to Africa (Katz, 1976, 1982; Marshall, 1969; Sawada, 1997; Woodburn, 1959) and North and South America (e.g., Dobrizhoffer, 1822; Feit, 1997; Handleman, 1967; Henry, 1941; Hoebel, 1940; Hultkrantz, 1992; Kelly, 1978; La Flesche, 1925; Landes, 1937; Levi, 1978; Linton, 1935; Loeb, 1926; Opler, 1947; Ray, 1963; Spott & Kroeber, 1942).

It is of interest that shamanistic practices also continued among hunter-gatherers after they sedentarized in Japan (Atuy, 1997; Ikeya, 1997; Irimoto, 1997; Obayashi, 1997; Ohnuki-Tierney, 1980) and on the American Northwest Coast (Amoss, 1978; Barbeau, 1958; Eells, 1889; Haeberlin, 1918; Park, 1938). Furthermore, shamans are found widely in tribal horticulturist societies (e.g., Chagnon, 1983) and in peasant societies. They also may exist in urban contexts.

Given this sampling of the field studies, I shall make some tentative generalizations in the discussion that follows. In doing so, I must acknowledge that there is considerable cultural diversity in this type of medical practice, but at the same time I emphasize that there are definitely some universal features to be found (see Dow, 1986; Harner, 1990; Kleinman, 1980; Marshall, 2003).

There can be wide variation in the types of spiritual connections, in specific practices, and in the degree to which herbal remedies are used, but basically a group's shamans are specialists in healing—in both supernatural and "practical" ways. The social role expectation is that the shaman is an altruistic helper, and most are, although in some cases they expect to be rewarded for their services. However, this altruistic dimension depends heavily on the individual shaman's personality. For instance, Balikci (1970) reports a cunning shaman's manipulating supplicants to gain sexual favors, and the vast literature I cited above has numerous examples of shamans using their powers to harm enemies or, sometimes, to dominate their peers (see Boehm, 1993).

Basically, though, as gifted specialists, shamans perform valuable services for all members of their groups. I emphasize that, in the case of nomadic bands which are typical of prehistoric foragers, these predictably contain unrelated families, and this makes some of the shamans' work altruistic.

Because shamans work by means of supernatural agencies, one might question their realistic effect as curers. However, there are two things that affirm the efficacy of their medical practice. One is that they obviously help at the level of psychosomatic medicine, by providing a sense of support and confidence. The other is that they often practice herbalism as well.

· Herbal curing is not regularly described in comparison with shamanism, which invariably captures the anthropological imagination. However, we do have various reports from Africa (e.g., Shostak, 1983), Australia (e.g., Blainey, 1976), Asia (e.g., Peterson, 1978), and North America (e.g., Llewellyn & Hoebel, 1941). In the last work cited, learning herbal lore is included in a Cheyenne shaman's training, and we may assume that this combination of skills is widespread.

SHAMANISTIC ALTRUISM

Which of our evolutionary models fits best with this shamanistic type of helping behavior? First, where gifts are given to shamans, Trivers's (1971) reciprocal altruism model explains the behavior as being essentially selfish, genetically. Where shamans are not at all self-seeking, and where they help relatives and nonrelatives alike, the help to nonkin might be explained by group selection's having operated in the Pleistocene. In this connection, the psychosomatic and herbal benefits of shamanistic curing would have helped significantly to maintain the size and vitality of hunting groups, while the individual practitioner's costs would have been fairly negligible.

Our first piggybacking model offers an alternative selection scenario. Assume that shamanistic medical assistance using séances and herbs helps kin and that the proximate mechanism that motivates such help is social bonding. It is natural to extend these services from kin to nonkin if the nonkin are friendly members of the same band. The genetic piggybacking assumption is that a shaman's inclusive fitness will gain so much from helping kin that the slight losses in helping nonkin will be readily sustained.

Next, we have Simon's model. If shamans are good cultural learners, their docility will lead them to accept the cultural definition of shamans as altruistic helpers. This curbs their selfish and nepotistic tendencies, and as a result they help nonkin as well as kin. The genetic costs of their doing so are offset by the very large benefits accrued from being docile.

Then, there's the cultural issue of coercive social control. An individual may well be inclined to seek selfish gain, and even political dominance, in performing shamanistically. However, because his group will punish him if he acts too selfishly, out of fear he conforms to its expectations and behaves as an altruist. There are, in fact, Inuit, Australian, and California Indian cases of extremely selfish shamans being executed (see Boehm, 1993), so this fourth model helps to explain the appearance of altruism in shamanistic practice when a shaman has strong selfish tendencies.

Finally, we have the now-developing intrinsic reward theory to help us further in explaining the altruism of shamans. Here, we're talking about the satisfaction that comes from helping another human being in a life-threatening situation and the health benefits that accrue to the helper.

We now have five rather different ways of explaining the altruism of shamans, but we are not obliged to choose among the models for, in any given instance, all could be working in unison. The problem with relying solely on group selection models is that this level of selection is likely to operate quite weakly in comparison with the selection taking place within groups. However, any or all of these other effects could be helping group selection along.

By combining these five models, we have the possibility that sometimes what are taken to be self-sacrificial helping behaviors in effect are cost-free, and therefore are selectively neutral rather than being altruistically costly. If that is the case, even weak group selection effects must be taken very seriously (see Sober & Wilson, 1998), as forces that can help to shape human nature.

ALTRUISTIC STRESS REDUCTION

We now turn to a very different type of altruistic behavior, which also has an effect on health. This combines conflict intervention and conflict resolution, behaviors that are prominent among nomadic hunter-gatherers and also are found in the three great apes that live in Africa.

When two chimpanzees, bonobos, gorillas, or humans fight, if they are bonded members of the same group they are likely to reconcile afterward through some form of bodily contact. This contact visibly eases tensions between the two (see de Waal, 1996), and we may count it as a selfish or genetically egoistic behavior in the sense that both parties should have potentially unhealthy tensions erased.

In less-tractable fights, a higher-ranking individual intervenes because the fight seems to be escalating. Our descriptions of this behavior in bonobos are sketchy (e.g., Kano, 1992), but silverback gorillas routinely use a "disciplinary" pig-grunt (Fossey, 1983), and chimpanzee alpha males display aggressively, straight at the protagonists, or employ a number of other tactics to fulfill the same strategy, which is to stop the fight and keep the adversaries separated until their hostile feelings die down (see Boehm, 1994; de Waal, 1982).

It is this third-party intervention behavior that I believe involves altruism. The physical benefits are palpable: Individuals fighting can be wounded and can die from infections afterward. If not so readily measurable, the psychosomatic benefits are obvious enough: A serious fight creates very high immediate stress levels, and the more serious it is, the more likely it is that future meetings between the pair will result in further fighting and stress. Protracted stress will also affect other group members, and I have suggested that humans are evolved to be conflict aversive as a result (Boehm, 1999, 2000).

In considering the more immediate psychological motives that spur these third-party mediators into action, there would appear to be two main considerations. One is that the individuals involved could hurt each other, so protective feelings would be activated. The other is that the conflict per se is sufficiently irritating that the individual who is powerful enough to stop it does so in order to improve the overall quality of social life in his group—which reduces his own stress.

Conflict interventions are definitely altruistic in chimpanzees, insofar as the high-ranking individual who intervenes (usually the alpha) is impartial in his intervention strategy: He favors neither kin nor allies, victims nor aggressors (see Boehm, 1994; de Waal, 1982). Although because of high rank there is little chance of his being wounded, the charging display is a drain on energy, and, in the wild, often fight stopping takes time away from feeding. As a partial compensation, the intervention reinforces his high status, but I would still judge it to incur some net costs to fitness, making it altruistic.

That the intention is to make peace is clear from the fact that a number of different tactics are used, including charging, prying apart, and herding the adversaries in different directions in order to stop a conflict. This is also clear from the fact that the peacemaker monitors the situation once the adversaries have separated to make sure that they don't resume the conflict. When a chimpanzee peacemaker is confident they have calmed down, he often leaves the scene.

Chimpanzees actually seem to recognize the value of this role behavior, for in captivity de Waal (1996) has documented a case in which a female coalition supported a male's ambition to be alpha—but his rival, whom they opposed, won the contest. Even so, they refused to let this new alpha mediate their conflicts, and they would attack him if he tried. Instead, they permitted their losing alpha candidate to perform this valuable service for them. More broadly, de Waal (1996) speaks of "community concern," suggesting that, as individuals, captive chimpanzees are concerned about conflict and the problems it raises and are prone to become active in addressing this problem.

Conflict interventions in bonobos and gorillas are not nearly as well studied, but it would appear that impartial strategies may prevail there, as well. One reason for this is that if you intervene on behalf of one party, it may become emboldened because of the support and redouble its efforts to attack. This negates the intention of peacemaking.

Nomadic hunter-gatherers know that they cannot rely on their "leaders" to intervene, because they regularly suppress any strong leadership or authority (see Boehm, 1993). However, they do show community concern. Precisely because they can't forcefully stop escalating fights once they become intense, they work hard to head off conflicts before they escalate. Humans explicitly acknowledge the need for evenhanded approaches. They employ persuasion, distraction, and preaching in favor of harmony (see Fry, 2000), along with staging duels that allow adversaries to express some of their aggression in a structured context that will inhibit escalation. It is of interest that when foragers try to resolve conflicts, they are very likely to set aside considerations of right and wrong and ask the parties to split their differences in the name of group harmony—even if one is more the culprit than the other. This amounts to impartiality of the type that is so well documented for chimpanzees.

Humans, like the three other African apes, are innately aversive to conflict. We manifest this by "massaging" conflicts and sometimes by restraining the adversaries physically. One proximate mechanism that helps to trigger these practical measures surely is a rising stress level experienced by third parties, as they are exposed to angry words—and as they see their fellows about to harm each other. As empathetic beings, it is predictable that they would want to protect the individuals, and as individuals who are evolved to avoid unhealthy levels of stress, it is predictable that they would also seek to terminate this extreme type of disruption.

The role of stress in causing unhealthy levels of cortisol activity is well documented in a variety of problem areas (e.g., Chrousos & Gold, 1992; Gold & Chrousos, 2002; Shanks et al., 1998), and studies have shown that noise-induced cortisol increases can pose health problems (Spreng, 2000). Hunter-gatherer band life tends to be generally tranquil with occasional minor disagreements (e.g., Lee, 1979; Thomas, 1959), but when a major conflict is ongoing, people tend to take sides, arguments become loud, and the overall stress becomes great. This includes both irritatingly noisy quarrels and also exposure to angry, hostile feelings that poison a band's social relations.

In the absence of effective intervention, the consequence is that either the group must endure continually high rates of stress, or else the band has to split so the two sides can completely avoid each other (see Knauft, 1991). The first is bad for everyone's health, while fissioning can create two small bands that may experience difficulties in making a living because of too few hunters.

If we consider active peacemaking in the light of exactly how altruistic it is, certain individuals put much more energy and time into this activity than do others, and the main beneficiaries are the disputants. As with shamanism, a cost-benefit ledger based on our first four selection models must be adjusted to include the fifth model: This involves the health benefits that peacemakers gain simply from the experience of being helpful. This applies not only when individuals help to manage conflicts, but when collective intervention takes place and succeeds. We must assume that such benefits redound to all of the participants when their collective peacemaking is effective.

CONCLUSIONS

In thinking about how altruistic behaviors like medical healing and third-party conflict management could have been sustained over evolutionary time, it is clear that these behaviors are very complex and that they have been held in place not only by group selection forces, which were likely to be modest, but by inclusive fitness effects when they became involved with two types of genetic piggybacking. Sometimes social control, as a cultural force, shaped behavior in altruistic directions as well. And then there could have been automatic health benefits that were built into behaving altruistically, which provided altruism with a significant head start.

Thus, the roots of genetic altruism that affect health are not only ancient, but by definition they are heavily involved with our evolved human nature. It is for this reason that both the healing of others and the mediation of conflicts are found universally among hunter-gatherers, and they also are found in more modern societies. We are evolved to be altruistic in these ways, and our altruism impinges significantly on our own health and that of others.

The evolution of altruism has been controversial in evolutionary biology, largely because group selection theory has been overworked as a supposedly necessary agent for true genetic altruism to persist. Here, in an attempt to widen the discussion, I have looked to other paradigms, in the form of genetic piggybacking and social control, and also to the hypotheses developed elsewhere in this book, which hold that altruists automatically improve their own health.

If altruistic acts, in and of themselves, bring health benefits to the donors, then this could greatly reduce the burden of other paradigms for explaining the persistence of altruistic traits in the gene pools of our species.

REFERENCES

Akerman, K. 1979 Contemporary Aboriginal Healers in the South Kimberley. Oceana 50:23–30.

Amoss, P. 1978 Coast Salish Spirit Dancing: The Survival of an Ancestral Religion. Seattle: University of Washington Press.

Ashford, R. W., G. D. Reid, & R. W. Wrangham. 2000 Intestinal Parasites of the Chimpanzee *Pan Troglodytes* in Kibale Forest, Uganda. Annals of Tropical Medicine and Parasitology 94:173–179.

Atuy, M. T. 1997 Coexistence With Nature and the "Third Philosophy": Learning From the Spirit of the Ainu. *In* Circumpolar Animism and Shamanism. T. Yamada & T. Irimoto, eds. Pp. 3–7. Sapporo, Japan: Hokkaido University Press.

Balikci, A. 1963 Shamanistic Behavior Among the Netsilik Eskimos. Southwestern Journal of Anthropology 16:380–396.

Balikci, A. 1970 The Netsilik Eskimo. Garden City, NY: Natural History Press.

Barbeau, M. 1958 Medicine-Men on the North Pacific Coast. National Museum of Canada Bulletin No. 152 (Anthropological Series No. 42). Ottawa: Department of Northern Affairs and National Resources.

Blainey, G. 1976 Triumph of the Nomads: A History of Aboriginal Australia. Woodstock, NY: Overlook.

Boehm, C. 1981 Parasitic Selection and Group Selection: A Study of Conflict Interference in Rhesus and Japanese Macaque Monkeys. *In* Primate Behavior and Sociobiology. A. B. Chiarelli & R. S. Corruccini, eds. Pp. 161–182. New York: Springer-Verlag.

Boehm, C. 1993 Egalitarian Society and Reverse Dominance Hierarchy. Current Anthropology 34:227–254.

Boehm, C. 1994 Pacifying Interventions at Arnhem Zoo and Gombe. *In* Chimpanzee Cultures. R. W. Wrangham, W. C. McGrew, F. B. M. de Waal, & P. G. Heltne, eds. Pp. 211–226. Cambridge, MA: Harvard University Press.

Boehm, C. 1997 Impact of the Human Egalitarian Syndrome on Darwinian Selection Mechanics. American Naturalist 150:100–121.

Boehm, C. 1999 Hierarchy in the Forest: The Evolution of Egalitarian Behavior. Cambridge, MA: Harvard University Press.

Boehm, C. 2000 Conflict and the Evolution of Social Control. Journal of Consciousness Studies 7:79–183. Special issue on Evolutionary Origins of Morality. L. Katz, ed.

Boehm, C. 2002 Variance Reduction and the Evolution of Social Control. Paper presented at Santa Fe Institute, 5th Annual Workshop on the Co-Evolution of Behaviors and Institutions, Santa Fe, NM.

Borré, K. 1994 The Healing Power of the Seal: The Meaning of Inuit Health Practice and Belief. Arctic Anthropology 31:1–15.

Boyd, R., & P. J. Richerson. 1992 Punishment Allows the Evolution of Cooperation (or Anything Else) in Sizable Groups. Ethology and Sociobiology 13:171–195.

Caldwell, M. C., & D. K. Caldwell. 1966 Epimeletic (Caregiving) Behavior in Cetacean Whales, Dolphins and Porpoises. *In* Whales, Dolphins, and Porpoises: International Symposium on Cetation Research. K. S. Norris, ed. Pp. 755–785. Berkeley: University of California Press.

Cawte, J. 1974 Medicine Is the Law: Studies in Psychiatric Anthropology of Australian Tribal Societies. Honolulu: University Press of Hawaii.

Chagnon, N. 1983 Yanomamo: The Fierce People. New York: Holt, Rinehart and Winston.

Chrousos, G. P., & P. W. Gold. 1992 The Concepts of Stress System Disorders: Overview of Behavioral and Physical Homeostasis. Journal of the American Medical Association 267:1244–1252.

de Waal, F. 1982 Chimpanzee Politics: Power and Sex Among Apes. New York: Harper and Row.

de Waal, F. 1996 Good Natured: The Origins of Right and Wrong in Humans and Other Animals. Cambridge, MA: Harvard University Press.

Dobrizhoffer, M. 1822 An Account of the Abipones, an Equestrian People of Paraguay, in Three Volumes. Vol. 2. London: John Murray.

Dow, J. 1986 Universal Aspects of Symbolic Healing: A Theoretical Synthesis. American Anthropologist 88:56–69.

Eells, M. 1889 The Twana, Chemakum, and Klallam Indians, of Washington Territory. Annual Report of the Smithsonian Institution for Year Ending 1887. Pt. 1, pp. 605–681. Washington, DC: Smithsonian Institution Press.

Elkin, A. P. 1977 Aboriginal Men of High Degree. New York: St. Martin's.

Fabrega, H. 1997 Earliest Phases in the Evolution of Sickness and Healing. Medical Anthropology Quarterly 11:26–55.

Feit, H. A. 1997 Spiritual Power and Everyday Lives: James Bay Cree Shaking Tent Performers and Their Audiences. *In* Circumpolar Animism and Shamanism. T. Yamada & T. Irimoto, eds. Pp. 121–150. Sapporo, Japan: Hokkaido University Press.

Fletcher, C. M. 1997 Spirit Work: Nunavimmiut Experiences of Affliction and Healing. Inuit Studies 21:189–208.

Fossey, D. 1983 Gorillas in the Mist. Boston: Houghton-Mifflin.

Fry, D. P. 2000 Conflict Management in Cross-Cultural Perspective. *In* Natural Conflict Resolution. F. Aureli & F. B. M. de Waal, eds. Pp. 334–351. Berkeley: University of California Press.

Gold, P. W., & G. P. Chrousos. 2002 Organization of the Stress System and Its Dysregulation in Melancholic and Atypical Depression: High vs. Low. Molecular Psychiatry 7:254–275.

Goodall, J. 1971 In the Shadow of Man. Boston: Houghton-Mifflin.

Goodall, J. 1986 The Chimpanzees of Gombe: Patterns of Behavior. Cambridge, MA: Belknap.

Gould, R. A. 1969 Yiwara: Foragers of the Australian Desert. New York: Scribner's.

Haeberlin, H. K. 1918 SBeTeTDA'Q: A Shamanistic Performance of the Coast Salish. American Anthropologist 20:249–257.

Handleman, D. 1967 The Development of the Washo Shaman. Ethnology 6:444–464.

Harner, M. J. 1990 The Way of the Shaman. 3rd ed. San Francisco: Harper & Row.

Henry, J. 1941 The Jungle People. Locust Valley, NY: Ausgustin.

Hoebel, B. A. 1940 The Political Organization and Law-Ways of the Comanche Indians. Memoirs of the American Anthropological Association, No. 54.

Huffman, M. A. 2001 Self-Medicative Behavior in the African Great Apes: An Evolutionary Perspective Into the Origins of Human Traditional Medicine. Bioscience 51:651–661.

Huffman, M. A., & M. Siefu. 1989 Observations on the Illness and Consumption of a Possibly Medicinal Plant *Vernonia Amygdalina* by a Wild Chimpanzee in the Mahale Mountains National Park, Tanzania. Primates 30:51–63.

Huffman, M. A., & R. W. Wrangham. 1994 Diversity of Medicinal Plant Use in Wild Chimpanzees. *In* Chimpanzee Cultures. R. W. Wrangham, W. C. McGrew, F. B. de Waal, & P. G. Heltne, eds. Pp. 1–18. Cambridge, MA: Harvard University Press.

Hultkrantz, Å. 1992 Shamanic Healing and Ritual Drama: Health and Medicine in Native North American Religious Traditions. New York: Crossroad.

Hutton, R. 2001 Shamans: Siberian Spirituality and the Western Imagination. London: Hambledon and London.

Ikeya, K. 1997 Bear Rituals of the Matagi and the Ainu in Northeastern Japan. *In* Circumpolar Animism and Shamanism. T. Yamada & T. Irimoto, eds. Pp. 55–63. Sapporo, Japan: Hokkaido University Press.

Irimoto, T. 1997 Ainu Shamanism: Oral Tradition, Healing, and Dramas. *In* Circumpolar Animism and Shamanism. T. Yamada & T. Irimoto, eds. Pp. 21–46. Sapporo, Japan: Hokkaido University Press.

Kano, T. 1992 The Last Ape: Pygmy Chimpanzee Behavior and Ecology. Stanford, CA: Stanford University Press.

Katz, R. 1976 Education for Transcendence: !Kia-Healing with the Kalahari !Kung. *In* Kalahari Hunter-Gatherers: Studies of the !Kung San and Their Neighbors. R. B. Lee & I. DeVore, eds. Pp. 281–301. Cambridge, MA: Harvard University Press.

Katz, R. 1982 Boiling Energy: Community Healing Among the Kalahari Kung. Cambridge, MA: Harvard University Press.

Kelly, I. 1978 Coast Miwok. *In* Handbook of North American Indians, Vol. 8, California. R. F. Heizer, vol. ed., W. C. Sturtevant, gen. ed. Pp. 414–425. Washington, DC: Smithsonian Institution Press.

Kelly, R. L. 1995 The Foraging Spectrum: Diversity in Hunter-Gatherer Lifeways. Washington, DC: Smithsonian Institution Press.

Kleinman, A. 1980 Patients and Healers in the Context of Culture. Berkeley: University of California Press.

Knauft, B. M. 1991 Violence and Sociality in Human Evolution. Current Anthropology 32:391–428.

Kuroda, S. 1997 Possible Use of Medicinal Plants by Western Lowland Gorillas (*G. g. gorilla*) and Tschego Chimpanzees (*Pan t. troglodytes*) in the Ndoki Forest, and Pygmy Chimpanzees (*P. paniscus*) in Wamba. *In* Proceedings of the Sixth International Symposium on Traditional Medicine in Toyama, pp. 155–162. Shiga: University of Shiga Prefecture.

La Flesche, F. 1925 The Osage Tribe: The Rite of Vigil. Bureau of American Ethnology, Thirty-ninth Annual Report, 1917–1918. Pp. 31–630. Washington, DC: Smithsonian Institution.

Landes, R. 1937 The Ojibwa of Canada: Cooperation and Competition Among Primitive Peoples. M. Mead, ed. Pp. 87–126. New York and London: McGraw-Hill.

Lee, R. B. 1979 The !Kung San: Men, Women and Work in a Foraging Society. New York: Cambridge University Press.

Levi, J. M. 1978 Wii'ipay: The Living Rocks: Ethnographic Notes on Crystal Magic Among Some California Yumans. Journal of California Anthropology 5:42–52.

Linton, R. 1935 The Comanche Sun Dance. American Anthropologist 37:420–428.

Llewellyn, K. N., & E. A. Hoebel. 1941 The Cheyenne Way: Conflict and Case Law in Primitive Jurisprudence. Norman: University of Oklahoma Press.

Loeb, E. M. 1926 Pomo Folkways. University of California Publications in American Archaeology and Ethnology 19:149–405.

Marshall, L. 1969 The Medicine Dance of the !Kung Bushmen. Africa 39:347–381.

Marshall, M. 2003 Healing the Body, Healing the Spirit, Healing the Community. Reviews in Anthropology 32:315–325.

Michael, H. N., ed. 1963 Studies in Siberian Shamanism. Anthropology of the North: Translations From Russian Sources, No. 4. Toronto: University of Toronto Press.

Mikhailowskii, V. M. 1894 Shamanism in Siberia and European Russia. Journal of the Royal Anthropological Institute of Great Britain and Ireland 24:62–100, 126–158. Translated from the Russian original, published 1892.

Murphy, J. M. 1964 Psychotherapeutic Aspects of Shamanism on St. Lawrence Island, Alaska. *In* Magic, Faith, Healing. Ari Kiev, ed. New York: Free Press.

Obayashi, T. 1997 The Ainu Concept of the Soul. *In* Circumpolar Animism and Shamanism. T. Yamada & T. Irimoto, eds. Pp. 9–20. Sapporo, Japan: Hokkaido University Press.

Ohnuki-Tierney, E. 1980 Shamans and Imu: Among Two Ainu Groups. Ethos 8:204–228.

Opler, M. E. 1947 Notes on Chiricahua Apache Culture 1: Supernatural Power and Shamanism. Primitive Man 20:1–14.

Park, W. Z. 1938 Shamanism in Western North America: A Study of Cultural Relationships. Northwestern University Studies in the Social Sciences, No. 2. Evanston and Chicago: Northwestern University.

Peterson, J. T. 1978 The Ecology of Social Boundaries: Agta Foragers of the Philippines. Illinois Studies in Anthropology, No. 11. Chicago: University of Illinois Press.

Popov, A. A. 1968 How Sereptie Djaruoskin of the Nganasans (Tavgi Samoyeds) Became a Shaman. *In* Popular Beliefs and Folklore Traditions in Siberia. V. Diószegi, ed. Pp. 137–145. English translation revised by Stephen P. Dunn. Bloomington: Indiana University Press, and The Hague: Mouton.

Rasmussen, K. 1929 Intellectual Culture of the Iglulik Eskimos: Report of the Fifth Thule Expedition 1921–24, Vol. 7, No. 1. Copenhagen: Gyldendalske Boghandel, Nordisk Forlag.

Ray, V. F. 1963 Primitive Pragmatists: The Modoc Indians of Northern California. Seattle: University of Washington Press.

Rodriguez, E., & R. W. Wrangham. 1993 Zoopharmacognosy: The Use of Medicinal Plants by Animals. *In* Phytochemical Potential of Tropical Plants. K. R. Downum et al., eds. Pp. 89–105. New York: Plenum.

Sawada, M. 1997 Shamanic and Animistic Aspects of African Pygmies' Cultures. *In* Circumpolar Animism and Shamanism. T. Yamada & T. Irimoto, eds. Pp. 297–307. Sapporo, Japan: Hokkaido University Press.

Shanks, N., M. S. Harbuz, D. S. Jessop, P. Perks, P. M. Moore, & S. L. Lightman. 1998 Inflammatory Disease as Chronic Stress. Annals of the New York Academy of Sciences 840:599–607.

Shostak, M. 1983 Nisa: The Life and Words of a !Kung Woman. New York: Vintage.

Simon, H. 1990 A Mechanism for Social Selection and Successful Altruism. Science 250:1665–1668.

Smith, E. A. 1988 Risk and Uncertainty in the "Original Affluent Society": Evolutionary Ecology of Resource Sharing and Land Tenure. *In* Hunters and Gatherers, Vol. 1: History, Evolution, and Social Change. T. Ingold, D. Riches, & J. Woodburn, eds. Pp. 221–251. Oxford: Berg.

Smythe, C. W. 1984 Native Doctors Among the Australian Aborigines. Alaska Native News 2:6–11.

Sober, E., & D. S. Wilson. 1998 Unto Others: The Evolution and Psychology of Unselfish Behavior. Cambridge, MA: Harvard University Press.

Spencer, W. B., & F. J. Gillen. 1927 The Arunta: A Study of a Stone Age People. 2 vols. London: Macmillan.

Spott, R., & A. L. Kroeber. 1942 Yurok Narratives. University of California Publications in American Archaeology and Ethnology 35:143–256.

Spreng, M. 2000 Possible Health Effects of Noise Induced Cortisol Increase. Noise and Health 2:59–64.

Thalbitzer, W. C. 1931 Shamans of the East Greenland Eskimo. *In* Source Book in Anthropology. A. L. Kroeber & T. T. Waterman, eds. Pp. 430–436. Cambridge, MA: Harvard University Press.

Thomas, E. M. 1959 The Harmless People. New York: Knopf.

Trivers, R. L. 1971 The Evolution of Reciprocal Altruism. Quarterly Review of Biology 46:35–57.

Turner, E. 1989 From Shamans to Healers: The Survival of an Inupiaq Eskimo Skill. Anthropologica 31:3–24.

Turner, E. 1992 Psychology, Metaphor, or Actuality? A Probe Into Iñupiaq Eskimo Healing. Anthropology of Consciousness 3:1–8.

Warner, W. L. 1958 A Black Civilization: A Social Study of an Australian Tribe. Rev. ed. New York: Harper.

Wilson, D. S., & E. Sober. 1994 Reintroducing Group Selection to the Human Behavioral Sciences. Behavior and Brain Sciences 17:585–654.

Wilson, E. O. 1975 Sociobiology: The New Synthesis. Cambridge, MA: Harvard University Press.

Winterhalder, B. 1986 Diet Choice, Risk, and Food Sharing in a Stochastic Environment. Journal of Anthropological Archaeology 5:369–392.

Woodburn, J. C. 1959 Hadza Conceptions of Health and Disease. *In* East African Institute of Social Research: One Day Symposium on Attitudes to Health and Disease Among Some East African Tribes. Pp. 89–94. Kampala, Uganda: Makere College.

Wrangham, R. 1987 African Apes: The Significance of African Apes for Reconstructing Social Evolution. *In* The Evolution of Human Behavior: Primate Models. W. G. Kinzey, ed. Pp. 51–71. Albany: State University of New York Press.

Wrangham, R. 1995 Leaf-Swallowing by Chimpanzees, and Its Relationship to Tapeworm Infection. American Journal of Primatology 37:297–303.

Wrangham, R. W., & J. Goodall. 1989 Chimpanzee Use of Medicinal Leaves. *In* Understanding Chimpanzees. P. Heltne & L. Marqardt, eds. Pp. 22–37. Cambridge, MA: Harvard University Press.

Wrangham, R. W., & T. Nishida. 1983 *Aspilia*: A Puzzle in the Feeding Behavior of Chimpanzees. Primates 24:276–282.

Wright, R. 1994 The Moral Animal: Why We Are the Way We Are: The New Science of Evolutionary Psychology. New York: Vintage.

Yamada, T. 1997 The Concept of Universe and Spiritual Beings Among Contemporary Yakut Shamans: The Revitalization of Animistic Belief and Shamanic Tradition. *In* Circumpolar Animism and Shamanism. T. Yamada & T. Irimoto, eds. Pp. 207–228. Sapporo, Japan: Hokkaido University Press.

19 Altruistic Love, Resiliency, Health, and the Role of Medicine

Gregory Fricchione

In this chapter, the notions of stress, allostasis and allostatic loading, health strengthening, and resiliency will be reviewed against the backdrop of brain evolution and implications for the medical mission. A model based on the directed selection pressure of social attachment behavior on the evolution of the human brain and the subsequent variant effects of successful and unsuccessful attachment on the inborn need to maintain allostasis while reducing allostatic loading will be presented. Too much allostatic loading leads to metabolic wear and tear on the organism and a propensity to develop illness. The naturally selected human capacity to love, a product of secure attachment in both its reception and provision, would be expected evolutionarily to stimulate the brain's motivation circuitry. This circuitry's mesocortical terminal zones are sculpted in the earliest attachment experiences of the individual and go on to have top-down control responsibilities for the stress response systems.

Traditionally, researchers have investigated the positive effects of receiving social support. For some time, however, there have been hints that compassionate love can have salutary effects not only on the recipient but also on the provider. The threshold for illness may be raised by the creation of a loving bond between people. Being a resilient, loving person, in the context of creating a social support community, adds to the resiliency and health of said person and others in the community.

Such a construct has potentially important ramifications for the medical profession. Patients are products of eons of evolutionary pressure and years of individual development all designed to create a being that works best in a milieu characterized by empathetic bonding and compassionate love. While evidence-based medicine is important, it is not medicine at all unless physicians embody the kind of altruistic love that allows them to truly care for those with illness.

ALTRUISTIC LOVE AND THE MEDICAL MISSION

The old-fashioned medical values of empathy and trust are the keys to maintaining the lifeblood and soul of clinical medicine, as Alfred T. Tauber, a Boston University professor of medicine and philosophy, has espoused in his "new medical ethic" (Tauber, 2002).

Modern science alone is ineffective when faced with the most important reasons for the patient's visit to the doctor in the first place. To quote Richard Horton, editor of the *Lancet*:

> It is neither a wholly mechanistic nor a wholly metaphysical question, yet it remains, for many patients, a deeply important one: what is this disease doing to me? Doctors tend to recoil from these more holistic matters. In asking the question, I am not seeking an ultimate final meaning of human disease, [a] teleology of illness so to speak, instead I am trying to find a way to make sense of what it is that disease does to us, not only as human bodies but also as human beings. It is a question of ontology as much as it is of pathology. (Horton, 2003, p. 18)

We must never forget that the patient comes to the doctor because he or she is suffering. According to Horton, it is this "dis-ease"—this sorrow, regret, disappointment, and grief—that motivates the patient to enter into relationship with the doctor.

Doctors overenamored with evidence-based medicine and clinical guidelines tend to put aside the mire of psychological and social concerns and to ignore the fears of separation that the patient often has when in the throes of serious illness. Nevertheless, those with illness experience a human reality of suffering, and medicine is increasingly "disembedded," to use sociologist Anthony Giddens's term, from this reality. This becomes the schism in modern medical practice. It is a separation challenge to medicine itself as a profession, and Horton intuitively sees the need for an attachment solution: "The solution is to discover a way to reconnect doctor to patient through a bridge of common understanding and shared ways of knowing about disease. We need nothing less than a new philosophy of medical knowledge" (Horton, 2003, p. 58). In some ways, this chapter is about the search for this new philosophy of medical knowledge. As we will see is the case with evolutionary development, the key is hidden in what Horton has suggested above: When there is a separation challenge, we must find attachment solutions.

Thus, anything that threatens the human doctor-patient relationship is fraught with danger for the patient and also for the future of the medical profession. The doctor-patient relationship is built on empathy, trust, and belief, and whatever basic medical science affords us as clinicians, that information must be reembedded in the clinical context, in the person-to-person trust and face-to-face commitment that is the mutual love of doctor and patient.

Love is an affective compassionate affirmation of the worth of the life of the other. In all of us, there is the need to be affirmed in the reception of another's love and the need to affirm others through the free gift of our love to them. In the life of the patient dealing with illness and a threat to self-worth and purpose, there is a heightened need for love. Compassionate love may be the most important factor in maximizing the effectiveness of the patient-doctor relationship, which is a key to healing. This may not be news to anyone who has experienced a serious illness requiring competent and compassionate medical care. Nevertheless, this concept has yet to be placed on a scientific and evolutionary basis.

THE BRAIN EVOLUTION PERSPECTIVE

A review of how and why the brain evolved offers us insight into why medical altruistic love, as it emerges from our attachment survival strategy, is essential for human healing.

The *brain* is an organ with sensory, analyzer, effector, and motor functions. It evolved from unicellular life as today is represented in the amoeboid existences of the monocyte that protects and the bacterial cell that invades us. Both the monocyte and the bacterium possess primordial intelligence. They optimize their behaviors in light of incoming data. In each instance, cell surface sensory receptors are attached to machinery inside the cell. This machinery effects a cytoskeletal motor change in a process called *chemotaxis*. Thus, the unicell "decides" to mobilize or immobilize in response to stimuli in the environment.

What is the vertebrate brain for? It uses its *sensory* thalamus, its *motor* basal ganglia, and its *analyzer-effector* cortex to make optimal immobilization-mobilization, avoidance-approach, and separation-attachment response selections in an environment of much noisy and often-conflicting information. The *body* is the apparatus available to immobilize or mobilize, avoid or approach, separate or attach. The *mind* is what the brain produces in interaction with its internal and external environments, in order to accomplish what the brain is for.

As mutation provided an extra area in a part of the reptilian brain called the *general pallium*, this territory was exapted in a reptile line destined to become mammals (therapsids) in order to provide survival advantage through more effective attachment solutions to separation challenges. Thus, when talking about the evolution of the brain, we uncover a leitmotif to which I have referred elsewhere as the *separation-attachment dialectic* (Fricchione, 2002). At the core of the dialectical approach, there are the basic opposing concepts of separation and attachment and tension-based movement. Therefore, if we take the primary thesis and antithesis to be attachment and separation, respectively, then synthesis involves the inseparable interconnectedness of them both—in essence, a higher synthesis of attachment.

With an appreciation of this dialectic, we come to a fuller understanding of how the directed selection pressure of separation threats biased cerebrotype evolution in the direction of structures capable of producing enhanced and refined attachment solutions. These solutions required certain underlying neuronal constructs that evolved in the form of segregated yet integrated basal ganglia (motor) thalamo (sensory)—cortical (analysis-effector) loops (Alexander et al., 1990).

These forms began with the *protolimbic circuit* of the amphibian and the reptile, containing an amygdala-centered, emotional, "hot" memory system balanced by a hippocampus-centered, cognitive, calming, "cool" memory system. These structures effectively mediate avoidance-and-approach decision making.

In a mammal-like reptile species faced with a significant separation challenge, such as a need to strengthen the care of endangered infants, this challenge would cry out, so to speak, for an attachment solution that would provide the kind of survival advantage favored by evolution. Such a demand would work its way through the biologies of the brains available. In some cases, the genotypic space of individuals would be conducive to design improvements in things like parental caring, the separation cry, and play (the mammalian behavior triad). These improvements required the coming on line of the *paralimbic circuit*. This particular circuit contains a new cortical analyzer-effector section consisting of the anterior cingulate (ACA) and the medial orbitofrontal (MOF) cortical area. The evolution of the paralimbic circuit in mammals enabled us to employ parent-offspring and social attachments as our survival strategies.

The *prefrontal cortical* (PFC) *circuit* later emerged, especially in higher mammals, with working memory and "memory of the future" capabilities (Ingvar, 1985). Through the PFC connection to the ACA, decision making could be done based on these capabilities plus a memory of the past and an error detection network. Motivation is of course also a key component in deciding to avoid or approach, and evolution provided a structure to enhance this function. This is the mesocortical brain motivation dopamine circuitry: a group of neurotransmitter-laden neurons traveling in a fiber tract called the medial forebrain bundle from the lower part of the brain called the *brainstem* up through the middle regions and exiting into the frontal regions of the PFC and ACA. Based partly on dopamine signals in the PFC and ACA, fear conditioning stemming from amygdalar flow can be dampened. With a resulting pleasurable reduction of fear, the decision to approach rather than avoid becomes easier.

The prefrontal cortex, working together with the paralimbic zones, enables us to plan and execute our attachment behaviors. All of these developments form a foundation for the eventual human capacity to cascade from empathy to compassion to other-directed love (see Figure 19.1). Empathy can thus be described as the emotional impact of an evolution that outfits the brain to successfully attach. This can result in compassionate love, which is the empathetic output we can focus on our fellow human beings. Thus, the brain can be viewed as a highly complex organ for finding attachment solutions to separation challenges. In order to accomplish this, the brain undergoes psychological development.

The human psychological environment of evolutionary adaptedness is one of secure base attachment (Bowlby, 1969). Given the key cornerstone survival value of security and protection that a caretaker provides, the child's attachment control system will be structured to perform most efficiently and to support healthy development when bonding can take place with a person who is effective, responsive, and deeply loving. The mutuality of this attachment relationship is inherently pleasurable to both parties as would be expected in an evolved system bestowing key survival value. In summarizing development, Bowlby states that children will be more likely to grow up to be cheerful, socially cooperative, effective, and resilient citizens when they have had the benefit of loving, responsive parents throughout infancy, childhood, and adolescence providing them with a secure base from which to explore the world. Encapsulated in this statement is the recognition that security based on fulfillment of *need love* will encourage the capacity for *gift love* of an altruistic kind and will contribute to the strengthening of resiliency.

The dialectical interplay between separation and attachment here gives rise to the paradoxical message of evolution. Humans individuate only in community. There is self-realization only in self-giving love. He who loses his life gains it. The evolutionary process that provides the attachment-caregiving program forms the basis for human empathy and compassion and also provides for the emergence of the human capacity to altruistically love.

STRESS

Whereas approach is mediated by the attachment behavioral system, avoidance anxiety is mediated by the fear behavioral system, which heralds the threat of separation from one's objects of attachment and love. These behavioral systems seek to maintain a relatively steady state relationship between individuals and their environmental attachments. Within the individual, there are physiological systems that are also best maintained in a relatively steady state. These external and internal homeostatic mechanisms are complementary. When an individual is satisfactorily connected to caring companions, she is more likely to be securely fed and protected, and thus her internal physiology will be less taxed than it would be in an environment of evolutionary maladaptedness. By the same token, an individual whose physiology is well maintained will be healthier and presumably better equipped to maintain himself within his familiar

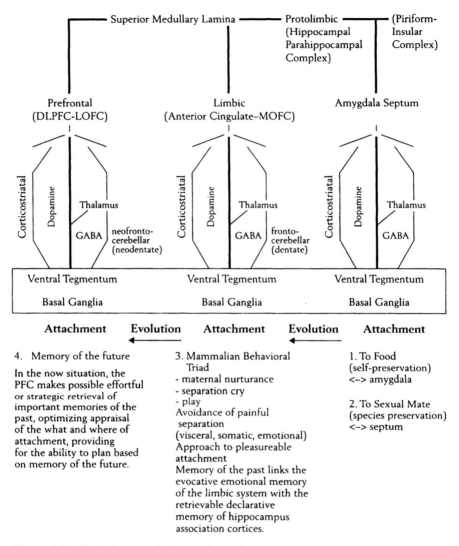

Figure 19.1. Brain loop evolution and attachment.

environment. These are Bowlby's *outer* and *inner* rings of life-maintaining systems that mutually support each other (Bowlby, 1973, p. 149).

Stress thus implies an outer ring separation challenge that ignites the fear behavioral system, requiring an inner ring physiological hyperarousal to be successfully met. This physiological hyperarousal is known as the stress/emergency or *fight-or-flight* response. Though designed to be helpful by protecting against acute separation events, stress may lead to the onset or progression of pathophysiological disease processes when the threat becomes unremitting or when an overwhelming acute stressor occurs.

The stress response starts when stimuli are perceived as stressful because they signify a discrepancy between what should be (the set goal variable of secure base attachment) and what actually is (the actual variable), reflecting a disturbance in the normal state of physical and mental affairs that will need attention and action (Ursin & Eriksen, 2004). This alarm system produces neurophysiological activation and arousal, which is necessary when the organism perceives danger. In this context, *stress* can be defined as a state of disharmony or threatened homeostasis (Chrousos & Gold, 1992). Biochemical (neurotransmitters, peptides, steroids), physiological (heart rate, blood pressure), and behavioral (anxiety, depression, tension) concomitants of stress may co-mediate a disease response.

The Stress Response Systems

There are two major stress response systems. One involves hormonal flow from the hypothalamus to the pituitary and down to the adrenal gland after threat alerts perceived up above are processed in the mesocortical and mesolimbic cortices. This hormonal system is called the *HPA axis* and includes the corticotrophin-releasing hormone (CRH) component with neurons projecting from lateral paraventricular hypothalamic nuclei (PVN). The other system is the neurotransmitter-based sympathetic nervous system (SNS) with norepinephrine-containing fibers arising in the locus coeruleus in the brainstem. These sympathetic neurons fire in response to signals from the lateral hypothalamus that arise in the context of amygdala-mediated conditioned fear. Large amounts of CRH will produce an anxiety-laden state as will output of the SNS (Chrousos & Gold, 1992). Other neurotransmitters and messengers also contribute to the stress response. Serotonin and acetylcholine stimulate both the HPA and the SNS systems while GABAergic, opioid, and glucocorticoid substances inhibit them. Immune activation causes an increase in HPA axis output.

There is also an intricate association of the stress systems with areas of the brain integral to memory, emotional tone, cognition, and planning (Chrousos & Gold, 1992). The amygdala and hippocampus interpret stressful signals and modulate the stress response (McEwen, 2003). Amygdala stimulation by the SNS is important for the recovery of affect-laden information and its emotional analysis. In the context of a fear-arousing stimulus, the central nucleus of the amygdala is important for the activation in turn of the HPA and SNS systems. The hippocampus performs an inhibitory function, dampening amygdala activity and the HPA system. The function of the corticosteroid receptors in the hippocampus and their regulation during stress and depression serves as another link.

As explained above, the mesocortical dopamine system projects to the prefrontal cortex, an area thought to be central to planning and cognition (Chrousos

& Gold, 1992). The mesolimbic system, with dopamine neurons traveling in the same bundle but exiting lower into the nucleus accumbens, is thought to be integral to the interaction between motivation and movement (via the mesostriatal dopamine system) and in reinforcement and reward. All of these dopaminergic networks are influenced by stress.

Allostasis

Allostasis, literally meaning "maintaining stability (or 'homeostasis') through change," refers to the capacity of our neural mechanisms to constantly modify physiological parameters in order to adjust to the anticipated demand of shifting environmental conditions (McEwen, 1998). Thus, in anticipation of an upcoming altercation, one's blood pressure may rise to meet the challenge. *Allostatic load* refers to the metabolic wear and tear that the body experiences due to repeated cycles of allostatic stress responses, as well as to the inefficient turning-on or shutting-off of these activated responses. It is the price we pay for adaptation.

Anxiety (the fear of separation) and depression (the mourning of attachment loss) are common mental disorders and may be conceptualized as stress induced allostatic load disorders that themselves lead to increased allostatic loading (Institute of Medicine, 2001). Allostatic loading secondary to these mood states has been associated with susceptibility to diseases such as coronary heart disease (CHD), the most disabling disease in our society, and it contributes to the onset or exacerbation of many other disabling diseases with high mortality and morbidity. Examples include hypertension, cardiomyopathy and heart failure, insulin-resistant diabetes, autoimmune diseases, and possibly HIV/AIDS and Alzheimer's.

Allostatic load can be considered a cumulative measure of the physiological burden borne by the body from attempts to adapt to life's stressors. It has predicted functional decline when a measure based on 10 physiological markers has been used (McEwen, 2003). Allostatic load contributes to the development of what is called the *metabolic syndrome*, now common in the United States, which consists of CHD, insulin resistance, hypertension, high cholesterol and triglycerides, and obesity (Illane-Parikka et al., 2004). Depression is often associated with hypercortisolism, which may predispose to the metabolic syndrome, which in turn may lower the threshold for CHD.

STRESS BUFFERING AND HEALTH STRENGTHENING

Can mind-body stimuli reduce allostatic loading, reversing the negative aspects of the stress response? The answer to this question appears to be yes.

Relaxation Response

The *relaxation response* (RR) is a self-induced stimulus that breaks the hold of a stress response. It is defined by a set of integrated physiological adjustments that are elicited when a subject engages in a repetitive mental or physical activity and passively ignores distracting thoughts. This response can be elicited through meditation, certain forms of prayer, tai chi, qi gong, yoga, autogenic training, etc., and is associated with rapidly occurring decreased oxygen consumption and carbon dioxide elimination (i.e., reduced metabolism) and lowered heart rate, arterial blood pressure, and respiratory rate. The RR can be thought of as the physiological counterbalance of the stress, or fight-or-flight, response (Benson, 1975). We may hypothesize that the RR functions as an innate protective mechanism against excessive stress. The RR has been shown to reduce stress-related anxiety and depression symptoms and to benefit several conditions, in addition to cardiovascular disease, which can be precipitated or exacerbated by allostatic loading.

Cognitive-Behavioral Therapy

This therapy teaches patients to substitute positive thoughts for anxiety- and depression-provoking ones and usually involves 6 to 12 weekly individual sessions. Patients record thoughts and feelings in diaries, noting situations that cause anxiety and depression and behaviors that relieve these mood states. Cognitive-behavioral therapy is effective for anxiety and depression and is being tried in patients with medical illnesses (Piette et al., 2004).

Social Support

Social relationships can have an impact on health-promoting behaviors, such as medical-treatment adherence, diet, and exercise, which in turn will influence health-relevant biological states resulting in physical health or disease propensities. At the same time, social relationships directly affect the health-relevant biology of the brain and contribute to the physical and mental status of the person. Social resources will influence the sequelae of perceived stress and will therefore lower vulnerability to physical and psychiatric disease.

Social stressors include isolation, marital and family discord, social conflict, job strain, unemployment, physical morbidity, retirement, and social inequalities, including pathological bias. The effects of social support on reducing disease activity and improving health have been shown in studies of CHD, systemic lupus erythematosus, irritable bowel disease, and anxiety and depression, among other diseases (Institute of Medicine, 2001). With what we have discussed in mind, we can now define a mind-body medicine equation:

$$\frac{\text{Stress-induced Allostatic Loading}}{\text{Social Support}} = \text{Propensity to Disease}$$

There appears to be a linkage between the circuitry responsible for mammalian separation distress and that for human sadness (Panksepp, 2003). These two feeling states both emerge from what Panksepp refers to as an "integrative emotional system for social affect" based on the common evolutionary antecedents of behavioral attachments and sensory modalities. A foundation of attachment comfort will predispose to social choice and approach behaviors that may pave the way for altruism. On the other hand, repeated separation distress will predispose to avoidance and ultimately to depression. Panksepp writes:

> [R]egions of the human brain activated during sadness . . . correspond to . . . areas activated during separation distress in animals. Localized electrical stimulation of many subcortical brain sites provokes separation cries in mammals. These sites include not only the anterior cingulate, but also the bed nucleus of the stria terminalis, . . . thalamus, and the periacqueductal central gray area of the brain stem. The latter two areas are known to control feelings of physical pain. Psychological pain in humans, especially grief and intense loneliness, may share some of the same neural pathways that elaborate physical pain. Given the dependence of mammalian young on their caregivers, it is not hard to comprehend the strong survival value conferred by common neural pathways. . . .
>
> Throughout history poets have written about the pain of a broken heart. It seems that such poetic insights into the human condition are now supported by the neurophysiological findings. Will the opposite also prove to be the case—that socially supportive and loving feelings reduce the sting of pain? A reasonable working hypothesis is that social feelings such as love are constructed partly from brain neural circuits that alleviate the feelings of social isolation. (Panksepp, 2003, p. 238)

Human love, founded on the evolutionary wisdom of social attachment, has the healing power to assuage the dis-ease of both physical and psychological pain. In the process, disease vulnerability and activity may be reduced.

BELIEF AND CONSCIOUS EXPECTATION

The belief a patient has in the ability of the doctor and the treatment to heal him or her is not inert. This positive conscious expectation of a return to wellness has the power to stimulate the brain reward/motivation circuitries in such a way that stress and allostatic loading, of the kind that emerges when a challenge to well-being is experienced, are reduced. Top-down control of the stress response systems is engaged when belief and positive expectation diminish dis-ease and provide solace.

In 2001, our research team suggested that the placebo response, which is based on belief and expectation, can be understood using insights gained from understanding of the RR (Stefano et al., 2001). We suggested that neural processes in the brain's mesolimbic-mesocortical reward/motivation circuitries are stimulated by the hopefulness and optimism inherent in a patient's belief in his or her doctor and the treatment offered, with the expectation that return of health will occur. A "memory" of future well-being leads to solace and a reduction in the stress response with salutary potential effects on end organs. These neural processes activate downstream signaling molecules that may stimulate constitutive nitric oxide release, which could result in a general reduction in neural, vascular, and immune overactivation syndromes.

In a recent study using positron emission tomography, when six patients with Parkinson's disease showed placebo benefit, there was a significant decrease in (^{11}C) raclopride binding potential, suggesting that endogenous dopamine (DA) was released synaptically in the caudate and putamen, dislodging the raclopride from the DA receptors (de la Fuente-Fernandez et al., 2001). Conscious expectations of benefit instigate a release of dopamine not only in the nigrostriatal system, but also from the ventral tegmentum cell bodies with output through the median forebrain bundle to the mesolimbic-mesocortical brain reward/motivation circuitries (de la Fuente-Fernandez et al., 2004).

To summarize, optimistic belief in a positive future may effect a change in prefrontal cortical activity, which will feedback to stimulate DA outflow in the medial forebrain bundle up from the ventral tegmentum. Receptors not only in the dorsal striatum (caudate and putamen) but also in the ventral striatum (nucleus accumbens) and further up the line in the anterior cingulate, medial orbitofrontal, and dorsolateral prefrontal cortices will record this change as pleasurable and motivating. This sets up a receptive field for the solace of being attached to a loving and protective caregiver. The result is relief of the pain-of-separation distress and a reduction in the stress response, which benefit end-organ functioning and the overall health of the individual.

RESILIENCY

The relaxation response, cognitive-behavioral therapy, social support, and belief and conscious positive expectation all have the potential to build resiliency through the mechanisms of reward and motivation, decreased fear responsiveness, and adaptive social behavior.

Maternal nurturance may lead to resiliency. High maternal nurturance, as reflected by rat pup licking, grooming, and nursing, increases glucocorticoid receptor (GR) gene promotion and expression in the offspring's hippocampus (Weaver et al., 2004). This is of great importance because the adult beneficiaries of this high nurturance show muffled responses to HPA axis stress overactivity. This resiliency against stress effects appears connected to hippocampal GR levels and improved feedback, resulting in reduced corticosterone levels in response to restraint. It is also known that high-nurturance mothering of rat pups stimulates lifelong amygdala benzodiazepine receptor increases, and these receptors are also important for reducing anxiety and improving resiliency (Caldji et al., 1998). These findings suggest a robust gene-environment mechanism for the long-term epigenetic effects of maternal nurturance on the offspring's genetic endowment.

Reward and motivation (hedonia and learned optimism), fear responsiveness (maintaining effective behaviors despite fear), and adaptive social behavior (altruism, bonding, and teamwork) are the neural mechanisms thought to be most relevant to resiliency traits (Charney, 2004).

Stress induces a reduction in DA-associated reward in the nucleus accumbens. Anhedonia and hopelessness may result. Activities and behaviors that increase DA function in the mesolimbic system will benefit resiliency.

Fear emerges in response to neutral conditioned stimuli after pairing with an aversive unconditioned stimulus. Resilience to severe stress is associated with the capacity to avoid the overinclusion of specific conditioned stimuli in the aversive category. Resiliency is further strengthened when there is an ability to reversibly store emotional memories with a reorganization of the original traumatic memory that is less fearsome. Moreover, an ability to quickly facilitate extinction of the learned fear will be a benefit to continued optimism and functioning in the stressful setting. This may be strengthened by a process of active responding with fear arousal diverted from the central to the basal nucleus of the amygdala with output to the motor circuitry.

Social behavior that emphasizes altruism and community support may also result in resiliency. Both being altruistic toward others and successfully attracting support for oneself are important resiliency factors. For this reason, it will be essential to further our understanding of the neural basis of altruism and other adaptive social behaviors if we want to uncover the secrets of resiliency. A recent study suggests that a gene variant on chromosome 11 may be linked to altruistic behavior measured by anonymous self-report questionnaire (Bachner-Melman et al., 2005). This polymorphism is responsible for boosting DA D4 receptor function and may be a source of the pleasurable feedback in the brain reward/motivation circuitries that accompanies and perpetuates altruistic behavior. In a recent twin study, approximately 42% of the variance for altruistic selfless behavior was estimated to be genetically produced; however, 58% was related to the familial and outside environments, suggesting gene-culture codevelopment of this phenotype (Rushton, 2004).

An important area of preclinical research has involved oxytocin (Uvnas-Moberg, 1998). In the vole model, oxytocin and another neuropeptide, vasopressin, play important roles in social engagement as well as in pair bonding (Insel et al., 1998). The montane variety of vole is genetically similar to the prairie vole, however, the more social and more nurturing prairie voles have higher levels of oxytocin receptors in the nucleus accumbens and basal lateral amygdala. This suggests that the neural mechanisms responsible for these neuropeptide social behavior effects are connected to the DA brain reward circuitry of the nucleus accumbens.

Oxytocin may also have potent antistress effects. In rats, when oxytocin is given, there are blood pressure declines, prolongation of withdrawal latency to heat stimuli, decreases in corticosteroid levels, and increases in insulin and cholecystokinin levels. And in a recent human study, intranasal oxytocin was given to 37 healthy men who were then exposed to a social stress test. Oxytocin, especially when paired with social support, was associated with increased calmness and reduced anxiety and salivary cortisol during stress (Heinrichs et al., 2003). Oxytocin released in response to social interaction is part of the neuroendocrine array of reactions that underlines the resiliency accompanying positive social experiences—whether it is the reception or the provision of social caregiving. This latter point is important when the health effects of altruistic love are considered. Charney concludes:

> Highly resilient children, adolescents and adults have exceptional abilities to form supportive social attachments. Individuals who demonstrate . . . courageous acts in the context of great personal danger are frequently characterized by unique altruism. Clinical studies in such individuals designed to examine the neural circuits related to social cooperation are now indicated. (Charney, 2004, p. 209)

ATTACHMENT, EMPATHY, ALTRUISM, AND HEALTH

Attachment theory focuses on the responses of others to one's needs (attachment behavioral system) but is also viewed as a valid way to view one's reactions to the needs of others (caregiving behavioral system) (Bowlby, 1969, 1973). Together, these systems interact to maintain a dynamic equilibrium of attachment security growing out of relationships. The caregiving behavioral system is propelled by an altruistic drive to relieve distress and suffering in others through the provision of protection and social support (Mikulincer et al., 2001).

Recent studies have shown that, when one has personal attachment security with the positive expectation that others will provide loving care in times of need, there is a greater likelihood of providing altruistic support to someone else who is in need of sensitive care (Collins & Feeney, 2000). Attachment security is built on (1) confidence in one's competencies; (2) the ability to manage stressors while maintaining a sense of optimism, control, and self-efficacy; and (3) less preoccupation with self-worth issues and self-focused needs.

Mikulincer and his colleagues (2001) examined 69 students (44 women and 25 men), ranging in age from 20 to 40, who were divided into three groups. In the attachment security priming condition, participants received a one-paragraph story of secure attachment. In the positive affect priming condition, the subjects were exposed to a series of jokes, and in the neutral priming condition, the subjects received mechanical instructions about radio installation. After filling out a mood assessment following the priming experience, the subjects all read a story about a person in need and then were asked to rate how much they had experienced empathy-derived and distress-related emotions while reading the story.

Results showed that attachment security priming strengthened empathy while decreasing distress. Empathy was found less often when attachment anxiety and avoidance were endorsed, while distress was associated with attachment anxiety. Avoidance suggests a lack of desire to be attached while anxiety reflects a fear of being rejected.

When one is securely attached, there will be more available resources to attend to others' needs and to provide adequate care to alleviate distress. Secure attachment allows one to perceive others not only as potential sources of security and support in an attachment behavioral system but also as human beings who may themselves need loving care in the caregiving behavioral system. Therefore, attachment security may promote a genuine concern for others' welfare and may facilitate altruistic helping in times of need. Positive working models of self and others promote altruistic reactions to others' needs. Empathy may involve a neural response in the anterior cingulate cortex activated in common for "self" and "other" conditions of pain (Singer et al., 2004). Encountering others' needs will elicit distress and thus activate affect-regulation strategies. Positive models of self, based in attachment security, will help to maintain a sense of control and confidence in coping with the needs of others (Batson, 1987). One's distress is reduced, freeing innate resources and fostering altruistic reactions to others' needs. When one cooperates altruistically it can activate the brain's reward and motivation circuitries and thus become reinforcing (Rilling et al., 2002).

When someone is securely attached and better equipped to provide altruistic caregiving for others in need, he or she will often be more resilient, displaying a profile of low stress and high social support. This conceptualization may help us to understand some recent studies on health outcomes of altruists.

For example, volunteer seniors for two or more organizations had a 63% lower mortality risk than did nonvolunteers during the 5-year study period (Oman et al., 1999). Indeed, being helpful was more important than exercise and weekly religious service attendance and only slightly less important than not smoking.

In another study, questionnaires designed to measure self-reported giving and receiving of aid, prayer, positive and negative religious-based coping, and physical and mental health were sent to 2,016 Presbyterian church members in the United States in order to evaluate whether altruistic behaviors are correlated with better health (Schwartz et al., 2003). While no association was found between giving or receiving help and physical health, giving was better correlated with mental health than was being the recipient of help.

Another research group studied 423 older couples over 5 years, asking them whether they were caregivers for family or friends, whether they had good social support networks, and what quality of emotional support they gave to each other (Brown et al., 2003). Surprisingly, the researchers found an association between giving help and a reduced risk of dying (by half) even after controlling for health, age, gender, and other factors. No such association was found between receiving help and reduced mortality. This report corroborates the results of Vaillant's Harvard Study of Adult Development. In his book *Aging Well*, Vaillant (2002) surmises that generativity and altruistic helping are predictors of health and longevity.

Anecdotal evidence from the Duke Heart Center Patient Support Program suggests that cardiac patients who voluntarily assist other cardiac patients can improve health outcomes for both the recipient of their caregiving and themselves (Sullivan & Sullivan, 1997). The altruistic act of volunteering, a process of active responding rather than a passive fear response, transforms someone who had previously been a victim of disease into an agent of positive change. This achieves both stress reduction and social integration.

Complete health is a construct of cross-classified physical and mental health characteristics in which people have a lack of physical illness and high mental well-being. Grzywacz and Keyes (2004) recently reported that volunteers were more likely than nonvolunteers to be completely healthy or at least completely mentally health and partly physically healthy. Positive psychological effects have been noted for altruistic organ donors and for research volunteers. Some have called this behavior *adaptive altruism* in that it permits one to reset one's self-image as a giving person, and this can be health promoting if one's previous self-image was negative or defective (Seelig & Dobelle, 2001).

While altruism may directly contribute to health through effects on the brain's reward pathways, more work will be needed to tease apart the effects of preselection on our view of causality. Altruists may be healthier because they share the characteristics of attachment security, which provides them with resiliency based on stress reduction and social support. This resiliency provides a reservoir of caregiving energy so that altruistic behavior, when not overwhelming, can be personally healthful and gratifying as well as beneficial for others. In other words, altruism by itself may not directly cause the health benefit. It instead may be a marker for the underlying resiliency that correlates with better health outcomes.

Some may argue that, if altruistic caregiving benefits the caregiver, it may not be genuinely altruistic. Of course, not all altruistic caregivers will benefit, and those who love altruistically are not doing it to benefit themselves. Mothers caregiving for a chronically ill child who have high perceived stress or high chronicity of stress appear to shorten their telomere DNA-protein chromosomal cap lengths approximately 10 times faster than low-stress mothers. This accelerated telomere shortening in response to caregiving stress may be responsible for accelerated aging effects (Epel et al., 2004). However, some of the caregivers in this study appear to have had the resiliency to have normal telomere shortening rates, supporting the concept that resiliency may nurture the ability to be altruistic in a healthful way. Future studies might examine the effect of attachment security on telomere length in the setting of providing altruistic care.

HUMAN DIGNITY AND MEDICAL ALTRUISTIC LOVE

Dignity may be thought of as one's capacity to control one's environment while simultaneously preserving the dignity of others. Horton calls this *virtuous control* or *action*. Dignity involves one's inner worth but also the value of one's actions toward others. What Horton is restating here is that humans, because of our ontogeny and phylogeny, can only individuate in community, a reflection of the separation-attachment dialectical process (Fricchione, 2002). And with attachment security comes a greater ability to act altruistically for others.

Dignity can be described in three areas (Chochinov, 2002). The first involves illness-related concerns, including physical symptoms and psychological distress from the separation anxiety that illness ignites. Individuals worry simultaneously about the loss of independence and the loss of connectedness to loved ones. Second, those with illness focus on positive things that they can do and look for sources of spiritual comfort. These measures are taken to maintain a sense of dignity, autonomy, and hopefulness. Third, a social dignity inventory focuses on the level of social support that is available. When separation challenges are overwhelming, people seek dignity in their attachments to families and communities.

Dignity in society is built on a foundation of love and community. Individuals express their own dignity, Mary Wollstonecraft's "enlightened self love," through their love for others. So it is on the smaller scale of the clinical encounter. In essence, the dignity of the physician and his or her own enlightened self-love can only be expressed and manifested "in virtuous action," through the altruistic love of the patient. In the final analysis, as David Weatherall (1995) notes, medicine must return to an ethic of "the love of our patients."

Medicine has as its root the word *med*, meaning to take appropriate measures—in essence, to make good response selections and to virtuously act. In Latin, *med* gives rise to *mederi*, which means to look after others and to heal their suffering. Etched on the the wall of the Massachusetts General Hospital lobby are the words of Dr. Edward Churchill, said over 60 years ago, "Charity, in its broad spiritual sense, that is[,] our desire to relieve suffering is the most prized possession of medicine." In looking after the dignity of others in medicine, it is our altruistic love that relieves suffering and truly heals.

Osler was referring to this sentiment when he talked of the two virtues of the effective physician. There is *imperturbability*: keeping one's head when all about one are losing theirs. Osler saw this as a hard-nosed love. Physicians work like soldiers to defeat the enemies—disease and dis-ease. They are meant to work long hours, to sacrifice personal comforts, to risk defeat and scorn, and to be hard-nosed, single-minded, and tough in their love for their patients. The medical altruistic love of patients is no more namby-pamby than the soldier's altruistic love of country and his fellow soldiers.

And then there is *equanimity*, "an infinite patience" and "an ever-tender charity." This is another aspect of medical altruistic love, which must not go missing, for it speaks to the core dialectic of human dignity, the Golden Rule if you will, that we must love one another as we would be loved. Horton writes at the end of his book a hint of what this chapter has been about: the separation-attachment dialectical process and its core importance for an individual with illness and for society: "Yet it is the interplay between the individual and the group—dialectical tacking once again—that creates the conditions for dignity to be protected and fostered" (Horton, 2003, p. 510).

Dignity represents the capacity of human beings to make the choice for loving attachment in the face of separation not expressly for their own benefit but for the benefit of others.

SUMMARY

The brain evolved to enable us to optimize our avoidance-approach responses. In psychological terms, this becomes separation-attachment decision making and experience. Our brain has the structures and systems that enable us to deal with the stress of basic separation anxiety—the worst distress a social mammal can experience—and to attempt to reestablish the security of attachment. If these systems fail in the context of excessive or enduring stress, and if excessive allostatic loading persists, resiliency may sag and genetically based disease vulnerability may be uncovered, leading to illness.

In this chapter, I have presented evidence to support Bowlby's idea that because of the way we have evolved, our environment of evolutionary adaptedness is one of secure base attachment. With attachment security comes resiliency based on less stress reactivity and better social support in life, which in turn strengthen belief and positive expectation, further adding to resiliency and health. Furthermore, attachment security and the resiliency it affords the individual will be associated with an increased likelihood that the person will perform altruistic acts for others. Health benefits occur when people learn to mitigate against stress overload, strengthen their social support, develop a hopeful, positive belief in their futures, and perhaps, armed with resiliency, act altruistically with regard to others.

It is clear that evolution has made the calm security of the meditative state and of social support rewarding and desirable. But it may also be rewarding and pleasurable in a fulfilling way to be the one to provide altruistic support to someone in need. This would be reasonable from an evolutionary point of view. Selection pressure that would sculpt a species that survives on social attachment would likely lead to biological reinforcement of the reception *and* the provision of loving social support.

Knowing what we now know, we can make a strong case that not only is it virtuous for medicine to be based on an ethic of altruistic love, it is medically indicated if we want to optimize our patients' outcomes. In addition, we can make the public health case that more effort should be given to building resiliency through the approaches outlined in this chapter. We are at the point where undertaking prevention studies aimed at teaching the relaxation response, changing negative habitual cognitions, improving social supports, and encouraging belief and positive expectations based on altruistic love is indicated, especially when it comes to children in society. Altruistic caretaking of children increases their chances of becoming resilient adults with the capacity for altruistic caregiving.

Therefore, in both clinical medicine and in public health, virtuous loving altruistic action, which emphasizes this full understanding of the individual patient and the community and what can be done to maximize the opportunity for health and for relief of suffering, should be studied, taught, and practiced.

REFERENCES

Alexander GE, Crutcher MD, DeLong MR. Basal ganglia-thalamocortical circuits: parallel substrates for motor, oculomotor, "prefrontal" and "limbic" functions. Prog Brain Res. 1990;85:119–46.

Bachner-Melman R, Gritsenko I, Nermanov L, Zohar AH, Dina C, & Ebstein RP. Dopaminergic polymorphisms associated with self-report measures of human altruism: A fresh phenotype for the dopamine D4 receptor. Mol Psychiatry 2005; epub ahead of print.

Batson CD. Prosocial motivation: Is it ever truly altruistic? In L. Berkowitz (Ed.),

Advances in experimental social psychology (Vol. 20, pp. 65–122). New York: Academic, 1987.

Benson H. The relaxation response. New York: Morrow, 1975.

Bowlby J. Attachment and loss. Vol. I. Attachment. New York: Basic, 1969.

Bowlby J. Attachment and loss. Vol. II. Separation, anxiety and anger. New York: Basic, 1973.

Brown SL, Nesse RM, Vinokur AD, & Smith DM. Providing social support may be more beneficial than receiving it: Results from a prospective study of mortality. Psychol Science 2003;14:320–327.

Caldji C, Tannenbaum B, Sharma S, Francis D, Plotsky PM, & Meaney MJ. Maternal care during infancy regulates the development of neural systems mediating the expression of fearfulness in the rat. PNAS 1998;95:5335–5340.

Charney DS. Psychobiological mechanisms of resilience and vulnerability: Implications for successful adaptation to extreme stress. Am J Psychiatry 2004;161:195–216.

Chochinov HM. Dignity conserving care: A new model for palliative care. JAMA 2002;287:2253–2260.

Chrousos GP, & Gold PW. The concepts of stress and stress system disorders: Overview of physical and behavioral homeostasis. JAMA 1992;267:1244–1252.

Collins NL, & Feeney BC. A safe haven: An attachment theory perspective on support seeking and caregiving in intimate relationships. J Pers Soc Psychol 2000;78:1053–1073.

de la Fuente-Fernandez R, Ruth TJ, Sossi V, Schulzer M, Calne DB, & Stoessl AJ. Expectation and dopamine release: Mechanism of placebo effect in Parkinson's disease. Science 2001;293:1164–1166.

de la Fuente-Fernandez R, Schulze M, & Stoessl AJ. Placebo mechanisms and reward circuitry: Clues from Parkinson's disease. Biol Psychiatry 2004;56:67–71.

Epel ES, Blackburn EH, Lin J, Dhabhar FS, Adler NE, Morrow JD, Cawthon RM. Accelerated telomere shortening in response to life stress. Proc Natl Acad Sci U S A. 2004 Dec 7;101(49):17312–5.

Fricchione G. Separation, attachment and altruistic love. The evolutionary basis for medical caring. In SG Post, LG Underwood, JP Schloss, & WB Hurlbut (Eds.), Altruism and altruistic love: Science, philosophy and religion in dialogue. New York: Oxford University Press, 2002. pp. 346–361.

Giddens A. The consequences of modernity. Cambridge: Polity Press, 1990.

Grzywacz J, & Keyes CLM. Toward health promotion and social behavior in complete health. Amer J Health Behav 2004;28:99–111.

Heinrichs M, Baumgartner T, Kirschbaum C, & Ehlert U. Social support and oxytocin interact to suppress cortisol and subjective responses to psychosocial stress. Biol Psychiatry 2003;54:1389–1398.

Horton R. Health wars: On the global front lines of modern medicine. NY Review of Books, 2003; pp. 18–19.

Illane-Parikka P, Eriksson JG, Lindstrom J, et al. Prevalence of the metabolic syndrome and its components: Findings from a Finnish general population sample and the Diabetes Prevention Study cohort. Diabetes Care 2004;27:2135–2140.

Ingvar DH. Memory of the future: An essay on the temporal organization of conscious awareness. Human Neurobiol 1985;4:127–136.

Insel TR, Winslow JT, Wang Z, Young LJ. Oxytocin, vasopressin, and the neuroendocrine basis of pair bond formation. Adv Exp Med Biol. 1998;449:215–24.

Institute of Medicine. Health and behavior: The interplay of biological, behavioral and societal influences. Washington, DC: National Academy Press, 2001.

McEwen BS. Protective and damaging effects of stress mediators. N Engl J Med 1998;338:171–179.

McEwen BS. Interacting mediations of allostasis and allostatic load: Towards an understanding of resilience in aging. Metabolism 2003;52:10–16.

Mikulincer M, Gillath O, Halevy V, Avihou N, Avidan S, & Eshkoli N. Attachment theory and reactions to others' needs: Evidence that activation of the sense of attachment security promotes empathic responses. J Personality Soc Psychol 2001;81:1205–1224.

Oman D, Thoresen CE, & McMahon K. Volunteerism and mortality among the community-dwelling elderly. Journal of Health Psychology 1999;4:301–316.

Osler W. Aequanimitas. NY: McGraw-Hill, 1953.

Panksepp J. Feeling the pain of social loss. Science 2003;302:237–239.

Piette JD, Richardson C, & Valenstein M. Addressing the needs of patients with multiple chronic illnesses: The case of diabetes and depression. Am J Managed Care 2004;10:152–162.

Rilling JK, Gutman DA, ZehTR, Pagnoni G, Berns GS, Kilts C. A neural basis for social cooperation. Neuron 2002;35: 395–405.

Rushton JP. Genetic and environmental contributions to pro-social attitudes: A twin study of social responsibility. Proc R Soc Lond B 2004;217:2583–2585.

Schwartz C, Meisenhelder JB, Ma Y, & Reed G. Altruistic social interest behaviors are associated with better mental health. Psychosom Med 2003;65:778–785.

Seelig BJ, & Dobelle WH. Altruism and the volunteer: Psychological benefits from participating as a research subject. ASAID Journal 2001;47:3–5.

Singer T, Seymour B, O'Doherty J, Kaube H, Dolan RJ, & Frith CD. Empathy for pain involves affective but not sensory components of pain. Science 2004;303: 1157–1162.

Stefano GB, Fricchione GL, Slingsby BT, & Benson H. The placebo effect and relaxation response: Neural processes and their coupling to constitutive nitric oxide. Brain Res Rev 2001;35:1–19.

Sullivan GB, & Sullivan MJ. Promoting wellness in cardiac rehabilitation: Exploring the role of altruism. J Cardiovasc Nurs 1997;11:43–52.

Tauber AT. Confessions of a medicine man. Cambridge, MA: MIT Press, 2002. p. 114.

Ursin H, & Eriksen HR. The cognitive activation theory of stress. Psychoneuroendocrinology 2004;29:567–592.

Uvnas-Moberg K. Oxytocin may mediate the benefits of positive social interaction and emotions. Psychoneuroendocrinology 1998;23:819–835.

Vaillant GE. Aging well: Surprising guideposts to a happier life from the landmark Harvard Study of Adult Development. Boston: Little, Brown, 2002.

Weatherall D. Science and the quiet art. New York: Norton, 1995.

Weaver IGC, Cervoni N, Champagne FA, et al. Epigenetic programming by maternal behavior. Nature Neurosci 2004;7:847–854.

20 Monogamy, Motherhood, and Health

C. Sue Carter

In the late 1970s, I had my first encounter with a small rodent known as the prairie vole. Field studies and then laboratory work suggested that prairie voles were "monogamous" (Carter et al., 1995). Prairie voles showed a complex suite of behavioral traits, including the capacity to form social bonds and develop extended families based on a male, a female, and their offspring. These unexpected findings led to a series of investigations that continue to this day. As the story unfolded, the concept of sexual monogamy had to be reconsidered. However, the social components of monogamy—including the capacity of prairie voles to show lifelong pair bonds, male parental behavior, and the formation of extended families—were real. By studying prairie voles, it became possible to explore the neural basis of the behaviors that characterized what is now being called " social monogamy." Prairie voles and their relatives can be seen as organic Rosetta stones. Embedded in their tiny brains and simple lives are clues to the origins of human sociality.

The second factor that has motivated my research was my personal experience with childbirth and lactation, which began about 25 years ago. Motherhood left me fascinated by the hormonal basis of human behavior and the transformations that could be attributed to a uniquely mammalian hormone known as oxytocin. The outcome of these studies revealed that neural systems, including those underlying social communication, relationships, and emotions, are based on ancient biological substrates that we share with other mammals. In addition, the same neural substrates that are necessary for social bond formation play a pivotal role in the capacity of mammals to manage the stress of life.

Humans tend to believe that our elaborate systems of morals, values, and cognitive processes distinguish us from other living creatures. This is only partially true. Assumptions about the cognitive nature of love, monogamy, social bonds, parental behavior, and even benevolence can be challenged in light of new knowledge regarding evolution and endocrinology. In addition, through a deeper understanding of mammalian neurobiology, we have begun to appreciate the importance of social bonds and the chemicals that allow such bonds to form for human health and happiness.

THE MONOGAMY PARADOX

Humans are obsessed with monogamy. Societies pass laws to regulate it; many religions demand it. Spousal disloyalty can disrupt families, dynasties, and governments. The slaying of an unfaithful spouse may be condoned as justifiable homicide. Nothing stimulates controversy or gossip more than monogamy or, more precisely, failures of monogamy. In spite of laws, religious codes, and good intentions, sexual monogamy sometimes fails.

Although patterns and durations of social relationships vary, what dictionary.com calls "the practice of having one mate" (monogamy, n.d.) emerges across cultures as the most accepted pattern of marriage for adult humans. Attempts to win social sanction for other forms of relationships, including polygamy (many spouses) or same-sex marriage, are rarely successful. Monogamy as a lifestyle or social system is so accepted that it was once called a cultural "universal" (Fisher, 1992; Murdoch, 1949). Even among societies where polygyny (many wives) and polyandry (many husbands) are not forbidden, in practice heterosexual individuals may live much of their lives in pairs or extended families that are based on a male-female pair—sometimes even in the face of open sexual adultery. Infidelity and divorce are so common that monogamy is sometimes called a "myth" (Barash & Lipton, 2001).

So, are humans in fact monogamous? If monogamy is not merely about sexual fidelity, then what is it? The answers to these questions are based on a new awareness that monogamy is fundamentally, perhaps first and foremost, a social system. Monogamy is a way of living that promotes, but does not always guarantee, sexual fidelity.

Monogamy can be a very successful reproductive strategy, especially in hard times. If a male abandons his sexual partner after mating, he cannot defend her from other suitors and thus has less confidence of paternity. Also, pair bonding and having two or more caretakers may have benefits for the young reared under these conditions (Hrdy, 1999, 2005). Investment by parents of both sexes can help to assure the survival of socially monogamous or cooperatively breeding species. Social and emotional bonds facilitate survival and reproduction, promoting safety and a sense of emotional security. Social bonds and the giving and receiving of love are essential components of human existence (Carter et al., 2005). But what do we really know about the processes that motivate social behavior?

Within any attempt to understand monogamy are interrelated issues, some semantic, others cultural and economic, and still others with roots in biology and the evolution of the nervous system. As we have sought to untangle this Gordian knot, something even more interesting than the solution to the paradox of monogamy has emerged. In the effort to understand monogamy, scientists also have unearthed ancient secrets about the physical essence of human nature.

By examining prairie voles and the neurobiology of social monogamy, we are gaining knowledge of complex human concepts such as love, benevolence, social bonding, compassion, and altruism (Carter, 1998; Carter et al., 2005). We may even gain insights into human disorders such as autism (Carter, 2006; Insel et al., 1999). Prairie voles and other monogamous mammals also have interesting physiological and behavioral adaptations that promote lifelong social bonds. There is reason to believe that knowledge of prairie vole monogamy contains essential clues to the biological basis of health and longevity.

THERE IS MORE TO MONOGAMY THAN SEX

The Greek origins of the word *monogamy* focus on the concept of "one spouse." For some people, monogamy is used only in reference to a sexually exclusive relationship. If absolute sexual fidelity with a single mate across the entire lifespan is required, then only a fraction of modern humans would be called "monogamous." This is also true of most mammals. Lifelong sexual monogamy is rare.

Monogamy also refers to a lifestyle that is based around a social or emotional bond and in some cases shared parental responsibilities. Using this broader definition, the majority of humans spend some part of their lives in socially monogamous relationships.

Adding to the confusion, biologists have used the term monogamy to describe a kind of syndrome of social and physical traits. Based primarily on behavioral observations, scientists attempted to divide species according to the family structure and presumed sex life of the majority of the members of that species. Historically, most attempts to understand the social life of animals were grounded in natural history. Naturalists watched animals, whenever possible in their home environments. Like humans, other animals were usually discrete regarding their sex lives. The scenarios extracted from such observations were not necessarily complete pictures. It was often assumed that when adult animals of the opposite sex lived together, they were also mating and that these relationships were sexually exclusive interactions. Most attempts to define an animal species as monogamous were actually based not on paternity or even maternity, but rather on human interpretations of these rough estimates of social interactions.

Using this type of indirect evidence, whole species of animals were classified as monogamous, and other species were not. Based on a set of primarily behavioral criteria, about 3% of mammalian species were described as monogamous (Kleiman, 1977). These monogamous mammals included groups as taxonomically and geographically diverse as African wild dogs, certain species of South American primates, and even a few rodents, such as the remarkable prairie vole.

Members of species termed monogamous—by biologists—were observed living most of their lives as male-female couples or in families consisting of a heterosexual pair and their presumed offspring (Carter et al., 1995). When given a choice, these pairs showed a social preference for their familiar partner over a stranger. In some cases, members of these presumably monogamous species seemed behaviorally and physically distressed when unable to contact their preferred companion. When babies were born into a family, males of these species typically helped in the care of babies. Even males that had no sexual experience were spontaneously parental. Under natural conditions, older offspring often served as baby-sitters for other family members. The willingness of males to care for their own babies or other younger members of their own species also was used as a defining feature of monogamy.

Families from these monogamous species showed very high levels of social interactions and physical contact among all of the family members. Yet, at the same time, incest was rare. Incest taboos were based on the behavioral avoidance of sex within the family, but also involved physiological adaptations that made it difficult for young animals within a family to reproduce with each other or with their parents.

Members of monogamous species were not ubiquitously friendly. Males, and in some cases females, of these monogamous species might attack and even kill strangers (Winslow et al., 1993). Violence was most likely when the intruders were of the same sex (Bowler et al., 2002). This form of defensive aggression might protect the offspring, but it could also be in defense of the mate. Sexual behavior has reflexive components that are organized in ancient parts of the brain. When these reflexes are triggered, even the forces of social monogamy may not be powerful enough to assure sexual fidelity. Thus, mate guarding may be important to the capacity of socially monogamous pairs to regulate the sexual behavior of the partners. As with other features of social monogamy, specific neurobiological processes lie at the core of this aspect of the behavior of socially monogamous animals.

But major surprises were yet to come. In the 1980s, DNA fingerprinting became available. Using DNA samples from presumed parents and their presumed offspring, it was possible to prove or disprove paternity. Over and over again, among species that had been classified as monogamous, the genetic father was discovered to *not* be the resident male. Although some *individuals* were indeed sexually monogamous, viewed from the perspective of the whole species, sexual or genetic monogamy was actually rather rare.

MONOGAMY IS *NOT* A MYTH

The genetic evidence turned sexual monogamy on its ear. Dozens of articles and even a book with the title *Myth of Monogamy* (Barash & Lipton, 2001) appeared. DNA fingerprinting of the offspring from apparently devoted pairs left no doubt that sexual exclusivity was much less prevalent than previously assumed. If sexual exclusivity was *not* an essential trait of monogamy, was the concept of monogamy a meaningless myth?

Perhaps the problem with monogamy was simply semantic. Whatever the genetic, moral, religious, or social imperatives for sexual fidelity, it is only one piece of a complex pattern of behaviors. To grasp its importance, it was necessary to look beyond the use of the concept of sexual or genetic monogamy to examine the broader biological causes and purposes of monogamy.

Maybe monogamy had no biological equivalent and was simply an attempt to impose sexually restrictive human values on other animals. Perhaps only humans, and at that only some humans, were capable of sexual monogamy. Maybe monogamy really was a myth. However, as scientists continued to study species that had been classified as monogamous, it became clear that there was more to monogamy than sex. Species that had been identified by their tendency to live in pairs were in fact capable of selective social bonds, and in many cases males helped to rear the young.

Especially intriguing was the fact that among most pair-bonding species, males are not just passively parental. Males of species like the prairie vole seem drawn to babies, and often are even more willing than females to take on the tedious task of baby-sitting. In other cases, males are not actively parental, but instead seem to express their investment in the offspring by defending the family. This defense could be dramatic as animals might fight to the death to repel intruders. Especially in males, this seemed an extreme risk to take if—as DNA fingerprints had revealed—the male was not necessarily protecting his own offspring.

Outside of biology, monogamy typically has been treated as a cultural construct, and one that had to be reinforced by religions, codes, or laws. However, as with biological studies of monogamy, human research also did not distinguish between social and sexual monogamy. In humans, accurate estimates of sexual monogamy are difficult to obtain. However, the rate of break-up of sexual relationships and the incidence of divorce leave no doubt that lifelong monogamy in humans is somewhat uncommon. However, as with other mammals, humans do form emotional bonds. Human social bonds can be very complex, and emotional relationships can last for generations. Male humans also do have a well-developed capacity (not always expressed) to become involved in the care of young, providing direct care of children or, in some cases, indirect support in the form of resources and defense of the family.

All types of mammals show some degree of sociality. However, those species that spontaneously form social bonds seem to have nervous systems that are especially designed for sociality. Humans, even among individuals or cultures that do not adhere to the notion of sexual monogamy, usually do seek stable relationships and secure social bonds. Humans typically become emotionally attached to their children. When these bonds are not possible, especially during early childhood, the effects are typically negative. Why do social bonds exist? Why do disruptions in social bonds have such pervasive effects on all aspects of behavior and physiology?

MONOGAMY IS MORE THAN SKIN DEEP

Humans label nonspecific feelings with imprecise names such as "fear" or "anxiety." The cortex and other parts of the brain that are involved in cognition do an admirable job of improvising. However, the cortex is a fairly modern innovation and does not exert perfect control over emotional states. The problem of giving names to feelings, whether positive or negative, is exacerbated by the fact that the emotional core of our nervous system evolved long before the parts of the human brain, including the cortex, that give names to these experiences. Not only do we have problems decoding the vague messages from our bodies, but we find it difficult to talk back to our visceral core. Among those fuzzy emotional feelings that our cortex tries to interpret are "love," "attachment," and "social bonds."

Until recently, remarkably little was known regarding either the physical causes or the consequences of social bonds. Studies of human sexual and social behaviors or bonds are difficult to conduct. To explore the neural mechanisms of behavior, it is typically necessary to use animal models, the most common of which are mice and rats. However, neither mice nor rats show much evidence of the selective social or emotional relationships that characterize human social bonds. Social bonds, apparently similar to the bonds that exist in humans, have been recognized in some species of primate, such as South American titi monkeys and marmosets. But these animals are difficult and expensive to study. The discovery of monogamous rodents has permitted the physiological analysis of social monogamy, and from that analysis has developed a new perspective on monogamy.

Knowledge primarily derived from prairie voles convinced me that monogamy is not simply a cultural concept. Monogamy is rooted in biology, in the brain.

Studies of prairie voles have been especially helpful to the understanding of the behavioral effects of two brain hormones, known structurally as neuropeptides (Carter, 1998, 2003). Hidden from view and often inaccessible even to scientists, oxytocin and vasopressin are tiny molecules with crucial roles in defining what it means to be a mammal. Oxytocin sits at the center of a neuroendocrine network which coordinates ovulation, sexual behavior, social attachment, birth, breast feeding, maternal behavior, and responses to various kinds of stress. Vasopressin plays a role in social behaviors and also is a hormone of self-defense and adaptation, credited with helping us deal with both physiological stresses and psychological threats. Vasopressin is structurally similar to oxytocin and probably evolved from a common ancestral molecule. Working together and in the context of the rest of the nervous system, these ancient molecules allow individuals to manage apparently contradictory tasks, such as reproduction, forming social bonds, and at the same time self-defense in the face of a threat.

SEX DIFFERENCES ALSO ARE MORE THAN SKIN DEEP

Research with prairie voles has identified previously undiscovered differences between males and females. Superficially, male and female prairie voles are similar. Males and females are virtually identical in appearance, and both sexes take care of the babies. Because of this, we hypothesized that males and females would form pair bonds under similar behavioral and physiological conditions. This assumption was wrong (Carter et al., 1995).

Both male and female prairie voles produce the same basic hormones, including vasopressin and oxytocin. Both sexes are capable of responding to these hormones when they are given from an external source (Cho et al., 1999). However, in some areas of the brain, vasopressin production is androgen-dependent (De Vries & Villalba, 1997). In other brain regions, oxytocin production depends on the female hormone, estrogen. These and other sex differences in the brain suggest a new understanding of the subtle differences between males and females (Carter, 2006).

Particularly intriguing is the fact that stressful experiences and specific "stress" hormones seem to have very different effects on males and females (DeVries et al., 1995, 1996). When male prairie voles were exposed to a brief stressor (such as 3 minutes of swimming), they quickly formed new pair bonds, while females treated in the same manner seemed unable to form pair bonds, and in some cases even avoided familiar mates. Interestingly, stressed females, though unwilling to form pair bonds with males, do pair with other females. Male and female prairie voles form pair bonds under different conditions, and different endocrine mechanisms permit or facilitate pair bonding in males and females. Social psychologists have used these findings to argue that sex differences in the reaction to stressful experiences in humans are similar to those seen in voles (Taylor et al., 2000).

A MOTHER'S LOVE

By definition, female mammals lactate and most give birth to their young. It is usually the mother who provides food and primary care; the main source of nutrition for an infant mammal is its mother's milk. Newborn mammals, including humans, cannot survive without the help of a caring adult, typically the biological parent. The attachment between a mother and child also is the most accepted form of enduring social bond. In fact, the absence of maternal concern is considered pathological.

As with pair bonding, oxytocin is implicated in the bond between a mother and her infant. The mechanical effects of oxytocin, including its capacity to regulate labor and breast feeding, have been recognized for almost 100 years, and the idea that oxytocin might affect maternal behavior is not new. Oxytocin was one of the first candidates for a hormone of "motherhood." However, removal of the pituitary did not prevent females from becoming maternal. In addition, early attempts to induce maternal behavior in animals by injecting oxytocin into the bloodstream were unsuccessful. It eventually became apparent that oxytocin given in this manner did not easily enter the brain, and thus the absence of behavioral changes following injections was not surprising.

The exact mechanisms through which any hormone improves maternal behavior are still not fully understood, but several kinds of evidence suggest that oxytocin may decrease fear and increase a female's tolerance for stressful stimuli, such as those coming from a newborn. In rats, oxytocin can be used to inhibit anxiety toward a variety of fearful stimuli both related and unrelated to maternal behavior, and it can also reduce sensitivity to pain (Uvnas-Moberg, 1998). The interaction between oxytocin and stress hormones is particularly apparent in fear-sensing areas of the brain, such as the amygdala. It may therefore be the case that the exceptionally high levels of oxytocin released into the nervous system at birth orchestrate maternal responses that require activity throughout widespread areas of the brain.

When oxytocin reaches the brain, it does in fact facilitate maternal behavior, even in virgin female rats (Pedersen & Boccia, 2002). Sexually inexperienced female rats are subject to neophobia—the fear of new things—and they are normally quite anxious around other rats' pups. But less than 30 minutes after treatment with oxytocin, the reproductively naive females became fully maternal. Conversely, if postpartum mothers that would normally become maternal were treated with a drug blocking the effect of oxytocin, they did not become maternal and even avoided their pups. Since those original discoveries, support for a role for oxytocin in maternal behavior in rodents has continued to accumulate (Keverne, 2005).

It is logical to assume that oxytocin also plays a role in the powerful bonds that exist between mothers and their infants. However, the *selective* maternal behaviors that characterize human mothers and their infants are not found in rodents. Sheep, however, have provided an excellent prototype for analyzing the chemistry of selective mother-infant bonds (Keverne, 2005). Lambs are capable of walking immediately following birth, and each lamb must identify and follow its own mother. In addition, maternal responses in sheep are usually directed preferentially toward the ewe's own lamb, and females will not usually feed infants that are not their own. The period of maternal receptivity in sheep lasts just a few hours. Under normal conditions, a ewe will encounter only one lamb—her own—immediately postpartum. Once this bond is established, unfamiliar lambs will be physically rejected—literally butted and kicked away. The correct lamb is the one to which she has just given birth. The smell of amniotic fluid becomes attractive at the time of birth, and its presence on the newborn's wool is essential for the development of normal maternal behavior. As soon as the infant is born, its mother licks and removes the amniotic membranes and also gets a taste/smell of her own baby. As with maternal behavior in rats, the presence of oxytocin within the mother's brain is essential to maternal bonding in sheep. Without oxytocin (or if the mother is separated from her baby in the first hours after birth), she will later reject all lambs, including her own. Even in the absence of birth, a naive female can be encouraged to accept a foreign lamb either by giving her oxytocin, via an injection that reaches the nervous system, or by stimulating her cervix, thus causing her own body to release oxytocin. Research in sheep and various rodents leaves no question that oxytocin's behavioral actions are due to effects within the brain itself (Carter & Keverne, 2002; Pedersen & Boccia, 2002).

The parallels between maternal bonding in sheep and pair bonding in voles are striking. In both cases, the natural trigger to the formation of a bond involves genital stimulation, which, in turn, is known to release oxytocin. Blocking oxytocin's receptors or its release in the brain interferes with both types of bonding. In maternal ewes, as in voles, oxytocin opens an endocrine window of opportunity during which strong social relationships that may last a lifetime can form.

But does the oxytocin-bonding story apply to humans? In animals, it is possible to inject oxytocin directly into the nervous system. However, such experiments are not easily done in humans. We do know that as a woman breast feeds, oxytocin, primarily made by her own brain, rises in her blood. Mothers with higher levels of oxytocin are more sensitive to other people's feelings, more interested in pleasing others, and better at reading nonverbal cues than those with lower levels (Uvnas-Moberg, 1998)—obviously important traits when one is providing care to a newborn. Based primarily on the known effects of oxytocin in other animals and on studies of lactating women, it appears that oxytocin—made in the brain and acting within the brain—acts as a natural tranquilizer, lowering a new mother's blood pressure and heart rate, blunting her sensitivity to pain and stress, and reducing her anxiety. Indeed, under some conditions, oxytocin is amnesic, and it has even been suggested that this peptide may help women to forget the agony of childbirth.

Does this mean that oxytocin is necessary for maternal bonding? Perhaps humans with their complex nervous systems are less reliant on hormones to help assure good parenting and, where appropriate, parental bonds? The most obvious events associated with maternal behavior are birth and lactation. But, nursing or even birth are *not* required for human parents to become parental toward their children. A woman who delivers a baby by cesarean section without going through labor, for instance, and who then opts not to breast feed can still form a bond with her infant. Fathers and adoptive parents often report anxiety or fear prior to their exposure to a child. Yet these individuals as well as grandparents—people who have no opportunity to give birth or breast feed—also form lifelong attachments to their children and grandchildren. Very little is known regarding the release of oxytocin in humans who are not either giving birth or lactating. However, based again on recent research in male voles, we have found that it is possible for even brief exposure to an infant to release oxytocin and to inhibit the production of the adrenal hormone, corticosterone. In fact, brief pup exposure primes adult animals to form pair bonds more quickly (Carter et al., 2004).

While not essential for parenting, the elevation of oxytocin associated with birth and lactation may make it easier for a woman to be less anxious around her newborn and to experience and express positive feelings for her child (Altemus et al., 1995, 2001; Carter & Altemus, 1997). Taken together, research on humans and other animals suggests that oxytocin acts as a form of hormonal insurance, helping to guarantee that mothers, and perhaps fathers as well, will accept and care for their infants. The insurance is imperfect to be sure, but it is successful enough that we presume appropriate responses and receptiveness and make no effort to teach parents to love their infants. The biology of a new mother's selective memory (forgetting the intense pain of childbirth, for instance, but not forgetting the child) and the remarkable attachment between a mother and her infant provide insights into the mechanisms responsible for love. The biology of fatherhood, while less well understood, also may rely on the release of oxytocin and related neuropeptides, such as vasopressin (Bales et al., 2004). For example, vasopressin, which in the brain is androgen-dependent, may elevate the tendency of a male to be vigilant and defensive of his family, helping to assure the survival of his offspring. The behavioral role of vasopressin in females is in general poorly understood. However, recent evidence from animals suggests that females are less reliant than males on vasopressin for defensive responses (Carter, 2006).

As explained above, research in animals and also in lactating women suggests that oxytocin has the important capacity to down-regulate behavioral and emotional reactivity to stressful experiences. This hormone is well positioned within the brain to influence the behavioral and autonomic distress that typically follows separation from a mother, child, or partner (Carter, 1998). Oxytocin may even protect the vulnerable mammalian nervous system from regressing into the primitive states of lower brainstem dominance (such as the reptile-like freezing pattern with an associated shutdown of higher neural processes) that mammals are so carefully designed to avoid (Porges, 1998).

This is not to imply that oxytocin and vasopressin are the only brain chemicals that are important in social and reproductive behaviors. Various other neurochemicals have also been implicated in social, sexual, and maternal behavior in monogamous and nonmonogamous mammals. For example, prolactin, endorphins, and dopamine, to name only a few, may influence parental behavior and social attachment. These chemicals interact with and even regulate the release of oxytocin and vasopressin, and they may also have direct effects on the nervous system.

Of particular relevance to forming new relationships are the events that precede the social bond. Stressful experiences, including those associated with birth or puberty, may set the stage for a particularly powerful form of social bonding. Stress hormones play a role in social attachments, but alone are probably not responsible for the formation of social bonds. However, once a social bond is formed, by fulfilling our need for affiliation it also can contribute to the reduction of stress and to feelings of safety, love, and attachment.

EPIGENETICS AND THE ORIGINS OF SPECIES AND GENDER DIFFERENCES IN SOCIALITY

A deep understanding of behaviors such as those that characterize mammalian sociality and reproduction requires awareness of the factors that led to the development of the adult nervous system, including differences between males and females.

Sex differences are thought to be due to interactions among genetics and the hormonal and experiential histories of the individual. It was originally believed that most sex differences were due to the presence of male sex hormones, including testosterone, in males and the absence of this hormone in females. As we have now come to expect, research on monogamous mammals did *not* follow the pattern predicted from research on nonmonogamous species, such as rats. We also have discovered that male and female prairie voles respond in very different ways to both early social experiences and exposure to hormones (Carter, 2003, 2006). Males seem especially vulnerable to the negative effects of early experiences, possibly explaining the increased sensitivity of males to various developmental disorders (Teicher et al., 2003). For example, autism—defined in part by atypical social behaviors—is four to five times more common in males. Oxytocin production is defective in certain forms of autism (Green et al., 2001), and there is evidence that the oxytocin receptor is different in autistic and in nonautistic individuals (Wu et al., 2005). Neural mechanisms reliant on oxytocin may help to protect females from disorders such as autism. Alternatively, the androgen-dependence of vasopressin, particularly in early life and in certain brain regions such as the amygdala, may help to explain the increased vulnerability of males to this disorder (Carter, 2006). There is evidence from genetically manipulated mice that females are less behaviorally dependent on vasopressin than males (Bieksky et al., 2005). In addition, the gene responsible for the vasopressin (V1a) receptor is susceptible to evolutionary change (Hammond & Young, 2005). Reliance on vasopressin and a reduced availability of oxytocin might render males more vulnerability than to females to a variety of emotional and physical challenges (Carter, 2006).

Understanding of the origins of sex differences in the brain and in behavior also may help us to understand why males and females respond differently to children and to stressful experiences. Sex differences in the brain, and especially in neuroendocrine systems, also may help us understand why the two sexes are differentially susceptible to various physical and emotional disorders.

SOCIAL BONDS AND LOVE ARE POWERFUL MEDICINE, BUT WHY?

Love has traditionally been the domain of poets and novelists, and it is viewed by some as beyond the scope of experimental science. It is possible to study love and its biological origins, but it is necessary to carefully clarify the nature of our questions and the limitations of our scientific tools (Carter, 1998). Although love is a hypothetical construct with many dimensions and interpretations, for the purposes of science, love can be defined as a group of processes, experiences, and behaviors that promote and maintain social ties. Scientifically useful definitions of love also include the concept of selective attachment and assume the existence of social bonds.

Definitions of pair bonds in animals use apparently similar emotional and social behaviors: positive social behaviors; social selectivity rather than promiscuity; mate guarding or "jealousy"; stress or anxiety in the absence of the loved one. The object of these behaviors or feelings is not always a member of the opposite sex. It can be a child, a pet, or even an inanimate object. Ideally, love is reciprocal, but this is not essential. It is the feeling, emotions, and desires—the internal (emotional-visceral) state—of the individual doing the loving that define the experience of love.

Most research on social behavior began in the context of reproduction. However, the advantages of social living extend well beyond reproduction to the very roots of survival. Humans, like other social species, need social bonds. Children still need parents or loving caretakers. Adults need each other. Isolation is a powerful punishment and can unhinge even the most stable person.

Few of us grow all of our own food, find our own water, build our own homes, or rear a child alone. Traditional societies typically were designed around groups and often around extended families (Hrdy, 1999, 2005). Social bonds were virtually guaranteed by prolonged proximity. Mobility and modern economics have changed our culture in a few generations, but our physiology has not kept pace. Group living can provide easier access to food, warmth, and other essentials, and it reduces vulnerability to predation. Social interaction buffers individuals from the stress of life, and this effect is based on ancient physiological systems.

The subtle benefits and costs of social behavior are more important than most people realize. By examining the physiology of pair bonding, we have gained insight into another mysterious observation that has emerged from modern medical research. A wealth of evidence suggests that individuals with a perceived sense of social support survive illness and have longer lives than otherwise similar people who live alone or who, even in the presence of others, feel lonely. Demographic studies of human behavior reveal that "people who need people" are not only the "luckiest people in the world," but they are also the among the healthiest (Singer & Ryff, 2001; Uchino et al., 1996).

Modern medicine has sophisticated tools for discerning what makes us sick. But health is not solely the absence of illness. We remain exceptionally ignorant regarding the source of the good health that most humans enjoy for much of their lives. We do know that separation or grief can have devastating consequences for emotional and physical health. Knowledge of the scientific basis of sociality and social bonds allows a glimpse into mechanisms through which social relationships help to protect the human body.

Social support and trust appear to rely on a concoction of naturally occurring chemicals. As mentioned above, central to the neural mechanisms for social bonding and parental behavior are oxytocin and vasopressin. Although made in abundance in the mammalian brain, these hormones are released and become active only under special conditions. Oxytocin in particular may be inhibited by fear or stress (Carter, 1998; Neumann, 2001; Uvnas-Moberg, 1998). Both birth and lactation occur less readily when females feel vulnerable. The physiological and emotional circumstances that lead to social bonding and parental behavior are closely related to those necessary for general wellness and survival. Once more we ask, why? Research exploring the neurobiology of social behavior, and especially studies of the developmental effects of oxytocin and vasopressin, may suggest solutions (Carter, 2003, 2006).

But oxytocin and the neural systems that it helps to regulate also may counteract the tendency to be defensive or fearful. At the time of birth or during lactation and sexual behavior, women are especially vulnerable. At those times, oxytocin—released in large amounts—may help to allow these essential reproductive processes to occur. Men too can respond to oxytocin, and it has been shown that a single treatment with an intranasal oxytocin spray increases the willingness of humans to "trust" others, at least as measured in a computerized game (Kosfeld et al., 2005). Intranasal oxytocin also has direct effects on neural activation of the amygdala in response to fear-inducing stimuli (Kirsch et al., 2005). Oxytocin treatment also was associated with reduced coupling of the amygdala to brainstem regions that have been implicated in fear and autonomic arousal. Studies using oxytocin treatments in humans thus far have mainly been done in men. However, intranasal vasopressin has been given to both sexes and the reactions to slides of human facial expressions differed in men and women (Thompson et al., 2006). Men given additional vasopressin frowned more and rated unfamiliar, neutral facial expressions as more "unfriendly." In contrast, women given vasopressin actually smiled more and rated neutral expressions of others as more positive. Both oxytocin and vasopressin are central components of neural networks that are essential for adaptive social communication.

Oxytocin modulates reactivity to stress, reduces anxiety, reduces pain, and facilitates wound healing. Oxytocin has been called by others "the hormone of love" (Klopfer, 1971). Oxytocin may be essential for the formation of social bonds between mothers and their infants (Keverne, 2005) and between adults (Carter, 2005; Williams et al. 1994). Knowledge of the biology of love and the mechanisms through which it protects may be one of the lessons from prairie voles.

Simply put, social support and social bonds are powerful medicine. This is a cost-effective medicine with few side-effects. But it is also a medicine that modern culture can subvert. We can, perhaps for the first time in human history, actually survive, at least in adulthood, with almost no human contact. But the physiological and behavioral lessons from the prairie voles suggest that there may be unexpected prices for living with reduced human contact.

Atypical or disrupted social behaviors are a feature of many forms of mental illness, including schizophrenia, anxiety, and depression (Carter et al., 2001; Charney & Bremner, 2004). Animal research is allowing us to identify a central role for peptides in mental health and mental illness. Prairie vole social behavior, with its many parallels to human behavior, offers a unique opportunity to examine the interactive role of genetics and experience in the development and expression of mental disorders, including the mysterious developmental disorder called autism. The study of the biological basis of social behavior, even in animals such as voles, has much to teach us about mental health.

The desire to engage in positive behaviors and to express goodness, even under conditions where there are no obvious benefits to being good, may have archaic roots (Porges, 2003a, 2003b). Normal humans possess a need to form trusting relationships. Forced isolation can be devastating and even deadly. Mistreatment or denial of the existence of the social nervous system may increase the vulnerability of a child or adult to mental and physical illness (Teicher et al., 2003). Active mechanisms for the benefits of love and social support do exist, but they have been elusive. The study of social bonds allows us to understand the neurobiology of benevolence.

SUMMARY

The capacity to experience love and benevolence is a property of the human nervous system. Feelings of love are inherently motivating and rewarding. Love is good for your health. A knowledge of the social nervous system and the chemistry of social behavior helps to explain why people experiencing positive social environments live longer, recover more quickly from disease, and lead more successful, productive lives. Knowledge of these systems is now offering insights into mental health and mental illness.

The formation of strong social bonds is not a random occurrence. Social bond formation is especially prevalent around certain key life events, including birth, puberty, or periods of extreme duress when the survival of one individual depends on the presence of another. Neuroendocrine processes provide these windows of opportunity during which social bonds can form.

The characteristics of social bonds are expressions of physiological processes and are affected by interactions between genetics and developmental experiences. In addition, specific hormones—especially oxytocin and vasopressin—influence social behaviors and also have the capacity to influence stress and coping. Remarkably, exposure to these same hormones during early life can reprogram brain tissue, alter stress reactivity, and influence the same social behaviors that collectively define social monogamy (Carter, 2003; Weaver et al., 2004; Yamamoto et al., 2004). These studies suggest yet another mechanism through which social interactions, mediated by hormones, can influence behavior —in this case, producing changes that last a lifetime. Although experimental evidence for the role of hormones in human maternal behavior is still unavailable, we do know something about human endocrinology. Humans have the same basic bodily processes and hormones as are found in other mammals. We probably use those hormones for more or less the same general purposes.

Nature is quite economical. Well-designed chemicals are used over and over again. In the case of oxytocin, for example, we now know that this hormone occupies a uniquely integrative position within the nervous system. The same hormones and areas of the brain that serve the survival demands of the body also help us adapt to an ever-changing social and physical environment and to form social bonds.

The Greek philosopher Socrates proposed that the need of societies to do good arose from the desire of individuals to show goodness. Socrates argued that goodness or justice is associated with balance, harmony, and health. Modern neurobiology and the wisdom from prairie voles support this philosophy.

REFERENCES

Altemus, M, Deuster, PA, Gallivan, E, Carter, CS, & Gold, PW. (1995). Suppression of hypothalamic-pituitary-adrenal responses to exercise stress in lactating women. *Journal of Clinical Endocrinology and Metabolism*, 80, 2954–2959.

Altemus, M, Redwine, LS, Leong, Y-M, Frye, CA, Porges, SW, & Carter, CS. (2001). Responses to laboratory psychosocial stress in postpartum women. *Psychosomatic Medicine*, 63, 814–821.

Bales, KL, Kim, AJ, Lewis-Reese, AD, & Carter, CS. (2004). Both oxytocin and vasopressin may influence alloparental care in male prairie voles. *Hormones and Behavior*, 45, 454–361.

Barash, DP, & Lipton, JE. (2001). *Myth of monogamy: Fidelity and infidelity in animals and people*. New York: Freeman.

Bielsky, IF, Hu, SB, & Young LJ. (2005). Sexual dimorphism in the vasopressin system: lack of an altered behavioral phenotype in female V1a receptor knokcout mice. *Behavioural Brain Research*, 164, 132–136.

Bowler, CM, Cushing, BS, & Carter, CS. (2002). Social factors regulate female-female aggression and affiliation in prairie voles. *Physiology and Behavior*, 76, 559–566.

Carter, CS. (1998). Neuroendocrine perspectives on social attachment and love. *Psychoneuroendocrinology*, 23, 779–818.

Carter, CS. (2003). Developmental consequences of oxytocin. *Physiology and Behavior*, 79, 383–397.

Carter, CS. (2006). Sex differences in oxytocin and vasopressin: Implications for autism spectrum disorder? *Behavioural Brain Research*, in press.

Carter, CS, Ahnert, L, Grossman, KE, Hrdy, SB, Lamb, ME, Porges, SW, & Sachser, N. (Eds.). (2005). *Attachment and bonding: A new synthesis*. Cambridge, MA: MIT Press.

Carter, CS, & Altemus, M. (1997). Integrative functions of lactational hormones in social behavior and stress management. *Annals of the New York Academy of Sciences, Integrative Neurobiology of Affiliation*, 807, 164–174.

Carter, CS, Altemus, M, & Chrousos, GP. (2001). Neuroendocrine and emotional changes in the postpartum period. In C. Ingram & J. Russell (Eds.), *The maternal brain: Progress in brain research*, 133, 241–249.

Carter, CS, DeVries, AC, & Getz, LL. (1995). Physiological substrates of mammalian monogamy: The prairie vole model. *Neuroscience and Biobehavioral Reviews*, 19, 303–314.

Carter, CS, Epperson, PE, Kramer, KM, Ruscio, MG, & Bales, KL. (2004). The infant as a neuroendocrine manipulation in monogamous prairie voles. *Society for Neuroscience* Abstract No. 423.23. San Diego, CA.

Carter, CS, & Keverne, EB. (2002). The neurobiology of social affiliation and pair bonding. In D. Pfaff et al. (Eds.), *Hormones, brain, and behavior*, vol. 1. San Diego, CA: Academic (pp. 299–335).

Charney, DS, & Bremner, JD. (2004). The neurobiology of anxiety disorders. In DS Charney & EJ Nestler (Eds.), *The neurobiology of mental illness*. New York: Oxford University Press (pp. 605–627).

Cho, MM, DeVries, AC, Williams, JR, & Carter, CS. (1999). The effects of oxytocin and vasopressin on partner preferences in male and female prairie voles (*Microtus ochrogaster*). *Behavioral Neuroscience, 113*, 1071–1080.

DeVries, AC, DeVries, MB, Taymans, SE, & Carter, CS. (1995). The modulation of pair bonding by corticosterone in female prairie voles. *Proceedings of the National Academy of Sciences, 92*, 7744–7748.

DeVries, AC, DeVries, MB, Taymans, SE, & Carter, CS. (1996). Stress has sexually dimorphic effects on pair bonding in prairie voles. *Proceedings of the National Academy of Sciences, 93*, 11980–11984.

De Vries, GJ, & Villalba, C. (1997). Brain sexual dimorphism and sex differences in parental and other social behaviors. *Annals of the New York Academy of Sciences, 807*, 273–286.

Fisher, HE. (1992). *Anatomy of love: The natural history of monogamy, adultery, and divorce.* New York: Norton.

Green, L, Fein, D, Modahl, C, Feinstein, C, Waterhouse, L, & Morris, M. (2001). Oxytocin and autistic disorders: Alterations in peptide forms. *Biological Psychiatry, 50*, 609–613.

Hammock EA, & Young, LJ. (2005). Microsatellite instability generates diversity in brain and sociobehavioral traits. *Science, 308*, 1630–1634.

Hrdy, SB. (1999). *Mother nature: Maternal instincts and how they shape the human species.* New York: Ballantine.

Hrdy, SB. (2005). Evolutionary context of human development: The cooperative breeding model. In CS Carter, L Ahnert, et al. (Eds.), *Attachment and bonding: A new synthesis.* Cambridge, MA: MIT Press (pp. 9–32).

Insel, TR, O'Brien, DJ, & Leckman JF. (1999). Oxytocin, vasopressin, and autism: Is there a connection? *Biological Psychiatry, 45*, 145–157.

Keverne, EB. (2005). Neurobiological and molecular approaches to attachment and bonding. In CS Carter, L Ahnert, et al. (Eds.), *Attachment and bonding: A new synthesis.* Cambridge, MA: MIT Press, Vol. 1, pp. 101–117.

Kirsch, P, Esslinger, C, Chen, Q, Mier, D., Lis, S., Siddhanti, S, Gruppe, H, Mattay, VS, Gallhofer, B, Meyer-Linderberg, A. (2005). Oxytocin modulates neural circuitry for social cognition and fear in humans. *Journal of Neuroscience, 25*, 11489–11493.

Kleiman, D. (1977). Monogamy in mammals. *Quarterly Review of Biology, 52*, 39–69.

Klopfer, PH. (1971). Mother love: What turns it on? *American Scientist, 59*, 404–407.

Kosfeld, M, Heinrichs, M, Zak, PJ, Fischbacher, U, & Fehr, E. (2005). Oxytocin increases trust in humans. *Nature, 435*, 673–676.

monogamy. (n.d.). Dictionary.com Unabridged (v 1.0.1). Retrieved November 14, 2006, from Dictionary.com website: http://dictionary.reference.com/browse/monogamy.

Murdoch, GP. (1949). *Social structure.* New York: Free Press.

Neumann, ID. (2001). Alterations in behavioral and neuroendocrine stress coping strategies in pregnant, parturient and lactating rats. In C Ingram & J Russell (Eds.), *The maternal brain: Progress in brain research, 133*, 143–152.

Pedersen, CA, & Boccia, ML. (2002). Oxytocin links mothering received, mothering bestowed and adult stress responses. *Stress*, 5, 259–267.

Porges, SW. (1998). Love as an emergent property of the mammalian nervous system. *Psychoneuroendocrinology*, 23, 837–861.

Porges, SW. (2003a). The polyvagal theory: Phylogenetic contributions to social behavior. *Physiology and Behavior*, 79, 503–513.

Porges, SW. (2003b). Social engagement and attachment: A phylogenetic perspective. *Annals of the New York Academy of Sciences*, 1008, 31–47.

Singer, BH, & Ryff, CD. (Eds.). (2001). New horizons in health: An integrative approach. Washington, DC: National Academy Press.

Taylor, SE, Klein, LC, Lewis, BP, Gruenewald, TL, Gurung, RA, & Updegraff, JA. (2000). Biobehavioral responses to stress in females: Tend-and-befriend, not fight-or-flight. *Psychological Review*, 107, 411–429.

Teicher, MH, Andersen, SL, Polcari, A, Anderson, CM, Navlta, CP, & Kim, DM. (2003). The neurobiological consequences of early stress and childhood maltreatment. *Neuroscience and Biobehavioral Reviews*, 27, 33–44.

Thompson, RR, George K, Walton JC, Orr, SP, & Benson J. (2006). Sex-specific influences of vasopressin on human social communication. *Proceedings of the National Academy of Sciences USA*, 103, 7889–7894.

Uchino, BN, Cacioppo, JT, & Kiecolt-Glaser, JK. (1996). The relationship between social support and physiological processes: A review with emphasis on underlying mechanisms and implications for health. *Psychological Bulletin*, 119, 488–531.

Uvnas-Moberg, K. (1998). Oxytocin may mediate the benefits of positive social interaction and emotions. *Psychoneuroendocrinology*, 23, 819–835.

Weaver, IC, Cervoni, N, Champagne, FA, D'Alessio, AC, Sharma, S, Seckl, JR, Dymov, S, Szyf, M, & Meaney, MJ. (2004). Epigenetic programming by maternal behavior. *Nature Neuroscience*, 7, 847–854.

Williams, JR, Insel, TR, Harbaugh CR, & Carter, CS. (1994). Oxytocin centrally administered facilitates formation of a partner preference in female prairie voles (*Microtus ochrogaster*). *Journal of Neuroendocrinology*, 6, 247–250.

Winslow, JT, Hastings, N, Carter, CS, Harbaugh, CR, & Insel, TR. (1993). A role for vasopressin pair bonding in monogamous prairie voles. *Nature*, 365, 545–548.

Wu, S, Jia, M, Ruan, Y, Liu, J, Guo, Y, Shuang, M, Gong, X, Zhang, Y, Yang, X, & Zhang, D. (2005). Positive association of the oxytocin receptor gene (OXTR) with autism in the Chinese Han population. *Biological Psychiatry*, 58, 74–77.

Yamamoto, Y, Cushing, BS, Kramer, KM, Epperson, PD, Hoffman, GE, & Carter, CS. (2004). Neonatal manipulations of oxytocin alter oxytocin and vasopressin in the paraventricular nucleus of the hypothalamus in a gender-specific manner. *Neuroscience*, 125, 947–955.

PART IV

Altruism, Health, and Religion

Introduction

Stephen G. Post
Brie Zeltner

Let us assume that religious congregations serve the function of encouraging altruistic actions and emotions within the worshipping community and also toward the wider world. Can the purported association between religious service attendance and longevity be attributed to the disinhibition of altruism? We believe so.

Allen M. Omoto and Michèle M. Schlehofer, in "Volunteerism, Religiousness, Spirituality, and the Health Outcomes of Older Adults," assert that, since the 1980s, a growing body of literature indicates that there is little question that serving as a volunteer can produce health benefits for older adults. In addition to volunteerism, religiousness and spirituality have also been studied in relation to physical and mental health. Omoto and Schlehofer explore the interrelationships among volunteerism, religiousness, and health among older adults. Until this study, these components have only been studied separately. They attempt to provide evidence for possible connections among religiousness, spirituality, and volunteerism, as well as for their association with health among older adults. In their sample, religiousness and spirituality were significantly correlated with an array of mental health indicators, most consistently life satisfaction and (freedom from) depression. These associations are consistent with other research that has demonstrated the positive effects of religiousness and spirituality on mental health. They do find some evidence for the beneficial effects of volunteering on physical health and suggest that the narrow time period of their study limits their ability to reach more developed results. They do not conclude that there is no effect of volunteering on health, but do speculate that had their time frame been longer, their measures more sensitive and diverse, and the sample more variable in terms of health, they would have obtained stronger evidence for the physical health benefits of volunteerism. Suffice it to assert that these researchers are beginning the difficult process of teasing apart the simultaneous contributions of religion/spirituality and altruism on health. This is by no means an easy project.

Neal Krause, in "Altruism, Religion, and Health: Exploring the Ways in Which Helping Others Benefits Support Providers," suggests that, for those so inclined, a religious community in which altruism is prescribed might be useful. Krause discusses the ways in which formal places of worship provide opportunities for helping behavior and its associated health benefits to flourish. Because religions extol the virtues of loving others and helping those in need and offer both informal and formal ways of putting these virtues into practice, it is no surprise that more volunteer work is done through churches, synagogues, mosques, and so on than through any other organization. There are many ways in which religion promotes helping behavior, which all merit further study. Religion advocates empathy, compassion, and nonjudgmental concern, as well as evaluating the situation of others rather than judging them. Also, the church teaches the value of forgiveness, which itself has health benefits and can be considered to be a form of altruism. Last, Krause argues that the primary function of religion is to provide a sense of meaning to life and that helping others may be the best avenue for doing so. Next, the author reviews four major studies that address volunteering in the religious setting and concludes that a good deal of volunteer work takes place in this setting, and the benefits of volunteering may be the greatest for older adults who help within the church. This is primarily because the church often provides easy access to volunteering opportunities; there are more religious older adults than religious people in other age groups; and volunteering in old age may be especially critical to making the transition to a productive retirement lifestyle. In conclusion, Krause identifies four key issues to examine in the future study of this field: identifying the relative importance of altruistic attitudes versus concrete behaviors, the role of recognition of the volunteer's service to its health benefits, the relative benefits of helping a transgressor and the role of forgiveness, and finally, how to devise interventions that encourage altruistic behavior in all settings.

Harold G. Koenig, in "Altruistic Love and Physical Health," also highlights the ways in which prescribed altruism through religious communities may be helpful to those who are so inclined and could even explain the association between religious attendance and health. Altruistic love may improve both mental and physical health indirectly by increasing positive emotions and mediating the body's response to stress. The fight-or-flight response, a physiological reaction to internal and external stressors, has the immediate adaptive advantage of preparing the mind and body for survival. When exposure to stressors is prolonged, however, there are significant cardiovascular and immune costs to this response system. Evidence from a large number of high-quality studies has shown that stress and negative emotions (depressive symptoms) adversely affect physical health and survival through cardiovascular, immune, and endocrine pathways. Stress buffers, such as social support, religious beliefs and practices, and to a lesser extent, altruistic behaviors, have been shown to counteract stress and negative emotions and lead to positive health outcomes. Koenig reviews recent research on the mental and physical health effects of altruistic love, noting that there is more robust evidence of a positive effect on the former, but it is reasonable to predict that continued research will reveal positive physical health effects as well. This will likely be due to the fact that altruistic behaviors promote social integration, distract from the self, enhance a sense of meaning in life, increase self-efficacy and competence, and improve mood. Next, Koenig discusses the relationship between religion and health and the vast body of research that has shown that religious people are more loving and more likely to volunteer and that religious involvement is a strong predictor of both physical and mental health. It is possible that altruism is the mediator in this relationship, and researchers need to address this possibility. From a clinical standpoint, Koenig believes that altruistic love can go a long way toward healing the doctor-patient relationship and may even encourage trust and treatment compliance in patients, as well as job satisfaction and lower burnout for health care professionals. In conclusion, the author identifies potential directions for future research on altruism, religion, health, and their interrelations.

21 Volunteerism, Religiousness, Spirituality, and the Health Outcomes of Older Adults

Allen M. Omoto
Michèle M. Schlehofer

Helping and community service occur in a variety of contexts and across a range of activities, including donations of money and goods and participation in one-day events (such as walkathons or charity auctions). Volunteerism, in particular, is a special form of helping consisting of ongoing commitments to service. This form of helping typically involves people choosing to help others in need, often in organizational contexts (e.g., volunteer service organizations), and the acts of helping are ones that have been actively sought out. What's more, these acts of charity and assistance are often sustained over extended periods of time and can involve considerable expenditures of effort and finances by the volunteer. And, because volunteers typically help people with whom they have no prior contact or association, it is a form of helping that occurs without any bonds of obligation or commitment to the recipients of the volunteer services (e.g., Omoto & Snyder, 1995; Snyder, Clary, & Stukas, 2000; Wilson, 2000).

Every year, millions of people engage in volunteer activities of this nature. The U.S. Department of Labor (2004) reported that 64.5 million people, or 29% of the U.S. population, volunteered during 2004 alone. Although their rate of volunteering is less than non-elder adults, older adults, specifically those over age 65, volunteer at relatively high levels; approximately 25% are currently active volunteers (U.S. Department of Labor, 2004). Furthermore, those older adults who do volunteer tend to give the most time, with estimates ranging up to 2.5 times the commitments of volunteers aged 25 to 34 (Brown, 2000; U.S. Department of Labor, 2004). With projections indicating that older adults will make up an increasingly larger percentage of the population and that adults will live longer into postretirement, there are calls to encourage productive aging and continuing civic engagement through volunteering (e.g., American Psychological Society, 1993). Without doubt, there are many important theoretical and practical reasons to scientifically explore acts of volunteering among this population.

VOLUNTEERISM'S EFFECTS ON THE HEALTH OF OLDER ADULTS

Although better health may make it more likely that an older adult volunteers in the first place, there is little question that serving as a volunteer can, in turn, produce health benefits for older adults. Since the 1980s, a growing body of research has strongly suggested a link between volunteering and an array of positive health outcomes (Piliavin, 2005). Research has found, for example, that older adults who volunteer compared to those who do not believe they are in better physical health (Young & Glasgow, 1998). Volunteerism also has been related to greater longevity (Moen, Dempster-McClain, & Williams, 1992; Musick, Herzog, & House, 1999), including a mortality rate among elderly volunteers that is 63% lower than that of nonvolunteers (Oman, Thoresen, & McMahon, 1999). This lower mortality rate persists even after several alternative explanations, such as chronic conditions, physical mobility, health habits, social support, religious attendance, and mental health are controlled (Oman et al., 1999). Recently, the beneficial effects of informal help giving among older adults have been demonstrated in a 5-year longitudinal study (Brown, Nesse, Vonokur, & Smith, 2003). Specifically, older adults who informally helped others, such as friends and family members, by providing instrumental or emotional support lived longer, even after controlling for functioning, health satisfaction, and the extent to which they engaged in healthy behaviors. In this study, those older adults who did not provide social support to others were more than twice as likely than those who helped to die during the project period. Although this study focused on informal help and not volunteering per se, much of the assistance provided by individuals is likely to be similar to some of the tasks performed by volunteers in different contexts. Taken together, this emerging body of research on volunteerism and informal help provision by older adults offers impressive evidence of the benefit of doing good for others. Moreover, it appears that helping others is what is critical in producing these positive effects on longevity.

The health benefits of volunteering are not limited to physical health and longevity, but seem to extend to mental health as well. Several studies (Hunter & Linn, 1980–1981; Van Willigen, 2000) have revealed that older volunteers are more satisfied with their lives than older adults who do not donate their time to helping others. One meta-analysis (Wheeler, Gorey, & Greenblatt, 1998), for example, concluded that the strength of the relationship between volunteering and life satisfaction among older adults is moderate ($r = .25$; 95% CI = .194 to .310). Here, volunteerism was loosely defined to include both^sdirect and indirect helping roles. Furthermore, results from this same meta-analysis suggested that almost 85% of elderly adults who volunteered scored better on the various mental health measures (e.g., life satisfaction, depression) than elderly adults who did not volunteer.

A wide range of other mental health benefits has also been found to accrue for older volunteers. For example, compared to older adults who are nonvolunteers, older adult volunteers have a greater will to live, lower levels of anxiety and depression (Hunter & Linn, 1980–1981; Musick & Wilson, 2003), and higher morale, self-esteem, positive affect, and general well-being (Midlarsky & Kahana, 1991). And older adults who volunteer either formally or informally typically perceive their health to be better than those who do not, a finding that has emerged in data from both the United States (Van Willigen, 2000) and Japan (Krause, Ingersoll-Dayton, Liang, & Sugisawa, 1999). Clearly, then, research demonstrates the positive effects of volunteering and helping on physical and mental health, if not the precise mechanisms by which these effects occur.

RELIGIOUSNESS AND SPIRITUALITY AS PREDICTORS OF HEALTH

Besides volunteerism, the health implications of a number of other behaviors, activities, and practices have been investigated among older adults. Prominent among these other activities are those related to religiousness and spirituality. Like volunteerism and helping behavior, there is a fast-growing scientific literature on the interrelationships among religiousness, spirituality, and the physical and mental health of older adults.

Religiousness is a multifaceted construct that consists of both attitudinal (e.g., religious beliefs, religious identification) and behavioral (e.g., participation in religious services, prayer) components (Hill et al., 2000; Zinnbauer et al., 1997). In addition, religious behaviors can be delineated into those that are organizationally based (e.g., attending services at a church or other religious institution) and those that are not organizationally based (e.g., watching religious television programming). Furthermore, religiousness is not the same as spirituality. For example, recent conceptual and empirical work suggests that religiousness contains more interpersonal components than does spirituality (Schlehofer & Omoto, 2004; Zinnbauer et al., 1997). This research, conducted with both working adults (Zinnbauer et al., 1997) and older adults (Schlehofer & Omoto, 2004), suggests that spirituality is often thought of in personal or experiential terms. Religiousness, on the other hand, tends to also encompass participation in institution-related or organizational functions, including formal services, study groups, and potlucks. In short, although religiousness and spirituality appear to share conceptual overlap, there are distinct components that warrant exploration of their separate and possibly joint effects.

These limitations aside, some tentative claims about the links between religiousness (spirituality) and health can be made. Paralleling the literature on volunteering and helping, religiousness and spirituality appear to be strongly related to the mental and physical health of older adults. Older adults who regularly participate in church activities report greater life satisfaction and better overall mental health compared to those who do not (Pope, Beck, Shue, & Cook, 2003). Similarly, finding meaning in one's religion and participating in spiritual practices, such as meditation, are related to better mental health (Fry, 2000). Older adults who find meaning in their religion, regardless of the extent of their religious behaviors, are least likely to drink alcohol (Krause, 2003), and those who are religious are more likely than those who are not religious to use preventative health care services, such as flu shots, mammograms, and prostate screenings (Benjamins & Brown, 2003). Thus, religiousness and spirituality may directly and positively influence health and promote healthy or health-protective behaviors.

In this literature on health, the relationship between religiousness and health has not been separately examined from the relationship between spirituality and health. Rather, the research has tended to confound the effects of both constructs on health. At minimum, then, there has been a mismatch between the conceptual definition and the operationalization of these constructs, if not confusion about the specific set of beliefs or practices that relates to health.

It is possible that older adults who are healthier more readily take part in religious and spiritual activities. For example, older adults in poorer health have been found to engage in more private (e.g., watching religious television programming) than public (e.g., attending church) religious behaviors (Benjamins, Musick, Gold, & George, 2003). Thus, the very real possibility exists that the direction of the effects is reversed—that health outcomes may actually predict older adults' religiousness and spirituality.

A related limitation in this work is that the separate effects of the behavioral and attitudinal components of religiousness have not been thoroughly delineated. Religiousness is a multidimensional construct, consisting of both attitudinal and belief components and behavioral components. Furthermore, behaviors can be divided into those that are organizationally and nonorganizationally based. In qualitative research that we conducted with older adults living in retirement communities, we asked participants to separately define both religiousness and spirituality. An analysis of these interviews revealed that participants saw a relationship with both concepts as encompassing a relationship with a higher power. Where they diverged was that religiousness, but not spirituality, was viewed as including interpersonal components and affiliation with a religious community. In short, older adults in our research provided broader and more complex definitions of religiousness than of spirituality (Schlehofer

& Omoto, 2004; see also Schlehofer, Omoto, & Adelman, 2006)). It remains to be seen if these two concepts exert different effects on older adults' mental and physical health.

So far, we have reviewed evidence for the health benefits of volunteering and religiousness (or spirituality). However, we have also noted limitations to the work in this area that prevent definitive conclusions from being drawn. We have been struck by the parallels in the research in these areas, as well as a little surprised that, with only a few notable exceptions, the joint influences of volunteering and religiousness have not been carefully investigated. Many older adults formally or informally volunteer their time through the context of a religious group or organization (Krause, Ingersoll-Dayton, Liang, & Sugisawa, 1999; Musick, Herzog, & House, 1999). Furthermore, there is research evidence that suggests that the beneficial effects of volunteering on the health of older adults may be stronger or enhanced for those who are also more religious (Musick & Wilson, 2003; Oman et al., 1999). In one study, for example, volunteering was generally related to decreased depression among older adults, but those who volunteered for religious causes were the ones who received the most mental health benefits from their work (Musick & Wilson, 2003; see also Oman et al., 1999).

Having identified a provocative pattern of findings, we decided to explore more closely the interrelationships among volunteerism, religiousness, and health among older adults. Precisely because many studies have examined these components separately, we sought to study their simultaneous influences. Furthermore, we sought to include separate measures of spirituality and religiousness, including measures that took account of the multidimensional nature of these constructs. To explore these issues, we drew from an existing data set of older adults that contained measures for some of the constructs of interest (see Omoto, 2004). Although this project was not specifically developed to investigate the interrelationships that are the focus of this chapter, it included data that made it possible to conduct preliminary tests of the interrelationships among these constructs. The data set also contained a short-term longitudinal component, with some measures collected over a 6–month time frame. Thus, we were in a position to explore the predictive, rather than simply the concurrent correlational, nature of these interrelationships.

PSYCHOLOGICAL RESEARCH ON OLDER ADULTS

As part of the project, 141 residents from four different retirement communities in Los Angeles County, California, took part in a survey that contained items on volunteering, religiousness, spirituality, and mental and physical health (see Omoto & Aldrich, 2007, for more on participants' lives in these retirement communities). For three of the retirement communities from which participants were recruited, admittance was contingent on meeting age and income requirements. The admittance requirement for the fourth community included having spent at least 20 years working for the Christian church (e.g., missionaries, denominational leaders, YMCA directors, etc.). Across participants, there was thus a wide range of religious involvement, although the extent of this involvement tended to be confounded with the communities in which participants lived.

The sample was primarily female (69.5%) and White (91.5%). The average age of the participants was 80.47 years ($SD = 6.21$), with a range of 62 to 94 years. Overall, the sample was well educated, with 83.2% having attained at least a bachelor's degree and 49.6% having obtained a graduate degree. The majority (47.5%) of participants was married, with 38.8% widowed, 10.1% single having never married, and 3.6% divorced or separated.

To recruit participants, members of our research team made presentations at each of the retirement communities about the research, and we distributed flyers and posters around the campuses. Volunteers were sought from the general population of retirement community residents, all of whom were compensated for taking part in the different studies. Participants completed the survey at two points in time, 6 months apart. We were successful in obtaining follow-up measures from 91.4% ($N = 129$) of our initial questionnaire sample.

At the initial assessment, participants completed measures of religiousness, spirituality, and volunteerism. Specifically, *religious identity* was assessed with three items on a 5-point Likert scale (1 = "strongly disagree" to 5 = "strongly agree"; ± = .83). A sample item is "My religious faith defines who I am as a person." *Spiritual identity*, likewise, was measured on the same 5-point Likert scale with three items (± = .90), such as "I consider spirituality a driving force in my life." Finally, participation in *organizationally based religious practices* (two items; ± = .77) and *nonorganizationally based religious practices* (four items; ± = .80) was measured by having participants rate on a 5-point Likert scale (ranging from 1 = "never" to 5 = "very often") the extent to which they did several different behaviors, including "How often do you attend organized religious services?" (organizationally based religious practices) and "How often do you watch or listen to religious programs on TV or radio?" (nonorganizationally based religious practices).

Participants also completed several measures of their volunteering behavior at this initial assessment. First, they self-reported the average number of hours a week they volunteered. Second, participants indicated on a 5-point Likert scale (1 = "not at all," 3 = "moderately," 5 = "extremely") how active they were as volunteers in 10 different types of organizations: church, other faith-based, civic or neighborhood, health-related, political, professional/employment, school or youth-related, seniors, service or philanthropic, and social (collapsing over all of these organizations, ± = .53). We broke down this measure further so as to tap volunteering activity in church or other faith-based organizations ($r = .28$,

$p < .001$) separately from volunteering activity in other types (nonchurch or non-faith-based) of organizations ($\pm = .45$).

Six months later, participants completed multiple-item measures of their mental health, many of them abbreviated versions of widely used scales or assessment instruments. Specifically, participants completed the Satisfaction With Life Scale (see Pavot & Diener, 1993), which assesses life satisfaction at three points in time: once for their past (two items; $\pm = .82$; sample item: "If I had the past to live over, I'd change little"), present (three items; $\pm = .84$; sample item: "I am satisfied with my current life"), and future life satisfaction (two items; $\pm = .87$; sample item: "The conditions of my future life will be excellent"). Participants also completed a 6-item scale of age-related anxiety that tapped concerns and potential problems associated with aging (Kafer, Rakowski, Lachman, & Hickey, 1980; $\pm = .68$; sample item: "The older I become, the more alone I feel"), self-esteem (five items from Rosenberg, 1965; $\pm = .59$; sample item: "At times I think I am no good at all"), and depression (five items from the CES-D; Radloff, 1977; $\pm = .53$; sample [reverse-coded] item: "I feel full of energy"). All items were measured on a 5-point Likert scale ranging from 1 = "strongly disagree" to 5 = "strongly agree." It should be noted that some of the scales have relatively low reliability, perhaps partially due to the limited number of items used for each scale. Finally, participants' physical health was assessed in two complementary ways. Specifically, participants reported physical health problems by checking which, if any, of 15 health problems that often afflict older adults they currently experienced (e.g., hypertension, poor vision). They also rated the frequency that they experienced limitations in their functioning across 9 different domains (e.g., limitations walking, limitations carrying moderately heavy items). These ratings were made on a scale with 1 = "never" and 4 = "very often." Scores from the health problems checklist and the limitations ratings were combined into a single indicator of physical health by first standardizing the scores and then averaging them together for each participant.

Cross-sectional Findings

We first examined the relationships between religious and spiritual identities and volunteering behavior. To do so, we started with participant responses to the question about the number of hours a week they volunteered, and grouped them as being less-frequent volunteers (volunteering no more than 5 hours a week; $N = 94$) or frequent volunteers (volunteering more than 5 hours a week; $N = 47$). Next, we compared these groups on their average scores on the measures of religious identity, spiritual identity, engagement in organizationally based religious practices, and frequency of nonorganizationally based religious practices. Confirming our expectations about the connections between volunteering and religiousness and spirituality, retirees who currently volunteered and spent considerable time doing so tended to have stronger religious identity, $t(135)$ = 1.77; $p < .10$. They also claimed significantly greater spiritual identity and engaged in more organizationally based religious practices, $ts > 2.56$; $ps < .05$. However, they did not engage in significantly more nonorganizationally based religious practices, although the means were in the expected direction, $t(136)$ = 1.31, ns.

Utilizing a continuous measure of volunteer hours revealed consistent, but less compelling results. Specifically, the number of volunteer hours was positively but weakly (and nonsignificantly) related to religious identity and frequency of organizationally based and nonorganizationally based religious practices $(.11 < r < .16)$. The association between volunteer hours and spiritual identity was positive and statistically reliable, $r = .27$; $p < .01$. Retirees who rated themselves as having stronger spiritual identities also tended to report more hours spent volunteering per week. Whereas the majority of participants in our sample claimed religious and spiritual identities and consistently engaged in religious practices, the ratings of these identities and practices were even higher among the retirees who volunteered more hours each week.

To refine our analyses further, we examined only those retirees who reported being a volunteer ($N = 121$) and their ratings of volunteer activity. As with the whole sample, we first divided this subset of participants into "less-active" and "more-active" volunteering groups, this time using the group median as a cutoff. As with the overall analyses, the results were quite clear: Participants who reported greater volunteer activity relative to less-active volunteers reported stronger spiritual identities and also more frequently engaged in organizationally based religious practices, $ts > 2.14$; $ps < .05$. They also tended to engage in more nonorganizationally based religious practices, although in a statistical test this difference was only marginally significant, $t(111) = 1.95$; $p < .06$. Surprisingly, the volunteering groups did not differ in their rated religious identities, $t < 1.32$, ns.

In correlational analyses, all of the associations between volunteer activity and the various religiousness and spirituality measures were positive and statistically significant, further supporting our expectations and other findings. Specifically, greater volunteering activity was related to stronger spiritual and religious identities ($rs > .238$; $ps < .01$). Volunteering was also related to the behavioral measures of religious engagement, with greater activity as a volunteer associated with more often engaging in both organizationally based and nonorganizationally based religious practices, $rs > .304$, $ps < .01$.

Taken together, these results provide support for the idea that volunteerism increases with both religiousness and spirituality, at least as tapped by our identity measures. Furthermore, the more frequently our sample of older adults participated in religious practices, either in organizational or nonorganizational contexts, the more time they spent volunteering each week and the more active they rated themselves as volunteers.

What is less clear from these results, however, is if these patterns of relationships hold for both those volunteer activities that are conducted within church or faith organizations and more general types of volunteer activities. It seems reasonable to expect that religious or spiritual individuals, or those who participate relatively frequently in religious practices, will also devote more hours to volunteer work in church or faith-based organizations. Of interest, though, is if religious and spiritual teachings and practices also encourage greater volunteer activity outside of religious contexts and organizations. In short, the question we posed was, is it the case that individuals with stronger religious or spiritual identities engage in more religiously based volunteering only or also in more general volunteering?

In order to begin to answer this question, we examined the data separately for volunteer activity conducted in church or faith-based organizations and volunteering activity in other types of organizations. In terms of volunteer activity in church or faith-based organizations, the picture that emerged was similar to the overall picture presented so far. That is, retirees who rated themselves as relatively more active in church or faith-based volunteering, in comparison with those reporting relatively less such activity, did indeed claim stronger religious and spiritual identities, $ts > 3.97$; $ps < .001$. And, as before, they also engaged in more organizationally based and nonorganizationally based religious practices, $ts > 4.52$; $ps < .001$. Furthermore, correlational analyses fully supported these patterns. Reports of volunteer activity in church or faith-based organizations was strongly associated with greater religious identity, stronger spiritual identity, more frequent participation in organizationally based religious practices, and more participation in nonorganizationally based religious practices, $rs > .446$; $ps < .001$. Looking at these results in another way, retirees who rated themselves as more religious or spiritual appeared to act on their beliefs by volunteering more in church or faith-based organizations.

However, the associations between volunteering and religiousness and spirituality disappeared when we examined volunteer activity *not* tied to church-related or faith-based organizations. In this case, there were no differences between more- and less-active volunteers in their rated religious and spiritual identities, nor in the extent of their organizational and nonorganizational religious practices, all $ts < 1.3$, *ns*. Even utilizing what could be considered to be more sensitive continuous measures of our constructs failed to produce significant relationships. None of the religiousness or spirituality variables were correlated with volunteer activity outside of church-related or faith-based organizations, all $rs < .144$, *ns*. In this context, the amount of volunteer activity was unrelated to any of the religiousness or spirituality constructs that we measured. That is, it appears that older adults who are religious and spiritual and who participate in organizationally and nonorganizationally based religious practices are more active volunteers in church or faith-based organizations. However, their relatively high rate of volunteer activity does not carry over to volunteering in nonreligious organizations; the degree of volunteering in these organizations is unrelated to religious or spiritual identities or to religious practices. Thus, it may be the case that being religious or spiritual works to influence the outlets through which people volunteer. Specifically, religiousness and spirituality seem to increase volunteering in church or faith-based organizations, but not necessarily in secular organizations.

Overall, the patterns of results from our analyses so far are intriguing and present a nuanced picture of the links between volunteering and religiousness and spirituality. First, the results provide initial evidence that retired individuals who volunteer more frequently tend to be more religious and spiritual and also to engage in more religious practices (both organizationally and nonorganizationally based) than retirees who do not volunteer or do not volunteer as frequently. However, this overall pattern actually seems to mask differences related to the context in which the volunteering occurs, specifically in differences between volunteer activity in church or faith-based organizations and volunteer activity in other organizations. Older adults who are more religious or spiritual volunteer more on average, but especially in the context of church or faith-based organizations. The degree of their volunteer activity in secular organizations does not differ from that of older adults who claim religious and spiritual identities to a lesser extent or who do not engage in religious practices as frequently.

This pattern of results is consistent with a dual process view of the links between religiousness and spirituality and volunteerism. First, religious or spiritual tenets and practices may encourage volunteer service so that individuals who more strongly claim religious identities or embrace religious practices are more likely to volunteer or to be more active volunteers than individuals with less religious identification or engagement. But religiousness and spirituality also appear to especially promote volunteering in church or faith-based contexts. It is possible that religious convictions promote volunteering and a sense of humanitarianism and that being involved in religious social networks—such as a church—provides readily available outlets through which to channel volunteering "energy" and propensities.

Longitudinal Findings

So far, we have reviewed evidence from a cross-sectional sample of older adults that suggests that older adults who volunteer more in church or faith-based organizations, compared to those who volunteer less in such organizations, are more religious and spiritual and engage in more organizationally and nonorganizationally based religious behaviors. However, the extent of volunteering in organizations *not* church-related or faith-based is unrelated to religiousness or spirituality. Next, we explored the implications of these patterns for health outcomes. In particular, we made use of our longitudinal data and explored the extent to which volunteering, religiousness, and spirituality were related to mental and physical health over a 6-month period.

Our analyses reveal that, in our sample of retired adults, volunteerism, religiousness, and spirituality are clearly related to later health, and especially to indicators of mental health. First, we computed correlations among participants' ratings of their religious and spiritual identities, their participation in organizationally and nonorganizationally based religious practices, and their 6-month mental and physical health. Initial religious identity was associated with greater past and future life satisfaction, as well as with less age-related anxiety and depression at 6 months, $rs > .16$; $ps < .10$. Spiritual identity, furthermore, was associated with more present and future life satisfaction ($rs > .24$; $ps < .05$), greater self-esteem ($r = .21$; $p < .05$), lower age-related anxiety ($r = -.24$; $p < .05$), and less depression ($r = -.20$; $p < .05$), all measured 6 months later. Thus, to the extent that retirees in our sample claimed stronger religious or spiritual identities, they also reported better mental health several months later.

Analyses of the religious behavior measures revealed similar findings. Specifically, greater participation in nonorganizationally based religious activities was positively related to later ratings of past and future ($rs > .17$; $ps < .05$) life satisfaction, and negatively correlated with 6–month age-related anxiety, $r = -.19$; $p < .05$. Furthermore, and in line with prior research (Pope et al., 2003), participation in organizationally based religious activities was associated with more past and future life satisfaction as reported at 6 months ($rs > .21$; $ps < .05$). These behaviors were also related to less depression later on, $r = -.26$; $p < .05$.

Contrary to the consistent positive and significant associations for the mental health measures, attempting to predict physical health (i.e., health problems and functional limitations) proved more elusive from our earlier measures of volunteering, religiousness, and spirituality. Although we correlated the religious and spiritual identity measures and both of the religious practices measures with the 6-month index of physical health, only one of these relationships was statistically reliable. Specifically, claims of stronger spiritual identity predicted better physical health 6 months later, although the magnitude of this association was actually relatively weak, $r = .19$; $p < .05$. Other research (e.g., Benjamins et al., 2003) has indicated that participation in nonorganizationally based religious activities may be related to being in poorer physical health, although the explanation for this effect may be that health problems and limitations prevent older adults from taking part in organizationally based religious activities. In our sample, however, participation in nonorganizationally based religious practices was simply unrelated to physical health, $r = -.06$, ns. We note, though, that our data were collected over a relatively short window of time (6 months) and from reasonably healthy individuals; either of these facts may account for our failure to replicate the findings from prior research.

In terms of the prospective health correlates of volunteering, our initial measure of hours per week spent volunteering was associated with later depression; more hours volunteering predicted less depression, $r = -.20$; $p < .05$. Likewise, higher self-rated activity as a volunteer was associated with more present life satisfaction and less depression 6 months later, $rs > .18$; $ps < .05$. The absolute magnitude of these correlations was not large, but the fact that they reveal reliable associations over a 6-month period in a relatively homogeneous sample suggests to us that the relationships are worthy of future study if not as targets for potential interventions.

As before, we examined volunteer activity in church and faith-based organizations separately from rated volunteer activity in other organizations. And, again, an interesting pattern of findings emerged when we attempted to predict 6-month health from the earlier assessment of volunteer activity in church and faith-based organizations. First, though, recall that greater volunteer activity (as well as more hours spent volunteering) in church and faith-based organizations was also related to greater religiousness and spirituality and that volunteering tended to predict better health 6 months later. In our analyses differentiating the types of volunteer activity, volunteering in church-related or faith-based organizations was related to more life satisfaction and less depression 6 months later, $rs > .19$; $ps < .05$. Volunteering in other types of organizations, aside from not being associated with the religiousness or spirituality measures, was also not associated with either of these later mental health indicators.

Clearly, the magnitude of all of these associations, and even the differences between them, were not that large. Nonetheless, they are consistent with theorizing that links volunteering, religious or spiritual identities, and health for many people. That is, to the extent that religiously inclined individuals volunteer, their later health is likely to be better. To the extent that their volunteer efforts are centered on the work of church-related or faith-based organizations, however, their short-term later health may benefit even more. We also note that these trends were more evident on our mental health measures than on the indicators of physical health. Contrary to our expectations and considerable past research, volunteering was unrelated to later physical health among our sample of older adults, $rs < .10$, ns.

CONCLUDING COMMENTS

We have attempted to provide evidence for possible connections among religiousness, spirituality, and volunteerism, as well as for their association with health among older adults. Although our findings are not definitive, they can be considered as a starting point for future research. They suggest that religiousness, spirituality, and volunteerism are interrelated and also predictive of the mental and physical health of older adults. In our sample, religiousness and spirituality were significantly correlated with an array of mental health indicators, most consistently life satisfaction and (lack of) depression. These associations are consistent with other research that has demonstrated the positive effects of religiousness and spirituality on mental health (e.g., Fry, 2000; Krause, 2003; Pope et al., 2003). Simply put, older adults who are religious or spiritual seem to benefit from improved mental health. Interestingly, the effects of religiousness and spirituality tended to parallel each other; we found few differences between them in their associations with our indicators of mental health. Attempting to replicate these effects and exploring why these constructs have similar effects on health despite their conceptual distinctiveness (Schlehofer & Omoto, 2004) would be useful directions for future work.

Our findings provide only limited evidence for the beneficial effects of volunteering on physical health. This could be for a variety of reasons. First, the relatively short time frame (6 months) in between surveys may not be enough to uncover changes in or effects on physical health. Indeed, the majority of research in this area utilizes a much longer time period to determine how volunteering affects physical health (Brown et al., 2003; Piliavin, 2005). Second, we assessed physical health via a checklist of health problems and a measure of functional limitations. A broader and more sensitive measure of physical health, including information on such things as number of medications, hospital visits, and number of colds experienced, might provide a clearer picture of the effects of volunteerism on health. Likewise, all of the measures in our research were self-report. It is possible that participants cannot or will not accurately report their health. Future research should examine not only self-report indices, but also medical records or other convergent (and, ideally, objective) indicators of health. Finally, our sample was relatively healthy. This limited variability in health likely compromised our ability to detect correlations. Rather than conclude that there is no effect of volunteering on health, then, we speculate that had our time frame been longer, our measures more sensitive and diverse, and the sample more variable in terms of health, we would have obtained stronger evidence for the physical health benefits of volunteerism.

We have suggested and empirically demonstrated that religiousness and spirituality are related to volunteering. Volunteering was associated with greater religious and spiritual identities and greater participation in both organizationally and nonorganizationally based religious practices. Further, religiousness and spirituality appear to be related to volunteering in church or faith-based organizations, but not in other types of organizations. Thus, it appears that those individuals who are more religious and spiritual volunteer more in church or faith-based organizations. Although self-selection is a concern here, these findings do provide insight into the types of volunteering activities to which individuals of different religious and spiritual identities are attracted and in which they actively engage.

Perhaps most important is our finding that volunteering in church or faith-based organizations is related to better mental health. Individuals who reported high volunteering activity in church or faith-based organizations, but not necessarily greater volunteer activity in nonchurch or non-faith-based arenas, demonstrated significantly better mental health 6 months later. Taken together, these results suggest that it may be the case that religiousness works to influence the types of volunteer activities engaged in, and it is involvement in these activities that translates into better mental health outcomes among older adults. This finding is also consistent with general functional theorizing in the volunteering realm, which posits that people receive the most benefit from serving as a volunteer when they are getting their specific needs met (Omoto & Snyder, 1995). In this case, religiously inclined individuals benefit more from volunteering in religious contexts. Alternatively, the results could also be taken to suggest that living a life informed by religion and volunteering, especially in religious contexts, simply leads to better health. Each of these possibilities is ripe for empirical exploration. Ultimately, investigations into these issues will help to answer questions about when and how doing good for others, specifically as a volunteer, can produce benefits for *both* helpers and recipients.

The research described in this chapter was supported by a grant from the Fetzer Institute and the Institute for Research on Unlimited Love. Direct correspondence to Allen M. Omoto, School of Behavioral and Organizational Sciences, Claremont Graduate University, 123 E. Eighth Street, Claremont, CA 91711; e-mail: allen.omoto@cgu.edu. The authors thank the following individuals for their assistance with this project: Anita Boling, Christina D. Aldrich, Anna M. Malsch, Viviane Seyrayani, Tanya Valery, and the participants who took part.

REFERENCES

American Psychological Society. (1993, December). Vitality for life: Psychological research for productive aging. *APS Observer (Special issue: Human capital initiative, Report 2)*. Washington, DC: American Psychological Society Press.

Benjamins, M. R., & Brown, C. (2003). Religion and preventative health care utilization among the elderly. *Social Science and Medicine, 58*, 109–118.

Benjamins, M. R., Musick, M. A., Gold, D. T., & George, L. K. (2003). Age-related declines in activity level: The relationship between chronic illness and religious activities. *Journals of Gerontology, 58B*, S377–S385.

Brown, E. (2000). The scope of volunteer activity and public service. *Law and Contemporary Problems, 62*, 17–42.

Brown, S., Nesse, R. M., Vonokur, A. D., & Smith, D. M. (2003). Providing social support may be more beneficial than receiving it: Results from a prospective study of mortality. *Psychological Science, 14*, 320–327.

Fry, P. S. (2000). Religious involvement, spirituality, and personal meaning for life: Existential predictors of psychological well-being in community-residing and institutional care elders. *Aging and Mental Health, 4*, 375–387.

Hill, P. C., Pargament, K. I., Hood, R. W., Jr., McCullough, M. E., Swyers, J. P.,

Larson, D. B., & Zinnbauer, B. J. (2000). Conceptualizing religion and spirituality: Points of commonality, points of departure. *Journal for the Theory of Social Behaviour, 30,* 51–77.

Hunter, K. I., & Linn, M. W. (1980–1981). Psychosocial differences between elderly volunteers and non-volunteers. *International Journal of Aging and Human Development, 12,* 205–213.

Kafer, R. A., Rakowski, W., Lachman, M., & Hickey, T. (1980). Aging opinion survey: A report on instrument development. *International Journal of Aging and Human Development, 11,* 319–333.

Krause, N. (2003). Race, religion, and abstinence from alcohol in late life. *Journal of Aging and Health, 15,* 508–533.

Krause, N., Ingersoll-Dayton, B., Liang, J., & Sugisawa, H. (1999). Religion, social support, and health among the Japanese elderly. *Journal of Health and Social Behavior, 40,* 402–421.

Midlarsky, E., & Kahana, E. (1991). *Altruism in later life.* Thousand Oaks, CA: Sage.

Moen, P., Dempster-McClain, D., & Williams, R. M., Jr. (1992). Successful aging: A life-course perspective on women's multiple roles and health. *American Journal of Sociology, 97,* 1612–1638.

Musick, M. A., Herzog, A. R., & House, J. S. (1999). Volunteering and mortality among older adults: Findings from a national sample. *Journals of Gerontology: Psychological Sciences and Social Sciences, 54B,* S173–S180.

Musick, M. A., & Wilson, J. (2003). Volunteering and depression: The role of psychological and social resources in different age groups. *Social Science and Medicine, 56,* 259–269.

Oman, D., Thoresen, E., & McMahon, K. (1999). Volunteerism and mortality among the community-dwelling elderly. *Journal of Health Psychology, 4,* 301–316.

Omoto, A. M. (2004, May). *Volunteerism, community, and compassionate acts among older adults.* Paper presented at the Compassionate Love Research Conference, Washington, DC.

Omoto, A. M., & Aldrich, C. A. (2007). Retirement community life: Issues, challenges, and opportunities. In J. B. James & P. Wink (Eds.), *Annual review of gerontology and geriatrics, Volume 26: The crown of life: Dynamics of the early post-retirement period* (pp. 283–303). New York: Springer.

Omoto, A. M., & Snyder, M. (1995). Sustained helping without obligation: Motivation, longevity of service, and perceived attitude change among AIDS volunteers. *Journal of Personality and Social Psychology, 68,* 671–686.

Pavot, W., & Diener, E. (1993). The affective and cognitive context of self-reported measures of subjective well-being. *Social Indicators Research, 28,* 1–20.

Piliavin, J. A. (2005). Feeling good by doing good: Health consequences of social service. In A. M. Omoto (Ed.), *Processes of community change and social action* (pp. 29–50). Mahwah, NJ: Erlbaum.

Pope, S. K., Beck, C., Shue, V. M., & Cook, S. C. (2003). The role of religion and forgiveness in the mental health of Arkansans attending senior citizens' centers. *Marriage and Family: A Christian Journal, 6,* 113–122.

Radloff, L. S. (1977). The CES-D scale: A self-report depression scale for research in the general population. *Applied Psychological Measurement, 1,* 385–401.

Rosenberg, M. (1965). *Society and the adolescent self-image*. Princeton, NJ: Princeton University Press.

Schlehofer, M. M., & Omoto, A. M. (2004, July). *Definitions of religion and spirituality among older adults*. Poster presented at the 112th Annual Convention of the American Psychological Association, Honolulu, Hawaii.

Schlehofer, M. M., Omoto, A. M., & Adelman, J. (2006). *How do "religion" and "spirituality" differ? Lay definitions among religious and spiritual older adults*. Unpublished manuscript, Claremont Graduate University, Claremont, CA.

Snyder, M., Clary, E. G., & Stukas, A. A. (2000). The functional approach to volunteerism. In G. R. Maio & J. M. Olson (Eds.), *Why we evaluate: Functions of attitudes* (pp. 365–393). Mahwah, NJ: Erlbaum.

U.S. Department of Labor. (2004). *Volunteering in the United States, 2004*. Bureau of Labor Statistics. Retrieved October 15, 2004, from http://www.bls.gov/news.release/volun.nr0.htm.

Van Willigen, M. (2000). Differential benefits of volunteering across the life course. *Journal of Gerontology: Psychological Sciences and Social Sciences, 55B*, S1–S11.

Wheeler, J. A., Gorey, K. M., & Greenblatt, B. (1998). The beneficial effects of volunteering for older volunteers and the people they serve: A meta-analysis. *International Journal of Aging and Human Development, 47*, 69–79.

Wilson, J. (2000). Volunteering. *Annual Review of Sociology, 26*, 215–240.

Young, F. W., & Glasgow, N. (1998). Voluntary social participation and health. *Research on Aging, 20*, 339–362.

Zinnbauer, B. J., Pargament, K. I., Cole, B., Rye, M. S., Butter, E. M., Belavich, T. G., Hipp, K. M., Scott, A. B., & Kadar, J. L. (1997). Religion and spirituality: Unfuzzying the fuzzy. *Journal for the Scientific Study of Religion, 36*, 549–564.

22 Altruism, Religion, and Health: Exploring the Ways in Which Helping Others Benefits Support Providers

Neal Krause

Some consider the classic poem by Alexander Pope (*An Essay on Man*, 1731/ 1965) to be one of the most succinct statements about human nature that has ever been written. Four lines in that poem speak directly to the notion, and the benefits, of altruistic behavior:

> Heav'n forming each on other to depend,
> A master, or a servant, or a friend,
> Bids each on other for assistance call,
> Till one Man's weakness grows the strength of all.
> (Pope, 1731/1965, p. 26)

Three main points emerge from these lines. First, we are by our very nature dependent upon others. Second, as a result, people cannot live without both giving and providing support. And third, in the process of helping others, support providers become stronger themselves. Simply put, assisting others benefits support providers as well as the recipients of help. Although these benefits may be manifested in a number of ways, one is especially important for the purposes of this chapter. A small but growing number of studies suggests that helping others tends to enhance the health and psychological well-being of support providers (Krause, Herzog, & Baker, 1992).

If these assumptions about helping behavior are correct, then it is important to identify the factors that promote the behavior and the constructs that link helping others with better health. One of the core tenets in sociology states

that social institutions shape the attitudes and behaviors of the people who inhabit them (Berger & Luckman, 1966). This suggests that one way to approach
the field involves focusing on the institutions that promote altruism and the ways
in which they make this possible. The main goal of the discussion that follows
is to explore the ways in which one particular type of institution—formal places
of religious worship—provides this important social function. Since most of the
work in the field has been done with Christians, specific references to churches
will be made below.

Churches may influence altruism and helping behavior in two broad ways:
through the informal social ties that tend to flourish in them and through more
formal mechanisms in the organizational structure, such as church-based volunteer programs. Both are examined below. Following this, a series of issues is
identified that may help to shape the agenda for future research on altruism and
health in religious settings.

INFORMAL SOURCES OF HELPING BEHAVIORS IN RELIGIOUS INSTITUTIONS

The basic precepts of virtually all of the religions in the world extol the virtues
of loving others and helping people who are in need. But it is important to reflect on how these specific supportive acts are fostered and how their health-
related effects become manifest. Toward this end, the discussion in this section
has three objectives: (1) to identify and define the different ways in which informal helping takes place in the church; (2) to speculate on the factors that
promote informal help giving and altruism in the church; and (3) to specify the
precise mechanisms linking informal helping behavior in religious institutions
with the health of the support provider.

The Essential Nature of Informal Church-Based Support

Church-based social support may be defined as informal assistance, in the form
of emotional, tangible, informational, and spiritual help, that is exchanged between people who are part of the same congregation. Krause (2002a) conducted
a program of research that produced a comprehensive set of measures to assess
religion. Among these measures was a detailed battery of items that assesses the
full range of informal support in the church. The dimensions of support that
emerged from this work are listed in Table 22.1.

As shown in Table 22.1, both giving and receiving support are evaluated.
Some well-known types of support, including emotional support (i.e., the provision of love, caring, and trust), tangible help (practical aid, such as help with

Table 22.1. Dimensions of Informal Support
in the Church

1. Church embeddedness
2. Support provided
    A. Emotional
    B. Tangible
    C. Informational
3. Satisfaction with support provided
4. Support received
    A. Emotional
    B. Tangible
    C. Informational
5. Satisfaction with support received
6. Anticipated support
7. Negative interaction with fellow church members
8. Informal support from the clergy

housework), and informational assistance (i.e., knowledge that helps people to help themselves, like passing along the name of a good physician to someone who is ill), are captured by these scales. But other types of support are less well known. Three need further clarification.

Church embeddedness is captured by items that assess the frequency of church attendance and how often people attend Bible study and prayer groups. In essence, these indicators reflect the degree to which a person is involved with a religious institution. These measures capture the structure but not the function of church-based support systems. Being embedded in a church or other place of worship is a necessary prerequisite for learning and implementing altruistic behavior.

Anticipated support in the church is a perceptual measure of support that refers to the belief that others in the congregation would be willing to provide assistance in the future should the need arise. By standing ready to help if it is needed, social network members help to provide a sense of security and impart a feeling that even though hard times may be encountered in the future, the resources necessary to deal with them are available. Research by Krause (1997a), which was conducted in secular settings, shows that anticipated support is more likely to enhance the psychological well-being of support recipients than support that has actually been provided. Moreover, this work reveals that it may also reduce the odds of dying (Krause, 1997b). Unfortunately, no research has appeared to date on anticipated support in the church and health. However, it may be important to do such research because letting people know that assistance will be available in the future represents an important way of expanding the temporal scope of altruistic behavior.

The last type of assistance described here is called spiritual support (Krause, 2002b). This refers to helping behaviors that are geared specifically toward bolstering and maintaining the religious beliefs and religious behaviors of the support recipient. Fellow church members provide this type of assistance by sharing religious experiences with a focal person and by helping him or her to find solutions to problems in the Bible. This type of church-based support is important because, as research by Krause (2002b) reveals, it is a better predictor of health than emotional support provided by fellow church members.

As the discussion above reveals, we know more about the benefits of receiving support than we do about the advantages of giving it. But it should also be evident that the different types of support listed in Table 22.1 may be given as well as received. Research is needed to determine which types of provided support are most beneficial for health and well-being. In addition, we also need to examine two closely related issues at this juncture. First, how does the church promote the giving of these various types of assistance, and second, how does giving this kind of help enhance the health and well-being of the support provider?

How Religion Promotes Helping Behavior

It is not sufficient to merely point out that the church encourages people to love one another and to help those who are in need. Instead, a better scientific understanding of this process requires that the specific mechanisms that promote altruism in the church be identified as well. The initial answer might be that altruism is promoted in the church through sermons at formal worship services, Bible study and prayer groups, and perhaps even role modeling by those who are in authority in the church, such as the clergy. But a closer examination of these factors reveals that they merely specify the conduits or vehicles of transmission, but not the content of the messages that are provided. Although the literature has relatively little to say about this key issue, some reasoned speculation may prove to be quite useful for developing a better understanding of church-based altruistic behavior.

At the most basic level, one person cannot provide effective help to another without first understanding the situation of the individual who is in need. Otherwise, assistance that is given may be inappropriate or, at best, ineffective. Some insight into what is needed in order to provide effective support may be found in the classic work of Cooley (1929). He maintained that in order to understand other people, we must enter into their minds sympathetically. The choice of words here is critical. It says that, in essence, we cannot fully grasp the situation and the needs of others without evaluating their objective circumstances with compassion. This approach to evaluating the situation of others is promoted in part by the teachings of the church. For example, one of the core tenets of the Christian faith warns the faithful to judge not lest they be judged. Moreover, the faithful are encouraged to approach others with a deep sense of love and compassion, even when others have been hurtful toward them. The research implications here are clear: Investigators must move beyond the mere assessment of helping behaviors per se to an evaluation of the underlying attitudes, motivations, and beliefs that support them. Feelings of empathy and compassion and a nonjudgmental concern are among the key attributes involved here. Unfortunately, these cognitions have yet to be evaluated empirically within the context of the church—but they should be.

Although the insights provided by Cooley (1929) provide a useful point of departure, identifying the empathetic or sympathetic underpinnings of altruistic behavior does not go far enough. We also need to know more about how these underlying motives are conveyed or communicated. One way to think about sketching out the research agenda involves thinking in terms of social skills. Often what is most helpful about an altruistic act is the way in which the assistance is provided—the way in which an underlying sense of concern, caring, and trust is conveyed. This often involves the assessment of nonverbal forms of communication, including a touch, a glance, and certain voice intonations. This type of communication skill is often modeled in the church. For example, in some congregations, people join hands when they pray together in groups. This adds a deeper, warmer, and more personal dimension to this religious activity.

Other formal teachings of the church promote helping behavior as well. Chief among these is forgiveness. One of the most central teachings of the Christian church has to do with forgiving others. A small but growing literature highlights the health-related advantages of doing so (McCullough, Pargament, & Thoresen, 2000). But we need to know more about how the potential benefits of forgiveness arise. One answer may be found by turning to a recent study by Krause and Ellison (2003). Their work indicates that forgiving others exerts a positive effect on a range of well-being measures, including depressive symptoms, life satisfaction, and death anxiety. But more important, this study reveals that how people go about forgiving others is critical. In particular, this study suggests that the beneficial effects of forgiveness arise only among those who forgive others right away, without requiring the perpetrator of a hurtful act to perform acts of contrition (e.g., make an apology, promise not to repeat the hurtful act, or make restitution). In contrast, feelings of well-being were diminished for those who required the perpetrator to perform acts of contrition. A key issue involves identifying the factors that encourage others to forgive automatically. The data provided by Krause and Ellison (2003) suggest that it is determined in part by believing that God has forgiven the sins of the person who offers forgiveness. Clearly, beliefs about being forgiven by God emerge primarily in the church. Forgiving others without requiring them to perform acts of contrition is among the most important behavior markers of altruism because it requires victims to put their own hurt feelings aside and do something that benefits not only them, but the perpetrator of the hurtful act as well. One might argue that forgiving those who have hurt us is the ultimate marker of altruism. Helping people who have not hurt or offended us is relatively easy.

But helping those who have hurt us is much more difficult and requires much more empathy, compassion, and selflessness.

There is a final way in which helping others in religious settings may enhance the health and well-being of the support provider, but this factor is more abstract and more elusive. Specifically, providing assistance to others through the church may help support providers to derive a sense of meaning in life. Reker (1997) defines *meaning* as "having a sense of direction, a sense of order, and a reason for existence, a clear sense of personal identity, and a greater social consciousness" (p. 710). This construct is important, because a recent study by Krause (2004) suggests that older people with a strong sense of meaning in life tend to enjoy better health. A number of investigators maintains that one of the primary functions of religion is to provide people with a sense of meaning in life. For example, Pargament (1997) argues, "In essence, religion offers meaning in life" (p. 49). Although religion may help people to find meaning in a number of ways, providing assistance to others may be one of the most critical avenues for doing so. As noted earlier, all of the major religions in the world extol the virtues of helping others. In essence, the need to help others is formally codified in religious norms. This is important because social psychologists have argued for decades that norms provide a number of important functions in society: They tell people what to do and what to expect, and they provide a basis for evaluating the adequacy of one's own behavior (Stryker, 2001). As a result, complying with socially sanctioned norms provides people with a sense of direction, purpose, order, and meaning in life (Thoits, 1991).

How Informal Helping in the Church Enhances the Health of the Support Provider

In his widely cited paper on helping behavior, Reissman (1965) spelled out how support providers benefit from giving assistance to those in need. Three factors figured prominently in his discussion. First, helping other people enhances the self-esteem of the support provider. Helping those who are unfortunate makes a clear and unambiguous statement about the support provider because it highlights aspects of his or her character that are admired by many in our culture. Second, helping others provides a psychological respite from the support provider's own difficulties: It shifts the focus away from the self and the problems with which one often grapples. Being able to escape from one's own problems for a while has been shown to have beneficial health-related effects. An important illustration of this basic principle within the context of religion was provided recently by Krause (2003). This study focused on the benefits of praying for others. Praying for others is often construed as a form of helping behavior in the church because it represents an instance where one person petitions God on behalf of another, with the intent of ultimately getting God to intervene.

This study showed that the deleterious effects of financial difficulty on health are reduced for older people who pray more often for others. Third, Reissman (1965) argues that seeing support recipients overcome their own problems tends to make support providers feel that their own difficulties may be overcome in the same way as well. This in turn tends to enhance their feelings of control. These intervening mechanisms are important because a large body of research conducted in secular settings indicates that self-esteem (Trzesniewski, Donnellan, & Robins, 2003), feelings of control (Skinner, 1996), and finding a respite from personal problems (Patterson, 2003) tend to exert beneficial effects on health and well-being.

As the discussion up to this point reveals, there are many ways that religion can encourage church members to help each other informally. But the church does much more than this. If people in this institution only provide help to other church members, then the organization becomes largely self-serving. In an effort to reach beyond its own boundaries and meet the needs of the wider community, the church often provides a number of formal ways to help people of other faiths as well as individuals who may not be religious at all. These formal mechanisms of church-based helping behavior are examined in the next section.

FORMAL MECHANISMS FOR HELPING OTHERS THROUGH THE CHURCH

In one of the most comprehensive studies to date, the Department of Labor (2002) examined volunteer work that was performed in a range of settings, including civic organizations, hospitals, community service organizations, and religious institutions. The findings from this nationwide survey reveal that more formal volunteer work is done through the church than through any other type of organization. More specifically, this study reveals that 33.9% of all volunteer work takes place through the church. The second most frequent volunteer setting was educational or youth service organizations, but only 22.7% of all volunteer work is done there. It is important to note that the Department of Labor (2002) study further indicates that people aged 65 and older are especially likely to perform volunteer work in religious settings. Fully 45.2% of all volunteer work performed by older adults takes place in religious institutions. This makes sense because research consistently shows that members of the current cohort of older adults are more deeply involved in religion than adults in younger cohorts (Gallup & Lindsay, 1999).

A number of studies have set out to evaluate the mental and physical health benefits of performing volunteer work. Two of these studies that look at mental health outcomes are especially noteworthy. The first is by Musick and Wilson (2003) while the second was conducted by Thoits and Hewitt (2001). Both used the same longitudinal data set: the Americans' Changing Lives Survey.

Three findings from the study by Musick and Wilson (2003) are especially important. First, these investigators report that performing volunteer work at the baseline survey is associated with fewer symptoms of depression at the Wave 3 follow-up, but these findings hold only for people aged 65 and older. Second, their results reveal that performing volunteer work in religious institutions exerts a more beneficial effect on depressive symptoms than performing volunteer work in secular organizations. But once again, this relationship is evident only among people who were at least 65 years of age. Finally, Musick and Wilson (2003) looked at the relationship between sustained volunteer work and depressive symptoms. Sustained volunteering was operationalized as a simple count of whether a study participant performed any volunteer work at Waves 1, 2, and 3. The findings reveal that performing sustained volunteer work benefited individuals in all age groups, but the effects were substantially greater for people aged 65 and older.

Consistent with the findings of Musick and Wilson (2003), Thoits and Hewitt (2001) found that volunteering exerts a positive impact on depressive symptoms, happiness, and life satisfaction. However, this work further reveals that people with an initially greater sense of well-being are more likely to subsequently perform more hours of volunteer work than individuals who had a diminished sense of well-being at the baseline interview. This suggests that a self-selection process may be at work whereby people with initially good mental health are more likely to become involved in volunteer work. But this finding might also be interpreted to suggest that instead of restoring a sense of well-being, volunteer work helps those who have relatively good mental health remain that way.

The physical health benefits of volunteering are perhaps most evident in two studies that examine the relationship between helping others in formal institutional settings and mortality. Both show that people who volunteer tend to live longer. The first was conducted by Musick, Herzog, and House (1999). Two important findings emerged from this work. First, the data suggest that people aged 65 and over who do volunteer work are less likely to die over an 8-year follow-up period than older individuals who do not do any volunteer work. Second, the findings indicate that the beneficial effects of volunteering are most evident among people who have relatively little informal contact with others. This suggests that volunteering may provide an important compensatory function because it tends to offset the otherwise noxious effects of social isolation.

The second study on volunteering and mortality was conducted by Oman, Thoresen, and McMahon (1999). Like Musick et al. (1999), Oman and his colleagues report that people aged 55 and over who do volunteer work tend to live longer than individuals who are not engaged in volunteering. Moreover, the work by Oman et al. (1999) further reveals that the beneficial effects of volunteering on mortality are especially evident among people who are more involved in religion.

Two major conclusions emerge from this research on formal volunteer work and health. First, the data indicate that a good deal of this work takes place in religious settings. Second, this research suggests that the health-related benefits of volunteer work may be greatest among older adults who provide help within religious settings. We need to know more about why this may be so.

The finding that formal volunteer work is especially likely to enhance the health of older people may be explained by focusing on the intersection of three factors. First, religious institutions encourage the faithful to help those who are in need, and they often provide the formal organizational structure to do so. Second, as noted earlier, research suggests that members of the older cohorts of adults are more involved in religion than are members of younger cohorts (Gallup & Lindsay, 1999). Third, providing volunteer work at age 65 may help older people to face a series of key life transitions. More specifically, many people retire around age 65, their children reach adulthood and move out of the home, and many experience the death of a spouse. This is one reason that Rosow (1976) defined aging as a "roleless-role." Perhaps volunteer work provides a way to meaningfully fill the social void that is encountered by many in late life.

ISSUES TO EXAMINE IN THE FUTURE

Although research on helping others in religious settings provides some valuable insight, a great deal of work remains to be done. Four key issues that may help flesh out this emerging field are discussed below.

First, altruism is often viewed as a combination of attitudes (e.g., loving others) and behaviors (e.g., helping others). But it is entirely possible that one may exist without the other. For example, an older person may help to feed the homeless through a formal program in the church, but the older help provider may not necessarily feel love toward those who are less fortunate. We need to know whether the health-related benefits of helping others is enhanced if the support provider loves as well as assists someone in need, or whether merely providing help without emotional involvement is sufficient. Stated the other way around, is merely loving others sufficient, or do the health-related benefits of altruism arise only when these attitudes are manifested in concrete helping behaviors?

Second, more research is needed on the role played by the recognition and gratitude for helping others in religious organizations. Does quiet, selfless, unrecognized, and unrewarded helping provide the greatest health benefits, or are the health-related benefits greatest when helping behavior is acknowledged and those who receive support express gratitude for it? Folklore suggests that more selfless forms of helping may be the most beneficial, but there have been no studies to date that evaluate this issue empirically within religious settings.

Third, many times it is hardest for one person to help another when conflict exists between them. Although the Christian faith has a great deal to say about the benefits of helping transgressors, we still don't know if the health-related benefits of helping people are greatest when help is provided within the context of interpersonal conflict. As discussed earlier, some studies suggest that forgiving others tends to enhance feelings of well-being in the person who forgives. But there do not appear to be any studies in the literature that assess whether actually helping a transgressor outside of forgiving the hurtful act itself provides the greatest health benefits. For example, does providing a transgressor with monetary assistance or help around the home engender even greater health benefits for the support provider? It appears as though helping a transgressor with his or her own problem would represent the ultimate demonstration of forgiveness and the ultimate expression of altruism, but this issue needs to be explored empirically.

Finally, if helping others benefits the support provider, then we need to know more about how to devise interventions aimed at encouraging this type of altruistic behavior. Unfortunately, this is likely to prove to be a difficult task. Writing in 1775, Samuel Johnson quipped, "Sir, Hell is paved with good intentions" (as quoted in Kaplan, 1992, p. 244). This suggests that loving another may not be enough and that certain social skills are needed in order to properly convey this emotion and to effectively assist those who are in need. Research reveals that some of the most painful experiences arise from well-intentioned but miscarried helping (Coyne, Wortman, & Lehman, 1988). At a minimum, potential help providers must learn how to listen carefully to those who need help; they must find out what potential recipients want; and they must determine when they want it. Moreover, help providers must find a way to deliver assistance that does not offend the recipient or bring some fault, deficiency, or weakness to the foreground. We need to know if religion helps to promote these attributes, and if it does, then we need to know precisely how this kind of information is conveyed. Some insight into these issues is provided in Wuthnow's (1994) study of small groups in the church, such as Bible study and formal prayer groups, but a good deal more work in this area is needed.

Loving others and finding ways to effectively help them is hard work. The church and other formal places of worship stand out as beacons that foster this type of altruistic behavior. Yet researchers have not fully exploited the rich possibilities offered by studying religion and altruism. Part of the problem arises from the fact that we don't know enough about how the two are related. Hopefully, the discussion provided in this chapter may encourage others to delve more deeply into this exciting yet largely unexplored field.

Address all communications to Neal Krause, Department of Health Behavior and Health Education, School of Public Health, University of Michigan, 1420 Washington Heights, Ann Arbor, MI 48109–2029. Phone: (734) 763–5583; fax: (734) 763–7379; e-mail: nkrause@umich.edu. Work on this chapter was supported by a grant from the National Institute on Aging (RO1 AG014749).

REFERENCES

Berger, P. L., & Luckman, T. (1966). *The social construction of reality: A treatise in the sociology of knowledge*. Garden City, NY: Doubleday.

Cooley, C. H. (1929). *Life and the student: Roadside notes on human nature, society and letters*. New York: Knopf.

Coyne, J. C., Wortman, C. B., & Lehman, D. R. (1988). The other side of support: Emotional overinvolvement and miscarried helping. In B. H. Gottlieb (Ed.), *Marshaling social support: Formats, processes, and effects* (pp. 305–330). Newbury Park, CA: Sage.

Department of Labor. (2002). *Volunteering in the United States*. Retrieved from http://www.bls.gov.cps.

Gallup, G., & Lindsay, D. M. (1999). *Surveying the religious landscape: Trends in U.S. beliefs*. Harrisburg, PA: Morehouse.

Kaplan, J. (1992). *Bartlett's familiar quotations* (16th ed.). Boston: Little, Brown.

Krause, N. (1997a). Anticipated support, received support, and economic stress among older adults. *Journal of Gerontology: Psychological Sciences, 52B*, P284–P293.

Krause, N. (1997b). Received support, anticipated support, social class, and mortality. *Research on Aging, 19*, 387–422.

Krause, N. (2002a). A comprehensive strategy for developing closed-ended survey items for use in studies of older adults. *Journal of Gerontology: Social Sciences, 57B*, S263–S274.

Krause, N. (2002b). Church-based social support and health: Exploring variations by race. *Journal of Gerontology: Social Sciences, 57B*, S332–S347.

Krause, N. (2003). Praying for others, financial strain, and physical health status in late life. *Journal for the Scientific Study of Religion, 42*, 377–391.

Krause, N. (2004). *Stressors in highly valued roles, meaning in life, and the physical health status of older adults*. Manuscript submitted for publication. *Journal of Gerontology: Social Sciences, 59B*: S287–S297.

Krause, N., & Ellison, C. G. (2003). Forgiveness by God, forgiveness of others, and psychological well-being in late life. *Journal for the Scientific Study of Religion, 42*, 77–93.

Krause, N., Herzog, A. R., & Baker, E. (1992). Providing support to others and well-being in late life. *Journal of Gerontology: Psychological Sciences, 47*, P300–P311.

McCullough, M. E., Pargament, K. I., & Thoresen, C. E. (2000). *Forgiveness: Theory, research, and practice*. New York: Guilford.

Musick, M. A., Herzog, A. R., & House, J. S. (1999). Volunteering and mortality among older adults: Findings from a national sample. *Journal of Gerontology: Social Sciences, 54B*, S173–S180.

Musick, M. A., & Wilson, J. (2003). Volunteering and depression: The role of psychological and social resources in different age groups. *Social Science and Medicine, 56*, 259–269.

Oman, D., Thoresen, C. E., & McMahon, K. (1999). Volunteerism and mortality among community-dwelling elderly. *Journal of Health Psychology, 4*, 301–316.

Pargament, K. I. (1997). *The psychology of religion and coping: Theory, research, and practice.* New York: Guilford.

Patterson, T. L. (2003). Interventions for caregiving in dementia: Physical outcomes. *Current Opinions in Psychiatry, 16,* 629–633.

Pope, A. (1965). *An essay on man.* New York: Macmillan. (Original work published 1731)

Reissman, F. (1965). The helper therapy principle. *Social Work, 10,* 27–32.

Reker, G. T. (1997). Personal meaning, optimism, and choice: Existential predictors of depression in community and institutional elderly. *Gerontologist, 37,* 709–716.

Rosow, I. (1976). Status and role change through the life span. In R. H. Binstock & E. Shanas (Eds.), *Handbook of aging and the social sciences* (pp. 457–482). New York: Van Nostrand Reinhold.

Skinner, E. A. (1996). A guide to the constructs of control. *Journal of Personality and Social Psychology, 71,* 549–570.

Stryker, S. (2001). Traditional symbolic interactionism, role theory, and structural symbolic interactionism: The road to identity theory. In J. H. Turner (Ed.), *Handbook of sociological theory* (pp. 211–311). New York: Plenum.

Thoits, P. A. (1991). Merging identity theory and stress research. *Social Psychology Quarterly, 54,* 101–112.

Thoits, P. A., & Hewitt, L. N. (2001). Volunteer work and well-being. *Journal of Health and Social Behavior, 42,* 115–131.

Trzesniewski, K. H., Donnellan, B., & Robins, R. W. (2003). Stability of self-esteem across the life span. *Journal of Personality and Social Psychology, 84,* 205–220.

Wuthnow, R. (1994). *Sharing the journey: Support groups and America's new quest for community.* New York: Free Press.

23 Altruistic Love
and Physical Health

Harold G. Koenig

This chapter examines the associations between altruistic or unconditional love and physical health. I examine the mind-body relationship and review recent research on the effects of negative emotions on medical outcomes, forming the basis for a model by which altruistic activities could indirectly influence physical health by modulating emotions. Next, I review research on the relationship between altruism and physical health, examine the relationship between altruism and religion, and explore whether the increasingly recognized effects of religion on physical health might be partly mediated by altruism. Finally, I address the implications of these findings for clinical practice and suggest directions for future research in this area. By *altruistic love*, I mean the kind of love that expects nothing in return, the kind that is given freely and generously with the other person's good in mind. By *health*, I mean a state of complete physical, mental, and social well-being that goes far beyond simply the absence of disease (World Health Organization, 1948). Included in this definition is the concept of completeness and wholeness.

Why should altruism or altruistic love be related to health, that sense of "complete physical, mental, and social well-being"? In particular, how is a person's kindness, charity, or generosity connected to his or her freedom from poor health? Since the 1970s, scientists have come up with a rational explanation for such an association.

MIND-BODY RELATIONSHIP

Harvard physiologist Walter Cannon in 1914 described the changes in the body that occur during periods of severe anxiety, fear, anger, or other negative emotions. He called the physiological changes in humans and lower animals evoked by the perception of danger the "fight-or-flight response," emphasizing the role of the adrenal medulla in producing epinephrine (Cannon, 1914). Austrian endocrinologist Hans Selye expanded the response to include the actions of the hypothalamus and pituitary (hypothalamic-pituitary-adrenal axis), calling these physiological changes the "general adaptation syndrome" (Selye, 1946).

In a highly simplified description of the fight-or-flight response, in the instant that danger is detected, nerve signals are sent to at least two special areas of the brain: the locus ceruleus and the hypothalamus (Rabin, 1999). Preganglionic sympathetic neurons have their cell bodies in the locus ceruleus. When activated, they immediately send signals down the spinal cord to masses of nerve cells (called ganglia) that lie alongside the spinal column. These neurons, in turn, connect to postganglionic nerve cells that send sympathetic nerve fibers throughout the body following blood vessels into the heart, stomach, intestines, and other vital internal organs. In addition to connecting to the ganglia alongside the spinal column, the preganglionic sympathetic neurons also extend their fibers directly into the adrenal glands. The firing of these nerves causes the adrenal glands to inject a large quantity of epinephrine and smaller amounts of norepinephrine into the bloodstream. These chemicals, called catecholamines, circulate throughout the body and together with stimulation by postganglionic sympathetic nerves cause the heart rate to increase, blood vessels to contract, and a host of other physiological changes all within an instant.

In addition, the hypothalamus is releasing a variety of hormonal substances, such as corticotropin releasing hormone (CRH), into the blood at the exact same time that the locus ceruleus is activating the sympathetic nervous system. In response to CRH, the pituitary gland releases adrenocorticotropic hormone (ACTH), which circulates through the blood to the adrenal glands once again. Stimulated by ACTH, cells in the adrenal cortex inject the hormone cortisol into the blood. The cortisol circulates to the large muscles in the arms, legs, and back, pumping them up and making them maximally effective in their efforts to help the person either escape from or fight whatever is attacking. Epinephrine and norepinephrine are also released from the adrenal glands resulting in an increase in heart rate, increase in blood pressure, and increase in alertness. These neuroendocrine changes are designed for one purpose: to prepare the body to defend itself against threats to its physical integrity. The result is that all of the body's resources in terms of its nervous system, musculoskeletal system, and cardiovascular system are directed to where they are most needed for escaping the threat or defeating it.

The immune system also changes in response to these nervous system and hormone changes (Rabin, 1999). Besides terminating in the adrenal glands, post-ganglionic sympathetic nerve fibers also innervate the spleen, thymus gland, lymph nodes, lymphoid tissue around mucous membranes, and bone marrow—the very heart of the immune system. It is here that T-lymphocytes are produced and provide help to B-lymphocytes. In response to physical or psychological threats to well-being, norepinephrine is released from these nerve endings and does a number of things, including slowing down the functioning and production of immune cells and proteins. At the same time, circulating cortisol is also slowing down immune function through a host of different mechanisms. Why? Because the immune system uses up a lot of energy, and when confronted with immediate threats to survival, we don't need our immune systems as much as we need our muscles and heart functioning at their maximum capacity.

These physiological changes of the fight-or-flight response are highly adaptive in response to short-term external threats to survival. If the threat continues for days, weeks, or months (as may occur in chronic stress or depression), then such changes may adversely affect the natural healing systems in the body, i.e., the immune and cardiovascular systems. Chronic activation of the fight-or-flight response weakens the body's natural defenses against viruses, bacteria, and fungi that are constantly trying to infect and destroy our bodies. In addition, the resulting immune system changes may make us more susceptible to the development and spread of cancer cells, which the immune system is designed to prevent.

The most important point here is that whether the threat is external (attack from a wild animal) or internal (any form of psychological stress), profound changes occur in the body that can alter its ability to fend off disease and illness.

This fight-or-flight response may be evoked by fear, anxiety, worry, or sense of time pressure; it may be triggered by aggressive emotions, such as anger, resentment, bitterness, or lack of forgiveness; or it may be set off by sadness, discouragement, loss of purpose, meaning, or hope, or even boredom. As a result, these negative emotions increase our susceptibility to disease and illness. The fight-or-flight response is entirely focused on preserving the physical or psychological self. It is completely and entirely *self*-directed.

STRESS, DISTRESS, AND PHYSICAL HEALTH

There is increasing evidence from mainstream science that emotional factors can influence physiological functioning and health outcomes. This then provides a basis for understanding how altruistic activities can affect physical health through their effects on mental health. I review here studies that examine the effects of psychological distress on immune function, cancer mortality, cardiovascular mortality and functioning, and overall survival.

Immune Function

The effects of chronic stress on immune system functioning have been examined. For example, investigators have found that the stress of caring for a loved one with Alzheimer's disease significantly elevates levels of interleukin-6 (IL-6) in the blood (Kiecolt-Glaser, Preacher, MacCallum, Atkinson, Malarkey, & Glaser, 2003). IL-6 is an inflammatory indicator and blood protein that reflects the health of the immune system. High levels indicate worse immune functioning or greater instability. Persons with AIDS, certain lymphomas, and other immune-system diseases have high levels of IL-6, reflecting impaired immune functioning. In the previously mentioned study, investigators found that the chronic stress of being a caregiver adversely affected IL-6 levels not only while participants were in the caregiver role but also for as long as 2 to 3 years after the loved one's death.

In another study, Rosenkranz and colleagues examined the effects of negative and positive moods on measures of immune functioning, using an experimental approach (Rosenkranz, Jackson, Dalton, Dolski, Ryff, Singer, Muller, Kalin, & Davidson, 2003). Investigators induced positive and negative emotional states in subjects by giving them different writing tasks. Electroencephalography and affect-modulated eye-blink startle were used to assess mood changes, and in vivo immune function was measured by determining subjects' antibody response to vaccination with influenza virus. Measures of negative mood predicted weaker antibody responses, indicative of poorer immune function. Investigators concluded that negative mood adversely affected immune responses and could therefore increase the risk of physical illnesses that result from immune dysfunction.

Even mild depressive symptoms may adversely affect immune functioning in older populations. In a sample of 119 older adults, Ronald Glaser and colleagues found higher interleukin-6 before and after influenza vaccination in those with depressive symptoms; furthermore, IL-6 levels were increased 2 weeks later in older adults with even low levels of depressive symptoms (Glaser, Robles, Sheridan, Malarkey, & Kiecolt-Glaser, 2003). Thus, anything that increases well-being in older persons may help to counteract immune impairments brought on by low levels of depression. Note that altruistic activities such as volunteering are consistently related to greater well-being and less depression in older adults (Morrow-Howell, Hinterlong, Rozario, & Tang, 2003; Musick & Wilson, 2003).

Cancer

The immune system plays an important role in both preventing cancer and containing the metastatic spread of cancer. If psychological stress affects immune function, then cancer outcomes may be influenced as well. Brown and colleagues followed a sample of 205 cancer patients over 10 years. They found that depressive symptoms were the most consistent of all predictors of poor survival, even after controlling for several known demographic and medical risk factors (Brown, Levy, Rosberger, & Edgar, 2003). This makes sense given the role that even mild depressive symptoms may have on immune function, as noted above.

Heart Disease

There is much research showing that psychological stress and negative emotions have an adverse effect on the heart. For example, James Blumenthal and colleagues followed 817 patients who underwent coronary artery bypass grafting at Duke University Medical Center for a period of up to 12 years (Blumenthal, Lett, Babyak, White, Smith, Mark, Jones, Mathew, & Newman, 2003). Depressive symptoms were measured before surgery and 6 months after surgery. Analysis of survival time, controlling for age, sex, number of grafts, diabetes, smoking, left ventricular ejection fraction, and previous myocardial infarction, revealed that those with moderate to severe depression at baseline were 2.4 times more likely to die ($p = 0.001$) and those with mild or moderate to severe depression that persisted from baseline to 6 months were 2.2 times more likely to die ($p = 0.015$) compared to patients without depression. Overall, 19% of depressed patients compared to 10% of nondepressed patients died during follow-up.

Negative emotions can also dramatically affect quality of life (QOL), even when QOL is largely measured by the physical ability to function and take care of oneself. For example, Bernice Ruo and colleagues examined factors affecting health-related quality of life in patients with coronary heart disease (Ruo, Rumsfeld, Hlatky, Liu, Browner, & Whooley, 2003). They found that depressive symptoms had more of an impact on physical functioning and QOL than did biological factors such as cardiac ejection fraction and coronary artery blood flow (standard measures of cardiac function). This suggests that emotional factors may have a greater impact on the actual functioning of persons with heart disease than does heart function itself.

Cerebrovascular Disease and Stroke

Psychosocial stress and negative emotions can also adversely affect blood pressure (Jonas, Franks, & Ingram, 1997), the development of vascular disease (Everson, Kaplan, Goldberg, Salonen, & Salonen, 1997), and the occurrence of stroke (Everson, Roberts, Goldberg, & Kaplan, 1998). For example, in the Kuopio Ischemic Heart Disease Risk Factor Study, Susan A. Everson and colleagues examined 942 middle-aged men in eastern Finland over a 4-year period to determine the effect that hopelessness might have on the progression of carotid atherosclerosis (measured by intima-media thickening of the arteries that supply blood to the brain; Everson, Kaplan, Goldberg, Salonen, & Salonen, 1997). Investigators found that those who felt hopeless or felt like a failure in life had a 20% greater measurable increase in atherosclerosis over the 4 years of follow-up. This level of risk is the same as that obtained when comparing a pack-a-day cigarette smoker to a nonsmoker.

At least three studies have now linked negative emotions to an increased risk of stroke (Everson, Roberts, Goldberg, & Kaplan, 1998; Jonas & Mussolino, 2000; Simonsick, Wallace, Blazer, & Berkman, 1998). For example, Bruce S. Jonas and Michael E. Mussolino from the Centers for Disease Control (CDC) in Hyattsville, Maryland, followed for 16 to 22 years a random national sample of 6,095 stroke-free adults aged 25 to 74 years old (Jonas & Mussolino, 2000). Elevated self-reported depressive symptoms at baseline increased the relative risk of having a stroke by 73% (95% confidence intervals 30% to 131%), even after adjusting for multiple other risk factors such as age, race, sex, education, smoking, body mass index, alcohol use, physical activity, cholesterol, history of diabetes, history of heart disease, and blood pressure.

Bereavement and Mortality

A number of early studies found an association between bereavement (loss of a spouse or other loved one) and mortality (Helsing & Szklo, 1981), findings that were backed up by documented immune system changes (Bartrop, Lazarus, Luckhurst, Kiloh, & Penny, 1977). Any controversy over the effects of bereavement on survival, however, were put to rest by Pekka Martikainen and Tappani Valkonen from Finland, who examined the effects of bereavement on mortality in the best and largest study ever done (Martikainen & Valkonen, 1996). These investigators conducted a retrospective cohort analysis of 1.6 million married Finish persons aged 35–84 years, who were followed from 1986 to 1991. Results indicated a clear excess of mortality among those who lost their spouse. The bereaved experienced a 50–150% increase in death from accidental, violent, and alcohol-related causes, a 20–35% increase in death from heart disease and lung cancer, and a 5–15% increase in death from other causes. Excess mortality was greater within 6 months of bereavement, was greater among younger rather than older bereaved persons, and was higher among men than among women.

Thus, there is evidence from multiple high-quality studies that psychological stress and negative emotions affect physical health outcomes and survival overall and that these effects are mediated by physiological mechanisms rooted in immune, endocrine, and cardiovascular changes. Anything that buffers against psychological stress or counteracts negative emotions, then, has the potential to reverse these stress-induced physiological changes that adversely affect physical health.

STRESS BUFFERS

A number of factors has been identified that may buffer against stress and thereby counteract the negative physiological changes that would otherwise result. Such factors include social support, religious practices such as meditation or prayer, and possibly altruistic behaviors such as unconditional love, compassion, and demonstrating care for others.

Social Support

There is ample research suggesting that social support acts as a buffering factor against psychological stressors and depression and may therefore influence the physiological changes involved in the fight-or-flight response. Social support has been directly linked with improved immune and cardiovascular functioning (Uchino, Cacioppo, & Kiecolt-Glaser, 1996).

Religious Beliefs and Behaviors

There is also evidence that meditation and religious practices such as prayer and involvement in religious community activities help to buffer against stress (Maton, 1989; Tix & Frazier, 1997), to counteract depression (Koenig, Cohen, Blazer, Pieper, Meador, Shelp, Goli, & DiPasquale, 1992; Koenig, George, & Peterson, 1998), and to relieve anxiety (Azhar, Varma, & Dharap, 1994), thereby having positive effects on cardiovascular and immune functioning (Alexander, Schneider, Staggers, Sheppard, Clayborne, Rainforth, Salerno, Kondwani, Smith, Walton, & Egan, 1996; Castillo-Richmond, Schneider, Alexander, Cook, Myers, Nidich, Haney, Rainforth, & Salerno, 2000; Koenig, Cohen, George, Hays, Larson, & Blazer, 1997; Woods, Antoni, Ironson, & Kling, 1999).

Altruistic Behaviors

By helping to alleviate boredom, by reducing depression, by providing a sense of purpose and meaning in life, and by enhancing well-being through a sense of being useful, altruistic activities that involve helping others may help to counteract negative emotions and psychological stress and thereby affect a person's physical health. Although research examining the effects of altruistic love (compassion, kindness, desire to help others) on physical health is not plentiful, there is growing evidence that altruism may have similar effects as social support and religious beliefs have on buffering the flight-or-flight response (Ironson, Solomon, Balbin, O'Cleirigh, George, Kumar, Larson, & Woods, 2002). Such an effect was anticipated more than 2,000 years ago: "There is no fear in love. But perfect love drives out fear" (1 John 4:18, New International Version).

ALTRUISM AND MENTAL HEALTH

A large literature exists on the mental health benefits of altruistic activities. One of the first studies to demonstrate this compared older adults who volunteered with those who were retired and did not engage in volunteering or other work activity (Hunter & Linn, 1980–1981). The researchers found that volunteers experienced significantly greater life satisfaction, a stronger will to live, and fewer symptoms of depression, anxiety, and somatization. There were no differences in demographic and other background variables between volunteers and nonvolunteers, leading researchers to conclude that it was the volunteer activity itself that helped to explain these mental health benefits. Note, however, that nonvolunteers spent significantly more days in the hospital, were taking more medications, and had a greater degree of sensory-motor impairment, which may have prevented them from volunteering and resulted in higher rates of depression, anxiety, and somatization. The apparent mental health benefits, however, persisted after controlling for social class and disability.

Many other reports have followed the Hunter and Linn study. Within the past 5 years, a flurry of studies has documented the positive effects that altruistic activities may have on mental health, including the enhancement of well-being and life satisfaction (Liang, Krause, & Bennett, 2001; Morrow-Howell, Hinterlong, Rozario, & Tang, 2003; Yuen, 2002), reduction of depression (Musick & Wilson, 2003), increased positive affect (Dulin & Hill, 2003) and promotion of other healthy psychological and mental traits (Krueger, Hicks, & McGue, 2001; Schwartz, Meisenhelder, Ma, & Reed, 2003).

ALTRUISTIC LOVE AND PHYSICAL HEALTH

As noted above, the evidence connecting altruism and physical health is more limited than the research linking altruism to mental health. However, because of the negative effect that poor mental health has on physical health and physiological functioning, there is a good rationale for expecting an association between altruism and better physical health. The limited evidence available also supports such a hypothesis.

I will now review the evidence that being selflessly attentive to the needs of others may affect physical health and medical outcomes. In her book *The Long-Living People of the Caucasus*, Sula Benet reports on her research with this remote group in the Russian Caucasus region (Benet, 1974). These are the people who supposedly live to an average age of 120 to 150 years. Although their birth dates have been subject to much speculation, these people do experience lifespans that far exceed those of the surrounding populations. According to her study, the keys to long life have to do with their devout religious beliefs, sense of extended family, which includes others in the community outside of their biological families, and efforts to help those who are poor and needy, a practice that is taught and modeled for them by family and other members in the community.

A more scientific approach has been taken by scientists at the University of California at Berkeley who studied 1,973 residents aged 55 or over living in Marin County, California (Oman, Thoresen, & McMahon, 1999). Residents were followed for 5 years between 1990 and 1995. Approximately one third of residents ($N = 630$) participated in some kind of volunteer activity, and about half volunteered for more than one organization. Investigators found that those who volunteered for two or more organizations experienced a 63% lower likelihood of dying during the study period than did nonvolunteers. After controlling for age, gender, number of chronic conditions, physical mobility, exercise, self-rated general health, health habits (smoking), social support (marital status, religious attendance), and psychological status (depressive symptoms), the effect on survival was only slightly reduced to 44%—still a highly significant effect.

Marc Musick and colleagues used data from a nationally representative sample to examine the effects of volunteering on mortality among persons aged 65 or over (Musick, Herzog, & House, 1999). They used Cox proportional hazards regression to examine these effects independent of other predictors of mortality. Results indicated a curvilinear relationship between volunteering and mortality, with volunteering associated with greater survival for those who volunteered for one organization or for 40 hours or less during the past year. They also found that the strongest positive effect on survival occurred among volunteers who reported low levels of informal social interaction. Researchers explained the curvilinear relationship between volunteering and mortality in terms of influences on self-identity, role strain, and purpose and meaning in life. In other words, volunteering may be helpful up to a certain level, but if people become too busy volunteering and this creates stress in their lives, then it may begin to have the opposite effect on their health and longevity.

Physiological changes have been reported immediately after volunteering and other helping behaviors. For example, the February 1987 issue of *Better Homes and Gardens* included an article about helping others. At the end of the article, the author asked readers to write to the journal about their own helping experiences and how it made them feel (Luks, 1988). The magazine received a total of 246 responses. Over two thirds (68%) indicated experiencing a distinct physical sensation while they were helping. About 50% reported that they experienced a "high" feeling, 43% felt stronger and more energetic, 28% felt warm, 22% felt calmer and less depressed, 21% experienced greater self-worth, and 13% experienced fewer aches and pains.

The physiological changes that occur in the body during the process of helping others, however, have not been subject to direct scientific study. There is evidence that brain chemicals called endorphins have the capacity to stimulate feelings of joy and happiness that sound remarkably similar to the highs reported by these volunteers. Furthermore, George Stefano and colleagues have theorized that cells in the skin contain a chemical called nitrous oxide that induces feelings of "warmth" in the body in response to positive emotions (Stefano, Fricchione, Glingsby, & Benson, 2001). This finding may help to explain the warm feelings reported above by those who help others, although clearly further work is needed to clarify such physiological responses and link them to altruistic acts.

In his book *Aging Well*, George Vaillant describes a 50-year prospective Harvard University study that examined the course of adult development (Vaillant, 2002). He reports that "generative helping behavior" (focused on the well-being of others) is one of the strongest predictors of study participants' health and longevity.

Most recently, a 5-year study involving 423 older couples was conducted at the University of Michigan's Institute for Social Research (Brown, Nesse, Vinokur, & Smith, 2003). Participants were asked about the type of practical support they provided for friends or relatives, about whether they could count on help from others when needed, and about the emotional support that they gave to one another. A total of 134 people died over the 5-year study. After controlling their analyses for age, gender, and physical and emotional health, the researchers found a significant association between giving help and a reduced risk of dying. However, there was no association between receiving help and reduced death risk. Participants who provided no instrumental or emotional support to others were more than twice as likely to die during the 5-year study as people who helped others. Although the findings could have been explained by the fact that healthier individuals were probably more able to help others, even after controlling for functional health, health satisfaction, health behaviors, age, income, and education level, the results still stood firm. They concluded: "If giving, rather than receiving, promotes longevity, then interventions that are currently designed to help people feel supported may need to be redesigned so that the emphasis is on what people do to help others" (p. 326).

There are at least five reasons that volunteering or giving help to others should benefit the helper's mental health and ultimately their physical health as well (Reisman, 1965). These include^senhancing their social integration, distracting persons from their own personal problems, enhancing the meaningfulness of their lives, increasing their perception of self-efficacy and competence, and improving mood or promoting a physically active lifestyle.

RELIGIOUS LOVE

Another kind of altruistic love is not directed toward a relationship with humans, but rather toward one's relationship with God. Epidemiologist Jeff Levin has done some fascinating work in this area. Levin has developed and validated an 8-item scale (based on the work of Sorokin) to assess what he calls "religious love"—the extent to which a person loves God and feels loved by God (Levin, 2001). He has now administered his scale to a sample of 205 family practice out-patients. Using hierarchical regression, Levin investigated the effect of religious love on a standard measure of self-rated health while controlling for other predictors of health. He hypothesized that several factors might mediate the relationship between religious love and self-rated health, including religious involvement, social resources, psychological resources, objective health status, and sociodemographic factors. As expected, he found a statistically significant relationship between religious love and self-rated health at baseline (beta = .33, $p < .001$).

In six successive models, Levin controlled for the effects of 15 other expected predictors. These other variables accounted for nearly 40% of the variance in self-rated health. However, even after controlling for these variables, Levin still found a statistically significant association between religious love and self-rated health (beta = .24, $p < .05$). He concluded that loving and being loved by God exerts a positive influence on persons' perceptions of their physical health.

ALTRUISTIC LOVE, RELIGION, AND HEALTH

The relationships among altruistic love, religion, and health raise some important questions. First, are the religious more charitable, generous, or philanthropic than the nonreligious? Second, are religious people healthier? Third, does greater altruism help explain the religion-health relationship?

Altruism and Religiousness

The Christian Bible says, "love is the fulfillment of the law" (Romans 13:10, New International Version). Is there any evidence that religious people are more loving? The answer is yes. This includes the giving of financial contributions and volunteering time and talents for the benefit of others. For example, of all variables, frequency of attendance at religious services is the best predictor of financial giving (Independent Sector, 2001). According to the Independent Sector, a nonprofit organization that monitors financial contributions and volunteering in the United States, regular attenders account for 80% of all giving in the

United States. Weekly attenders gave 2.8% of their incomes in 1998, whereas those attending less than weekly gave 1.6% and nonattenders gave 1.1%. Financial contributions, however, have dropped even among regular churchgoers. The figure of 2.8% for weekly attenders in 1998 was down from 3.8% in 1989.

Religion is also a major factor in volunteering, and volunteers are much more likely to have strong moral values about helping those who suffer (Hodgkinson, 1995). Only about one third of people who are not members of religious organizations volunteer compared to greater than 60% of church members (Lawson, 1999, p. 17). Likewise, nearly 50% of those who attend religious services do volunteer work, compared to 33% of those who do not attend services. Understandably, most of this volunteering is directed at meeting the needs of the religious community. Only 7–15% of volunteering done within religious organizations is carried out to meet needs within the nonreligious community (Lawson, 1999, p. 117).

Religious persons are more altruistic in other ways also. For example, the religious are more likely to donate their organs to others in need, even when there are no biological or emotional intimacy ties involved. At least two case reports exist in which proposed kidney donors conceptualized their offers exclusively in terms of their religious beliefs and not in terms of kinship or emotional ties with the recipients (Dixon & Abbey, 2000). Investigators were surprised to discover the negative reactions of some clinicians to these offers and felt that this revealed the readiness with which religious beliefs can be seen as pathological and one way in which biological relationships can unduly restrict the clinical understanding of healthy altruism. These clinicians couldn't understand why these religious donors would offer their kidneys for the benefit of others and assumed that there had to be a more sinister motive present.

Roberta Simmons and colleagues at the University of Pittsburgh also studied the self-image of individuals who donated bone marrow to strangers (Simmons, Schimmel, & Butterworth, 1993). They surveyed donors before donating ($N = 849$), shortly after donating, and a year after donating; they also conducted in-depth interviews of 52 donors by telephone at the same three points in time. Many of these donors believed that they were distinct from others in the importance they placed on helpfulness and generosity to others. This belief often resulted from a strong religious identity.

Religion and Health

If the religious are more altruistic, and altruism is related to better physical health, then perhaps the religious are healthier than others as well. There is growing evidence that this is indeed the case, whether it can be entirely attributed to greater altruism or not.

Religious activity has been correlated with lower blood pressure, better cardiovascular function, better immune function, a more positive hormonal milieu, and longer lifespans when compared to those who are less religious. More than 1,200 studies have now examined this relationship, nearly 400 for physical health alone, with the majority finding better health among those who are more religious (Koenig, McCullough, & Larson, 2001).

Altruism and the Religion-Health Relationship

There is evidence that altruism plays a role in the health benefits of religious faith. For example, Krause and colleagues at the University of Michigan studied a sample of 2,153 older adults in Japan, examining the relationships among religion, providing help to others, and health (Krause, Ingersoll-Dayton, Liang, & Sugisawa, 1999). They found that greater religious involvement was associated with providing help to others more often, especially among men. Those who provided more assistance to others, in turn, were significantly more likely to indicate that their physical health was better. The authors concluded that the relationship between religion and better health could be at least partly explained by the increased likelihood of religious persons helping others.

In the study that was discussed earlier, Doug Oman and Dwayne Reed studied the longevity of 1,973 residents aged 55 or over living in Marin County, California (Oman & Reed, 1998). They found that volunteering reduced mortality by 60% among weekly church attenders. Volunteering also reduced mortality among those participating in nonreligious social activities, but to a lesser degree. Thus, the positive effects of volunteerism on mortality may be particularly strong for those who are religiously involved. Frequent religious service attenders lived significantly longer than less frequent attenders, whether they volunteered or not. However, volunteering seemed to mediate at least some of this relationship.

Perhaps most relevant to the hypothesis that altruism helps to explain the religion-health relationship is a study by Gail Ironson and colleagues at the University of Miami (Ironson, Solomon, Balbin, O'Cleirigh, George, Kumar, Larson, & Woods, 2002). They compared the characteristics of long-term survivors with AIDS ($N = 79$) with those of persons who were HIV-positive but had been diagnosed for only a short while (control group; $N = 200$). Investigators found that the survivors with AIDS were significantly more likely to be religious compared to persons in the control group. Religiousness, then, appeared to be an important factor in enabling those with AIDS to survive as long as they had. However, the effect of religiousness became statistically nonsignificant when the analysis was controlled for "helping others with HIV." Thus, helping others (altruism) completely explained the relationship between religiousness and survival in this study. Thus, altruism may play an important role in mediating the relationship between religion and health, although it is premature to conclude that it can explain the entire relationship.

CLINICAL IMPLICATIONS

These findings have implications for how health professionals should provide health care to patients. Given the stress that physical illness causes, patients need the positive experience of altruistic love from their caregivers. Although little or no research exists directly on this topic, there is ample reason to suspect that altruistic love displayed by clinicians would have positive results on their patients. Feeling more deeply cared for, patients would likely develop greater trust in their care providers. We know that trust increases the likelihood that a patient will comply with the treatment plan that the health professional recommends (Thom, Kravitz, Bell, Krupat, & Azari, 2002; Thom, Ribisl, Stewart, & Luke, 1999). It is reasonable to expect, then, that compliance rates would likely increase as the caregiver showed more compassion and care. Patients would be more likely to take their medication, alter their lifestyle, and believe in the effectiveness of the medical treatments if they felt greater trust in their health provider. Greater compliance with the medical plan would influence health outcomes in a positive direction and probably even reduce health costs.

Greater altruistic love given to patients will also likely influence the health professional's experience with the care that he or she is providing. The problems of low staff morale and burnout are growing both in medicine and nursing, making it difficult to hire and retain staff and affecting the quality of patient care (Aiken, Clarke, Sloane, Sochalski, & Silber, 2002; Schroeder, 1992; Stechmiller, 2002). Having more positive experiences with patients would likely increase job satisfaction, and displaying more altruistic love in the health care setting would likely increase such positive experiences.

Given the potential health benefits of altruistic love, health professionals might also consider encouraging altruistic activities among their patients. Just as they encourage patients to pay attention to diet and exercise, health professionals might recommend that patients take up volunteering or otherwise use their talents to contribute to the lives of others in need. There is probably sufficient evidence even now—particularly in the mental health area—that altruism is beneficial to a patient's quality if not length of life. Having more research in this area, however, would help to justify such prescriptions.

FUTURE RESEARCH

The field of altruism and health is now in its infancy. Thus, the list of important research needing to be done is a long one. I divide this research into four types: (1) studies on altruism and physical health; (2) studies on the connection between altruism and religion; (3) studies on the clinical consequences of providing health care with altruistic love; and (4) studies on the measurement of altruistic love that go beyond self-report measures of attitudes or beliefs and instead focus on objective, observable behaviors.

First, there is a great need for studies on the physical health effects of altruistic activities such as volunteering, financial generosity, compassion, and caring —particularly when these activities are performed without expectation of reward. Despite subjective reports of feeling physiologically better after helping behaviors, no studies have yet examined the physiological changes that result, including changes in blood pressure, heart rate, immune function, nitrous oxide release, natural endorphin production, or cortisol and norepinephrine levels. This could help to establish a biological basis for the health effects associated with altruistic activities.

There are also studies needed on altruism and health outcomes over time, including the likelihood of developing high blood pressure, myocardial infarction, or cancer, and ultimately the effect of altruism on lifespan. There is every reason to think that these medical outcomes might be affected by the positive emotions experienced by those who express selfless care for others.

Second, studies are needed on the relationship among altruism, religion, and health. What are the particular doctrines in each world religion that encourage altruistic behaviors? Are members of world religions that emphasize altruism more generous, kind, and compassionate toward others—and in particular, are they healthier and happier, and do they live longer? Related to this is the question of whether altruistic attitudes and behaviors help to explain the relationship between religion and better health. Studies that examine the religion-health relationship should include measures of altruism (volunteering, for example, or financial giving) and then examine this as a possible mediator of health effects.

Third, studies are needed on the implications of clinicians providing health care with altruistic love (i.e., kindness, compassion, and selfless care for the individual sufferer). Studies are needed to better understand the effects this might have on patient satisfaction, compliance, and health outcomes. Studies on the health professional–patient relationship are needed to better understand how altruistic care influences patient-clinician trust, which is such a powerful predictor of compliance and medical outcomes. Likewise, studies are needed on how clinician altruism could influence how satisfied health professionals are with their jobs, absenteeism, and burnout rates.

Finally, new methodologies are needed to study altruistic behaviors, not just attitudes or beliefs. Many studies today depend on self-report measures of beliefs and attitudes or self-reported behaviors. These reports are often biased by how the person wants to be viewed and do not reflect the person's actual behaviors. New methods of objectively observing behaviors in particular settings are needed, perhaps experimentally setting up certain situations and observing behaviors. This has already been done with college students (see Daniel Batson's [1976] work on religion and altruism), but not in adult settings among those who are more mature. Furthermore, rather than questioning particular persons, it may be more accurate to question their family members, friends, and colleagues at work. Of course, altruistic behaviors may vary depending on the particular social context (for example, a person may be more altruistic with strangers than with family members), adding further complexity to such research.

SUMMARY AND CONCLUSIONS

There is evidence that negative emotions adversely affect physical health outcomes through the physiology of the fight-or-flight response. Altruistic behaviors that involve helping others without expectation of reward are associated with fewer negative emotions and more positive emotions. It is difficult to be angry, resentful, depressed, or fearful when one is showing selfless love toward another person. Such loving acts neutralize negative emotions that stimulate physiological responses known to adversely affect immune, endocrine, and cardiovascular functions. Religion may be a powerful motivating factor for altruistic acts, if not the *most* powerful motivator. A better understanding is needed of how religion affects altruism and whether the health benefits of religion are at least partly explained by altruistic attitudes and activities. The research that currently exists on the relationship between altruism and physical health is not well developed, making opportunities in this field virtually limitless.

REFERENCES

Aiken LH, Clarke SP, Sloane DM, Sochalski J, & Silber JH. (2002). Hospital nurse staffing and patient mortality, nurse burnout, and job dissatisfaction. *Journal of the American Medical Association* 288:1987–1993.

Alexander CN, Schneider RH, Staggers F, Sheppard W, Clayborne BM, Rainforth M, Salerno J, Kondwani K, Smith S, Walton KG, & Egan B. (1996). Trial of stress reduction for hypertension in older African Americans. II. Sex and risk subgroup analysis. *Hypertension* 28(2):228–237.

Azhar MZ, Varma SL, & Dharap AS. (1994). Religious psychotherapy in anxiety disorder patients. *Acta Psychiatrica Scandinavica* 90:1–3.

Bartrop RW, Lazarus L, Luckhurst E, Kiloh LG, & Penny R. (1977). Depressed lymphocyte function after bereavement. *Lancet* 1(8016):834–836.

Batson, CD. (1976). Religion as prosocial: Agent or double agent? *Journal for the Scientific Study of Religion* 15(1):29–45.

Benet S. (1974). *Abkhasians: The long-living people of the Caucasus.* New York: Harcourt Brace.

Blumenthal JA, Lett HS, Babyak MA, White W, Smith PK, Mark DB, Jones R, Mathew JP, & Newman MF, for the NORG Investigators. (2003). Depression as a risk factor for mortality after coronary artery bypass surgery. *Lancet* 362: 604–609.

Brown KW, Levy AR, Rosberger Z, & Edgar L. (2003). Psychological distress and cancer survival: A follow-up 10 years after diagnosis. *Psychosomatic Medicine* 65:636–643.

Brown SL, Nesse RM, Vinokur AD, & Smith DM. (2003). Providing social support may be more beneficial than receiving it: Results from a prospective study of mortality. *Psychological Science* 14 (4):320–327.

Cannon WB. (1914). The emergency function of the adrenal medulla in pain and the major emotions. *American Journal of Physiology* 33:356–372.

Castillo-Richmond A, Schneider RH, Alexander CN, Cook R, Myers H, Nidich S, Haney C, Rainforth M, & Salerno J. (2000). Effects of stress reduction [meditation] on carotid atherosclerosis in hypertensive African Americans. *Stroke* 31(3):568–573.

Dixon DJ, & Abbey SE. (2000). Religious altruism and organ donation. *Psychosomatics* 41(5):407–411.

Dulin P, & Hill R. (2003). Relationships between altruistic activity and positive and negative affect among low-income older adult service providers. *Aging & Mental Health* 7(4):294–299.

Everson SA, Kaplan GA, Goldberg DE, Salonen R, & Salonen JT. (1997). Hopelessness and 4–year progression of carotid atherosclerosis. The Kuopio Ischemic Heart Disease Risk Factor Study. *Arteriosclerosis, Thrombosis and Vascular Biology* 17:1490–1495.

Everson SA, Roberts RT, Goldberg DE, & Kaplan GA. (1998). Depressive symptoms and increased risk of stroke mortality over a 29-year period. *Archives of Internal Medicine* 158:1133–1138.

Glaser R, Robles TF, Sheridan J, Malarkey WB, & Kiecolt-Glaser JK. (2003). Mild depressive symptoms are associated with amplified and prolonged inflammatory responses after influenza virus vaccination in older adults. *Archives of General Psychiatry* 60(10):1009–1014.

Helsing KJ, & Szklo M. (1981). Mortality after bereavement. *American Journal of Epidemiology* 114:41–52.

Hodgkinson VA. (1995). Key factors influencing caring, involvement, and community. In P Schervish, V Hodgkinson, & M Gates (eds.), *Care in community in modern society* (pp. 21–50). San Francisco: Jossey-Bass.

Hunter KI, & Linn MW. (1980–1981). Psychosocial differences between elderly volunteers and non-volunteers. *International Journal of Aging in Human Development* 12:205–213.

Independent Sector. (2001). *The new non-profit almanac in brief: Facts and figures on the Independent Sector*. Washington, DC: Independent Sector. Available at http://www.independentsector.org/PDFs/inbrief.pdf.

Ironson G, Solomon GF, Balbin EG, O'Cleirigh C, George A, Kumar M, Larson D, & Woods TE. (2002). Spirituality and religiousness are associated with long survival, health behaviors, less distress, and lower cortisol in people living with HIV/AIDS: The IWORSHIP scale, its validity and reliability. *Annals of Behavioral Medicine* 24:34–48.

Jonas BS, Franks P, & Ingram DD. (1997). Are symptoms of anxiety and depression risk factors for hypertension? Longitudinal evidence from the National

Health and Nutrition Examination Survey: I. Epidemiologic follow-up study. *Archives of Family Medicine* 6:43–49.

Jonas BS, & Mussolino ME. (2000). Symptoms of depression as a prospective risk factor for stroke. *Psychosomatic Medicine* 62:463–471.

Kiecolt-Glaser JK, Preacher KJ, MacCallum RC, Atkinson C, Malarkey WB, & Glaser R. (2003). Chronic stress and age-related increases in the proinflammatory cytokine IL-6. *Proceedings of the National Academy of Sciences* 100(15):9090–9095.

Koenig HG, Cohen HJ, Blazer DG, Pieper C, Meador KG, Shelp F, Goli V, & DiPasquale R. (1992). Religious coping and depression in elderly hospitalized medically ill men. *American Journal of Psychiatry* 149:1693–1700.

Koenig HG, Cohen HJ, George LK, Hays JC, Larson DB, & Blazer DG. (1997). Attendance at religious services, interleukin-6, and other biological indicators of immune function in older adults. *International Journal of Psychiatry in Medicine* 27:233–250.

Koenig HG, George LK, & Peterson BL. (1998). Religiosity and remission from depression in medically ill older patients. *American Journal of Psychiatry* 155:536–542.

Koenig HG, McCullough M, & Larson DB. (2001). *Handbook of religion and health*. New York: Oxford University Press

Krause N, Ingersoll-Dayton B, Liang J, & Sugisawa H. (1999). Religion, social support, and health among the Japanese elderly. *Journal of Health & Social Behavior* 40:405–421.

Krueger RF, Hicks BM, & McGue M (2001). Altruism and antisocial behavior: Independent tendencies, unique personality correlates, distinct etiologies. *Psychological Science* 12(5):397–402.

Lawson DL. (1999). *More give to live: How giving can change your life*. San Diego, CA: ALTI.

Levin J. (2001). God, love, and health: Findings from a clinical study. *Review of Religious Research* 42:277–293.

Liang J, Krause NM, & Bennett JM. (2001). Social exchange and well-being: Is giving better than receiving? *Psychology & Aging* 16(3):511–523.

Luks A. (1988). Helper's high: Volunteering makes people feel good, physically and emotionally: And like "runner's calm," it's probably good for your health. *Psychology Today*, October:39, 42.

Martikainen P, & Valkonen T. (1996). Mortality after the death of a spouse: Rates and causes of death in a large Finnish cohort. *American Journal of Public Health* 86(8 Pt. 1):1087–1093.

Maton KI. (1989). The stress-buffering role of spiritual support: Cross-sectional and prospective investigations. *Journal for the Scientific Study of Religion* 28:310–323.

Morrow-Howell N, Hinterlong J, Rozario PA, & Tang F. (2003). Effects of volunteering on the well-being of older adults. *Journals of Gerontology Series B: Psychological Sciences & Social Sciences* 58(3):S137–145.

Musick MA, Herzog A, & House JS. (1999). Volunteering and mortality among older adults: Findings from a national sample. *Journals of Gerontology Series B: Psychological Sciences & Social Sciences* 54B(3):S173–180.

Musick MA, & Wilson J. (2003). Volunteering and depression: The role of psychological and social resources in different age groups. *Social Science & Medicine* 56(2):259–269.

Oman D, & Reed, D. (1998). Religion and mortality among the community-dwelling elderly. *American Journal of Public Health* 88:1469–1475.

Oman D, Thoresen CE, & McMahon K. (1999). Volunteerism and mortality among the community-dwelling elderly. *Journal of Health Psychology* 4:301–316.

Rabin BS. (1999). *Stress, immune function, and health: The connection.* New York: Wiley-Liss.

Reisman F. (1965). The "helper" therapy principle. *Social Work* 10:27–32.

Rosenkranz MA, Jackson DC, Dalton KM, Dolski I, Ryff CD, Singer BH, Muller D, Kalin NH, & Davidson RJ. (2003). Affective style and in vivo immune response: Neurobehavioral mechanisms. *Proceedings of the National Academy of Sciences* 100(19):11148–11152.

Ruo B, Rumsfeld JS, Hlatky MA, Liu H, Browner WS, & Whooley MA. (2003). Depressive symptoms and health-related quality of life: The Heart and Soul Study. *JAMA* 290:215–221.

Schroeder SA. (1992). The troubled profession: Is medicine's glass half full or half empty? *Annals of Internal Medicine* 116:583–592.

Schwartz C, Meisenhelder JB, Ma Y, & Reed G. (2003). Altruistic social interest behaviors are associated with better mental health. *Psychosomatic Medicine* 65(5):778–785.

Selye H. (1946). The general adaptation syndrome and the diseases of adaptation. *Journal of Clinical Endocrinology* 6:117–230.

Simmons RG, Schimmel M, & Butterworth VA. (1993). The self-image of unrelated bone marrow donors. *Journal of Health & Social Behavior* 34(4):285–301.

Simonsick EM, Wallace RB, Blazer DG, & Berkman LF. (1998). Depressive symptoms and increased risk of stroke mortality over a 29–year period. *Archives of Internal Medicine* 158:1133–1138.

Stechmiller J. (2002). The nursing shortage in acute and critical care settings. *AACN Clinical Issues: Advanced Practice in Acute & Critical Care* 13(4):577–584.

Stefano GB, Fricchione GL, Glingsby BT, & Benson H. (2001). The placebo effect and relaxation response: Neural processes and their coupling to constitutive nitric oxide. *Brain Research Reviews* 35:1–19.

Thom DH, Kravitz RL, Bell RA, Krupat E, & Azari R. (2002). Patient trust in the physician: Relationship to patient requests. *Family Practice* 19(5):476–483.

Thom DH, Ribisl KM, Stewart AL, & Luke DA. (1999). Further validation and reliability testing of the Trust in Physician Scale: The Stanford Trust Study physicians. *Medical Care* 37(5):510–517.

Tix AP, & Frazier PA. (1997). The use of religious coping during stressful life events: Main effects, moderation, and medication. *Journal of Consulting and Clinical Psychology* 66:411–422.

Uchino BN, Cacioppo JR, & Kiecolt-Glaser JK. (1996). The relationship between social support and physiological processes: A review with emphasis on underlying mechanisms and implications for health. *Psychological Bulletin* 119:488–531.

Vaillant GE. (2002). *Aging well.* Boston: Little, Brown.

Woods TE, Antoni MH, Ironson GH, & Kling DW. (1999). Religiosity is associated with affective and immune status in symptomatic HIV-infected gay men. *Journal of Psychosomatic Research* 46:165–176.

World Health Organization. (1948). Preamble to the Constitution of the World Health Organization as adopted by the International Health Conference, New York, 19–22 June, 1946; signed on 22 July 1946 by the representatives of 61 states (Official Records of the World Health Organization, no. 2, p. 100) and entered into force on 7 April 1948.

Yuen HK. (2002). Impact of an altruistic activity on life satisfaction in institutionalized elders: A pilot study. *Physical & Occupational Therapy in Geriatrics* 20(3–4):125–135.

INDEX

Bolded page numbers indicate authors of selections. Italicized page numbers refer to figures and tables.

CPSIA information can be obtained at www.ICGtesting.com
Printed in the USA
BVOW02*1723060813

327774BV00005B/105/P